# Physical Activity for Health and Fitness

Allen W. Jackson, EdD
*University of North Texas*

James R. Morrow, Jr., PhD
*University of North Texas*

David W. Hill, PhD
*University of North Texas*

Rod K. Dishman, PhD
*University of Georgia*

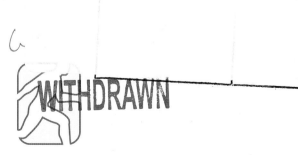
Human Kinetics

**Library of Congress Cataloging-in-Publication Data**

Physical activity for health and fitness / Allen W. Jackson . . . [et al.].
         p.  cm.
     Includes bibliographical references and index.
     ISBN 0-88011-599-8
     1.  Physical fitness--Health aspects.  2.  Exercise--Health aspects.  3.  Health--Physiological
aspects.  I.  Jackson, Allen W.
    RA781.P564  1999
    613.7--DC21
                                    98-43165
                                    CIP

ISBN: 0-88011-599-8

Permission notices for material reprinted in this book from other sources can be found on page viii.

Acquisitions Editors:  Richard Frey, Scott Wikgren
Writer:  Thomas Hanlon
Developmental Editors: Holly Gilly, Julie A. Marx
Assistant Editor: Laura Ward Majersky
Permissions Manager:  Terri Hamer
Copyeditor:  Joyce Sexton
Proofreader:  Ann Bruehler
Indexer:  Marie Rizzo
Graphic Designer: Keith Blomberg
Graphic Artist:  Judy Henderson
Cover Designer:  Jack Davis
Photographer (cover & interior):  Tom Roberts
Illustrator:  Tim Shedelbower

Printed in Hong Kong     10   9   8   7   6   5   4   3

**Human Kinetics**
Web site: www.humankinetics.com

*United States:* Human Kinetics, P.O. Box 5076, Champaign, IL 61825-5076
800-747-4457
e-mail: humank@hkusa.com

*Canada:* Human Kinetics, 475 Devonshire Road, Unit 100, Windsor, ON N8Y 2L5
800-465-7301 (in Canada only)
e-mail: orders@hkcanada.com

*Europe:* Human Kinetics, 107 Bradford Road, Stanningly
Leeds LS28  6AT, United Kingdom
+44 (0) 113 255 5665
e-mail: hk@hkeurope.com

*Australia:* Human Kinetics, 57A Price Avenue, Lower Mitcham, South Australia 5062
08  8277 1555
e-mail: liahka@senet.com.au

*New Zealand:* Human Kinetics, P.O. Box 105-231, Auckland Central
09-523-3462
e-mail: hkp@ihug.co.nz

# Contents

## Part I   Physical Activity and Fitness   1

### Chapter 1  The Physical Activity, Health, and Fitness Connection   3

▌ How much of health and fitness is related to heredity, and how much is directly affected by lifestyle choices?

▌ To what extent does being physically active affect how healthy you are and how you feel and look?

▌ Does physical activity make a substantial difference or just a minor difference?

### Chapter 2  Cardiorespiratory Fitness   17

▌ How much physical activity does it really take to notice cardiorespiratory fitness gains?

▌ How does aerobic activity affect fitness and oxygen consumption?

▌ What are the principles and components that go into designing an aerobic exercise program?

▌ What are the effects of exercise in different environments, such as heat, cold, and altitude?

### Chapter 3  Muscular Fitness   45

▌ Are the benefits of becoming stronger simply superficial, or are there additional fitness and health benefits?

▌ If you're not an athlete who *needs* to be more flexible to perform better, are there any reasons to work at increasing your ranges of motion?

▌ Do stretching exercises really help prevent injuries and enhance performance?

▌ Are there actual *health* benefits to becoming more flexible?

# Preface

This is a time in your life when you make many important decisions. You decide how you'll support yourself after college, which involves considerations about where you want to live, what kind of lifestyle you hope to have, how you want to spend your time, and with whom you want to live. The answers to those questions will map your life for the next several years as you leave college and begin to make your way in the world. But have you considered what you will be like when you're 40, or 60, or 80?

One of the most important decisions you need to make is how physically active you'll be in your life. You're young, you're busy, you're full of energy, and you're certain that you can put off health-related decisions until after your career and family are established. But mounting evidence shows that the quality of your later life is drastically affected by the way you live *right now*. We want to convince you to adopt a physically active lifestyle now—and we provide you with the information you need to adopt and maintain this healthier lifestyle so you can live the rest of your life with vigor and vitality.

We'll show you the medical evidence indicating that a lifetime of physical activity will improve your fitness and enhance the quality of your life, and we'll show you how to develop healthy habits. We'll help you understand the far-reaching effects of obesity on your own health and on the health of our nation, and we'll give you practical guidelines for maintaining a healthy body weight. We'll show you the undeniable links between sedentary living and the prevalence of a number of diseases and conditions that affect your quality of life as you age. Finally, we'll provide a framework for you to use to build your own healthful lifestyle that includes appropriate physical activity and good nutrition.

You may be tempted to put off the decision to be physically active. Our challenge is to make this such a practical and convincing book that you'll resist any such temptation. To do that, we use several elements to make the most important points obvious:

- *Healthchecks.* These are brief questions, with immediate answers, that will let you know if you're understanding us.
- *Key points.* These are the things we hope you'll remember for your whole life, not just for the time you're in this course.
- *Laboratories.* What would school be without schoolwork? Our labs are interesting, practical, and purposeful.

We aren't interested only in citing study after study to prove our points—but you need facts before you can make informed decisions. We're more interested in showing how the research results affect your lives now and in the future. We ask you to consider all the information and then make an educated decision about incorporating regular physical activity into your way of life, now and for your future.

# Acknowledgments

We wish to express our appreciation to the staff of Human Kinetics in the development of this book, especially Rainer Martens, Scott Wikgren, Holly Gilly, Thomas Hanlon, Julie Marx, and Laura Majersky. This was a cooperative project from its inception to its completion, and we truly believe this is a case where many minds produced a better product. Thanks also to chapter authors Ruth Carpenter (chapter 5) and Elaine Trudelle-Jackson (chapters 8 and 10) for their valuable contributions.

# Credits

**Lab 1: "Increase Your Awareness of Your Physical Fitness Status," p. 13**   Reprinted, by permission, from B.D. Franks and E.T. Howley, 1989, *Fitness facts* (Champaign, IL: Human Kinetics), 4.

**Lab 1: "Explore Your Goals for Physical Fitness," p. 14**   Reprinted, by permission, from B.D. Franks and E.T. Howley, 1989, *Fitness facts* (Champaign, IL: Human Kinetics), 6.

**Figure 1.2**   Reprinted from the 1994 revised version of the Physical Activity Readiness Questionnaire (PAR-Q and YOU). The PAR-Q and YOU is a copyrighted, pre-exercise screen owned by the Canadian Society for Exercise Physiology.

**Figure 2.1**   Adapted, by permission, from J. Wilmore and D. Costill, 1994, *Physiology of sport and exercise* (Champaign, IL: Human Kinetics), 173.

**Figure 2.5 and Lab 13: "Ratings of Perceived Exertion" RPE scale, p. 351**   Reprinted, by permission, from G. Borg, 1998, *Borg's perceived exertion and pain scales* (Champaign, IL: Human Kinetics), 47.

**Figure 2.7**   Reprinted, by permission, from B. Sharkey, 1997, *Fitness and health,* 4th ed. (Champaign, IL: Human Kinetics), 336.

**Lab 2: "Evaluate Your Aerobic Capacity," p. 41**   Adapted, by permission, from E.T. Howley and B.D. Franks, 1992, *Health fitness instructor's handbook,* 2d ed. (Champaign, IL: Human Kinetics), 160.

**Lab 3: Curl-Up Test, Trunk Lift Test, and Push-Ups Test, pp. 87-88**   Adapted, by permission, from J. Morrow, A. Jackson, J. Disch, and D. Mood, 1995, *Measurement and evaluation in human performance* (Champaign, IL: Human Kinetics), 255-256.

**Lab 4: Body Mass Index chart, p. 106**   Adapted, by permission, from J. Morrow, A. Jackson, J. Disch, and D. Mood, 1995, *Measurement and evaluation in human performance* (Champaign, IL: Human Kinetics), 224-225.

**Lab 7: "Evaluating Risks of Heart Attack," pp. 189-191**   From AMERICAN HEART ASSOCIATION'S YOUR HEART: AN OWNER'S MANUAL. Copyright © 1995 by American Heart Association. Adapted with permission of Prentice Hall. To contact the American Heart Association please call (800)AHA-USA1 or website address (www.americanheart.org).

**Lab 8: "Assess Your Risk of Developing Back Pain" questionnaire, p. 219**   Reprinted, by permission, from YMCA of the USA with Patricia Sammann, 1994, *YMCA healthy back book* (Champaign, IL: Human Kinetics), 31.

**Lab 8: "Perform Back Exercises" text, pp. 221-226**   Reprinted, by permission, from YMCA of the USA with Patricia Sammann, 1994, *YMCA healthy back book* (Champaign, IL: Human Kinetics), 31, 38-57.

**Chapter 10: "Physical Changes and Implications" text, pp. 254-260**   Adapted, by permission, from YMCA of the USA with Thomas Hanlon, 1995, *Fit for two* (Champaign, IL: Human Kinetics), 5-15.

**Lab 10: Contract and Release, Elevator, and Super Kegels exercises, p. 270**   Reprinted, by permission, from YMCA of the USA with Thomas Hanlon, 1995, *Fit for two* (Champaign, IL: Human Kinetics), 67.

**Figure 11.3**   Adapted, by permission, from P.H. Black, 1995, "Psychoneuroimmunology: brain and immunity," *Scientific American: Science and Medicine* 2 (6): 17.

**Lab 11: "Assess Your Level of Perceived Stress," p. 295**   Adapted, by permission, from S. Cohen, T. Kamarck, and R. Mermelstein, 1983, "A global measure of perceived stress," *Journal of Health and Social Behavior* 24: 385-396.

**Figure 12.5**   Adapted, by permission, from J. Wilmore and D. Costill, 1994, *Physiology of sport and exercise* (Champaign, IL: Human Kinetics), 428.

**Lab 12: "Health Risk Analysis," pp. 313-317**   Reprinted, by permission, from B. Sharkey, 1997, *Fitness and health,* 4th ed. (Champaign, IL: Human Kinetics), 61-66.

**Chapter 13: "Benefits of—and Barriers to—Physical Activity," p. 325**   Adapted, by permission, from M. Steinhardt and R. Dishman, 1989, "Reliability and validity of expected outcomes and barriers for habitual physical activity," *Journal of Occupational Medicine* 31: 536-546.

**Lab 13: "Consider Gains and Losses From Being Physically Active," p. 347**   Adapted from L. Wankel, 1984a, "Decision-making approaches to increase exercise commitment," *Fitness Leader* 2 (10): 21.

**Lab 13: "Setting goals," pp. 349-350**   Adapted from L. Wankel, 1984b, "Participant goals and leadership roles," *Fitness Leader* 2 (9): 17.

# Part I

# Physical Activity and Fitness

We know on the basis of scientific research that physical activity benefits health and lowers the risk of disease. In part I we'll examine how physical activity accomplishes these things. Through chapter 1 you'll develop an understanding of good and poor health and you'll learn of epidemiological evidence that exists for the health benefits derived from a lifetime of physical activity. You'll see the connection between physical activity and health-related physical fitness and gain insight into the importance of developing an active lifestyle early on in life. Most Americans don't engage in enough physical activity to improve their levels of fitness. This need to increase activity levels and fitness was a driving force behind the U.S. Department of Health and Human Services' *Healthy People 2000,* introduced in 1991, and *Physical Activity and Health: A Report of the Surgeon General,* published in 1996.

In chapter 2 you'll learn about aerobic exercise and develop the skills needed to design and evaluate an exercise program aimed at improving your cardiovascular endurance. You'll also learn the effects of exercising in various environments—like cold, heat, and altitude—and you'll examine how aerobic activity affects fitness and oxygen consumption. Chapter 3 provides insight into the fitness benefits of strength and flexibility. In all, part I provides a solid foundation for understanding how physical activity affects cardiorespiratory fitness, strength, and flexibility.

# Chapter 1

# The Physical Activity, Health, and Fitness Connection

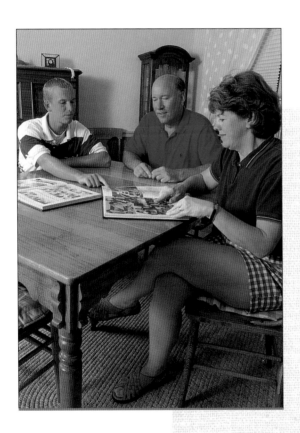

Last night my parents attended their 25th high school reunion. I had to wonder when my dad told me about Jake, who used to be the hotshot quarterback. Now Jake is 40 pounds overweight, and he had a mild heart attack last summer. Then my mom told me about a friend of hers who was shy, hated sports, and was a little overweight in high school—but now she's fit and trim and teaches jazz dance.

It made me think about what people will be saying about me at *my* 25th high school reunion. Will I be like Jake, or will I stay in good shape and be feeling and looking good? I guess I've taken my health and fitness for granted, but thinking about Jake makes me wonder if I should.

—Pat, 19-year-old sophomore

*W*hat *do you think?*

Pat's in relatively good health and shape right now. Does he have anything to worry about regarding his long-term health and fitness? Jake certainly was healthy in high school. What do you think were the reasons for his becoming overweight and having a heart attack? And what about the jazz dance teacher, who actually *lost* weight and became more fit? How much of health and fitness is related to heredity, and how much is directly affected by lifestyle choices, such as being physically active and eating a well-balanced diet?

It should come as no surprise that physical activity affects your health and fitness. But to what extent does being physically active affect how healthy you are and how you feel and look? Does physical activity make a substantial difference or just a minor difference?

This book explores how physical activity affects your health, your fitness, and your quality of life. As you explore, you'll

- examine the relationships between physical activity, health, and fitness;
- learn how to develop cardiorespiratory fitness, strength, and flexibility;
- understand the effects of obesity and nutrition on health;
- separate fact from fiction regarding weight control;
- discover how musculoskeletal health is affected by physical activity;
- explore the relationships between physical activity and disease, pregnancy, mental health, and aging; and
- consider how to use all this information to develop your own physical activity plan.

That final point is the bottom line: we want to show you the latest research, help you separate fact from fiction on a number of health- and activity-related issues, and allow you to make informed decisions about leading an active lifestyle that promotes health and fitness.

Keep in mind that fitness has no staying power of its own. You can be active and fit for a number of years, but if you stop being active, you'll lose a good portion of your fitness very quickly. The reverse is true, too: you can be relatively inactive for a number of years, and not very fit, but your fitness escalates rapidly when you become active on a regular basis. Being fit, as you'll learn, has many great benefits—and *you* are in control of how fit you are. The benefits are there for the taking, but you have to actively take them.

A good starting point is making sure we're all on the same page regarding some key terminology. Various definitions for *physical activity, health,* and *fitness* are encountered in a wide range of publications and in everyday usage. Next we give our definitions and key concepts for those three terms. After defining the terms we'll briefly mention another important element—nutrition—as it relates to health and fitness.

## PHYSICAL ACTIVITY

In simplest terms, *physical activity* means moving about. There are, of course, degrees of physical activity. Any physical activity is better for your health than none at all; some is better than a little; and more is better than some. When you increase your amount or level of physical activity, you will increase the benefits related to physical activity—to a point. Too *much* physical activity can result in overuse injuries, burnout, and other problems.

While physical activity may mean "moving about," we think such activity is more involved than simply choosing to walk to the television to change channels instead of using the remote control. According to the American College of Sports Medicine and the Centers for Disease Control and Prevention, adults should be moderately physically active for at least 30 minutes on most—and preferably all—days of the week. *Moderate physical activity* is roughly that which uses approximately 150 kilocalories of energy per day, or 1,000 kilocalories per week. You can accomplish this by taking part in a less vigorous activity for a longer period or a more vigorous activity for a shorter period (the ACSM recommends exercising five days a week doing moderate activity, or three days a week for vigorous activity). See "Everything in Moderation" for a description of what we mean by moderate physical activity.

**KEY POINT** Adults should take part in moderate physical activity for at least 30 minutes on most or all days of the week.

**HEALTHCHECK**

**If you walk moderately for 20 minutes five times per week, are you getting enough physical activity for good health?**

No. To maintain good health, you need at least 30 minutes of moderate activity five times a week, which would mean 150 minutes. Walking 20 minutes five times per week is only 100 minutes.

Now you have a description of physical activity, which may help you gauge how active you are. The lab at the end of this chapter will help you become even more aware of your physical fitness status. But knowing your status probably won't motivate you to *become* active if you're not already. Why should you become physically active, or maintain at least a moderate level of activity? There are two answers to the question, "What's in it for me?":

### Everything in Moderation

Okay, so you can't count walking to your TV or your refrigerator as moderate physical activity. But, as you can see from the following list (from the U.S. Department of Health and Human Services 1996), there are numerous activities you *can* count. And these are just the tip of the activity iceberg. Note that some activities need to be performed longer than others to be classified as "moderate."

▮ **15 minutes:** Stair walking; shoveling snow; running 1.5 miles (2.4 kilometers); jumping rope; bicycling 4 miles (6.4 kilometers)

▮ **20 minutes:** Playing basketball or wheelchair basketball; swimming laps

▮ **30 minutes:** Water aerobics; walking 2 miles (3.2 kilometers); raking leaves; pushing a stroller 1.5 miles (2.4 kilometers); fast dancing; bicycling 5 miles (8 kilometers); shooting baskets (basketball)

▮ **30-45 minutes:** Wheeling self in wheelchair (30-40 minutes); gardening (30-45 minutes); playing touch football (30-45 minutes); walking 1.75 miles (2.8 kilometers; 35 minutes)

▮ **45-60 minutes:** Playing volleyball (45 minutes); washing windows or floors (45-60 minutes); washing and waxing a car (45-60 minutes)

1. Plenty.
2. What do you want out of it?

In a moment we'll get to the benefits of physical activity (which are many). But first we want to acknowledge that different readers will have different motivations for being physically active. That stems, in part, from varied activity backgrounds. Taken as a whole, readers of this book represent a wide spectrum on a physical activity scale, ranging from not active at all to extremely active. With these varying backgrounds come an assortment of reasons for wanting to be physically active.

Just a sampling of those reasons, or motivations for being active, includes wanting to

- have fun,
- feel good,
- look good,
- feel healthy,
- *be* healthy,
- control body weight,
- interact with others,
- learn or improve sport or recreational skills,
- relieve stress, and
- increase energy level.

The list could go on and on. And most likely your interest in physical activity is spurred not just by one factor, but by several working together. You can use the lab at the end of this chapter to look more carefully at your own goals for physical fitness. The good news is that if you are active, no matter what your motivation, you'll be benefiting in a variety of ways. According to Heyward (1998), the health benefits of physical activity are substantial—they include reducing the risk of dying prematurely from heart disease and of developing diabetes, high blood pressure, and colon cancer. Physical activity has also been found to reduce blood pressure in people who have high blood pressure and to alleviate feelings of anxiety and depression. It also helps build and maintain healthy bones, muscles, and joints and helps develop strength and agility, not to mention helping to control weight and create a sense of psychological well-being.

These and similar benefits have been known for a long time—and we do mean *long*. Hippocrates, who lived 2,400 years ago, stated that "eating alone will not keep a man well; he must also exercise." Fast-forwarding 2,100 years, medical books in the 1700s were filled with the same terms you'll see in books on preventive health in today's bookstores: "self-help," "self-management," "self-regulation," "health behavior," and so on.

In more modern times, the relationship between physical activity and health can be traced from Jeremy N. Morris's study of London Transport Authority employees in the 1950s. Dr. Morris found that bus drivers (the sedentary group) had a significantly greater number of cases of coronary heart disease (CHD) than did bus conductors (the active group). This study paved the way for a variety of studies over the latter half of the century that clearly illustrate the relationship between physical activity and a number of causes of disease and death. And using several of these studies as a basis, many national organizations have developed position papers and statements on the links between physical activity, quality of life, and health.

---

### HEALTHCHECK

**Do more people in the United States die each year from (a) gunshot wounds, (b) unprotected sex, (c) car accidents, (d) alcohol abuse, or (e) disease related to lack of physical activity and appropriate nutrition?**

The answer is (e). In fact, disease related to lack of physical activity and appropriate nutrition—such as CHD, stroke, and cancer—accounts for more deaths than (a) through (d) combined!

---

## HEALTH

*Health* can be defined in many ways, in part because health can be related to physical, men-

## ◯ OF INTEREST

### Physical Activity and Health: National Issues

In the last decade the importance of physical activity to the public health of the United States has been officially recognized by the nation's leaders. In 1991, the U.S. Department of Health and Human Services (DHHS) implemented *Healthy People 2000: National Health Promotion and Disease Prevention Objectives,* a program whose overarching goals were to increase years of healthy life, reduce disparities in health among different population groups, and achieve access to preventive health services in the U.S. population. The first of the program's 22 priority areas was to increase physical activity and fitness by establishing 13 specific objectives to meet the overall established goal by the year 2000. Unfortunately, a review of the program in 1997 by the National Center for Health Statistics revealed that this goal and many of the specific objectives will not likely be met in this time frame. The DHHS and the Healthy People Consortium have already begun developing new national objectives to be achieved by 2010—*Healthy People 2010* will be released in January of 2000.

In addition, in 1996, the Office of the Surgeon General of the United States released *Physical Activity and Health: A Report of the Surgeon General,* which documented the health benefits of regular physical activity and improved physical fitness. Those benefits principally involved the decreased risk of a variety of chronic diseases, improved mental health and quality of life, and increased functional capacity for Americans of all ages. The report represents the most comprehensive examination available of the health benefits of physical activity and the need for increased physical activity in the American people if the risks of chronic disease are to be decreased.

Much of the information in this book is based on the public health messages provided in these landmark publications.

---

tal, emotional, social, and spiritual aspects of our lives. Many people think of good health as the absence of sickness or disease. This is in part true, but it doesn't tell the whole story. Good health, according to Nieman (1998), might be better defined as the presence of *"sufficient energy and vitality to accomplish daily tasks and active recreational pursuits without undue fatigue"* (p. 4).

While other factors are involved, people who are more physically active tend to be healthier than those who aren't very active. The greatest gains in health occur when a person goes from an inactive lifestyle to being moderately active. In other words, you don't have to train around the clock, trying to be a great triathlete, to experience the health benefits of physical activity. You just have to maintain moderate activity.

In fact, health gains often begin to plateau as one becomes very physically active, and can actually *drop* with excessive activity, in large part due to overuse injuries.

 You just have to maintain moderate activity to experience health benefits.

In practical terms, good health for you means that you can lead a full and active life day in and day out—attending classes, studying, participating in recreational activities, enjoying an active social life—without collapsing into bed each night, exhausted. And if you maintain your health through physical activity, you should be able to walk into your 25th high school reunion without having to refer back to the "good old days" when you used to look and feel fit.

As we mentioned, good health also is understood in terms of the absence of sickness and disease. People who are generally healthy and physically active tend to contract infectious disease less often, and they tend to be able to fight off infectious disease better than those who are sedentary. This affects not only your health today, but your health and quality of life in later years. Average life spans of Americans have increased from less than 48 years in 1900 to 73 years for men and 79 years for women in 1996, in large part because of improved medical practices that help us ward off once-deadly diseases. Physical activity can help make these additional years healthy ones.

Moreover, according to Blair (1993), the evidence linking certain diseases or conditions to a lack of physical activity and fitness is strong: this is the case for CHD, hypertension, obesity, colon cancer, diabetes, and osteoporosis. There is also some evidence linking a lack of activity and fitness to experiencing a stroke and to developing cancer of the breast, prostate, and lung.

What does all this mean for young adults? While it's true that children and young adults have very low rates of CHD, cancer, and stroke, it's *also* true that these diseases develop over time, and quite often *begin* developing in youth. Gilliam et al. (1977) studied risk factors for CHD in children ages 7 to 12, and found that

- 20% had high body fat,
- 11% had high cholesterol and low cardiovascular endurance,
- 25% had a family history of CHD, and
- 60% had one or two of the risk factors for CHD.

This study has been supported by many large-scale investigations in the intervening years. As we head into the millennium, children are not more active or fit than they were a quarter century ago.

All this points to the importance of choosing a healthy lifestyle. The fact that you *can* control how active you are and what you eat, and that these choices *do* directly influence your health—even to the point of whether you develop chronic and serious diseases—should be a great motivator for you to remain active and live a healthy life. And one of the results of making healthy lifestyle choices is that you become more fit along the way.

### The Changing Face of Death

In 1900, the most common causes of death—pneumonia, influenza, and tuberculosis—were contracted by *infection*. Because of vaccines and antibiotics that have since been developed through modern medicine, these and similar diseases, such as smallpox and polio, are typically no longer life-threatening.

Today, the most common causes of death—CHD and cancer—are *lifestyle- and age-related diseases.* In part we fall prey to CHD, cancer, and strokes because we are living longer. Heredity (which we obviously can't control) certainly plays a part in whether we develop these diseases. How we choose to live our lives, however, has a great influence on our health and our disposition for developing CHD, cancer, stroke, and other serious and potentially lethal diseases.

## HEALTHCHECK

**With all the emphasis on fitness and the greater understanding of how fitness affects health, why aren't children more fit today?**

The issue is complex, but in part children are less fit today because more sedentary diversions—television, video games, computers—pull them away from physical activity. Add to this the deemphasis on physical education in schools, past negative experiences in physical activity or sports, and—perhaps most critically—parents who are not active, and it's easy to see why many of today's children have adopted a more sedentary lifestyle.

## FITNESS

Fitness is another hard-to-define term. Its general description is similar to the description for health: if you're fit you have the stamina to perform your daily activities with energy and vigor, and you are less likely to develop chronic disease. Fitness can be further understood as having two aspects: health-related fitness and skill-related fitness.

*Health-related fitness* is focused on areas that affect our overall health and energy and our ability to perform daily tasks and activities. Its components include cardiorespiratory fitness, body composition, and musculoskeletal fitness—the latter including flexibility, strength, and muscular endurance. *Skill-related fitness* refers to our ability to perform specific skills required to take part in various activities and sports. Its components include agility, balance, coordination, speed, power, and quickness. Skill-related fitness has little to do with overall health. We'll focus our attention, then, on health-related fitness and its components (see figure 1.1).

Health-related fitness—including cardiorespiratory fitness, body composition, and musculoskeletal fitness—affects our overall health and energy and our ability to perform daily tasks and activities.

## ⬤ OF INTEREST

### "Look What Happened to Jim Fixx"

Jim Fixx was a noted author and runner who died of a heart attack during a jog in 1984. Well over a decade later, Fixx remains something of an icon for the "why sweat it?" crowd. "What's the use?" say those who continue to take a dim view of exercise. "Look what happened to Fixx."

Jim Fixx took up an active life at 36, the same age at which his father had experienced his first heart attack. Jim lived to be 52—nine years older than his father had been at his death—despite the fact he had several strikes against him from the start: aside from a bad family history, suggesting a genetic predisposition to heart disease, Jim had been overweight and had been an injudicious eater and a heavy smoker for years—during which plaque had been building up in his coronary arteries.

Most important for Jim, the years he lived after he took up exercise were better years. He described his own quality of life as much improved after he began running. He looked better, felt better, and was essentially asymptomatic up to his demise. In other words, he achieved what we should all hope to realize—an active, vigorous, fulfilling life.

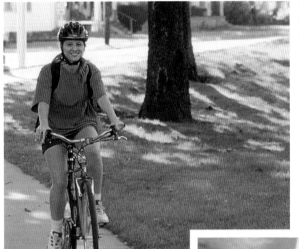

**Cardiorespiratory fitness:** Your circulatory and respiratory systems affect your ability to persist in strenuous tasks or moderate to vigorous activities for extended periods of time. Your cardiorespiratory fitness also affects how quickly you recover from such tasks or activities.

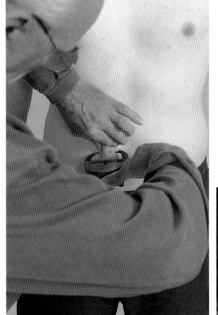

**Body composition:** Body composition refers to your relative amounts of body fat and lean body tissue or fat-free mass (muscle, bone, water, skin, blood, and other nonfat tissues). Your body composition is expressed in terms of percent body fat.

**Musculoskeletal fitness:** Musculoskeletal fitness includes flexibility, strength, and muscular endurance. Flexibility refers to the ability of your joints to move through full ranges of motion; strength entails how much force you can exert against resistance; and muscular endurance speaks of the ability of your muscles to maintain force during an activity or through a series of repetitions (such as lifting weights).

**FIGURE 1.1**   The three components of health-related fitness.

By focusing on all aspects of health-related fitness, you can work toward gaining total fitness through a well-rounded fitness program. Many people work only on their strengths and ignore their weaknesses. For instance, a person who is naturally strong may be inclined to further develop strength through lifting weights while ignoring a relative lack of cardiorespiratory fitness. And a person who has a considerable amount of cardiorespiratory fitness but who lacks upper body strength may focus exclusively on cardiorespiratory activities such as running and biking. It's best to pay attention to all three facets of health-related fitness (cardiorespiratory fitness, body composition, and musculoskeletal

fitness). And it's also wise to pay attention to another important element of health and fitness: nutrition.

## NUTRITION

Nutrition is, quite literally, the fuel through which we live. Good nutrition is important for health *and* for optimal performance, be it in recreational activities, daily living, or sports. Proper nutrition plays a vital role in how our bodies function; and the more we ask of our bodies, the more important it is, in terms of reaching optimal performance, that we provide our bodies with "high-performance fuel."

If you're like most college students, you're on your own for the first time and making more food choices than ever before. You also probably feel more pressed for time, and are tempted to eat fast foods and "junk foods" that are high in fat and calories and low in nutrition. If you begin to develop such habits while in college, you may find those habits hard to break once you're out—and you might end up like Jake, the star quarterback who was 40 pounds overweight at his high school reunion! In later chapters we'll explore what good nutrition is and offer ideas on how to choose foods that will fuel an active and healthy lifestyle.

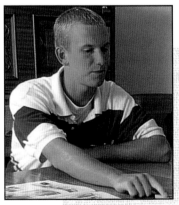

## Health Concepts

If you remember, Pat wondered what people would be saying about him at his 25th high school reunion, and whether he'd remain in good shape. He had always taken his health and fitness for granted, but realized—after hearing about Jake—that he probably shouldn't.

He's right. In fact, one thing is certain: if you aren't physically active as you grow older, your fitness will fade. You also open yourself up to health-related problems. It doesn't matter how healthy and fit you are right now—

if you don't *remain* physically active you will lose the fitness and you will risk loss of health.

The good news, of course, is that you can control how physically active you are. And that's what this book is all about—helping you to be healthy and fit by being physically active.

---

## SUMMARY

▌ Physical activity has a direct effect on your health and fitness. To reap the benefits of being physically active, you should take part in moderate physical activity for at least 30 minutes on most or all days of the week.

▌ The benefits of physical activity include reduced risks of dying prematurely from heart disease and reduced risks of developing diabetes, high blood pressure, or colon cancer. Being physically active can also help alleviate anxiety and depression; maintain healthy bones, muscles, and joints; and develop strength and agility. You can also help control your weight, relieve stress, and achieve a sense of psychological well-being through being physically active.

▌ The most common causes of death today are lifestyle- and age-related diseases (e.g., CHD, cancer, strokes). Physical activity reduces the risks of developing these and other serious and potentially lethal diseases.

▌ Health-related fitness can be described in terms of your cardiorespiratory fitness, body composition (percent body fat), and musculoskeletal fitness (flexibility, strength, and muscular endurance).

*Now that we've introduced you to the general topic of physical activity as it relates to health and fitness, we'll begin to explore in greater detail the effects of physical activity on fitness. First up, we'll look at one of the components of health-related fitness: cardiorespiratory fitness.*

---

## KEY TERMS

| | |
|---|---|
| health | physical activity |
| health-related fitness | skill-related fitness |
| moderate physical activity | |

# 1

# Determining Physical Fitness, Goals, and Readiness to Participate

**THE PURPOSES OF THIS LAB EXPERIENCE ARE TO**

▌ increase your awareness of your physical fitness status,

▌ explore your goals for physical fitness, and

▌ determine your readiness to participate in physical activity.

## Increase Your Awareness of Your Physical Fitness Status

The following two exercises (reprinted from Franks and Howley 1989) will help you determine your degree of satisfaction with different aspects of fitness.

*Circle the best number for each aspect of your fitness level, using this scale:*

4 = Very satisfied

3 = Satisfied

2 = Dissatisfied

1 = Very dissatisfied

| | | | | |
|---|---|---|---|---|
| Amount of energy | 4 | 3 | 2 | 1 |
| Cardiovascular endurance | 4 | 3 | 2 | 1 |
| Blood pressure | 4 | 3 | 2 | 1 |
| Amount of body fat | 4 | 3 | 2 | 1 |
| Strength | 4 | 3 | 2 | 1 |
| Ability to cope with tension/stress | 4 | 3 | 2 | 1 |
| Ability to relax | 4 | 3 | 2 | 1 |
| Ability to sleep | 4 | 3 | 2 | 1 |
| Posture | 4 | 3 | 2 | 1 |
| Low back function | 4 | 3 | 2 | 1 |
| Physical appearance | 4 | 3 | 2 | 1 |
| Overall physical fitness | 4 | 3 | 2 | 1 |
| Level of regular medication | 4 | 3 | 2 | 1 |

## Things That Bother Me

*List the things that bother you about yourself:*

Specific physical problem: _____

Appearance of particular part of body: _____

Ability to play a specific sport: _____

Risk of a health problem: _____

Other: _____

## Explore Your Goals for Physical Fitness

This table (reprinted from Franks and Howley 1989) will help you determine your plans to change various fitness-related behaviors.

*Circle your plans to change each area:*

| Behavior | Plan to change | | |
|---|---|---|---|
| Physical activity | Now | Soon | No plans |
| Weight | Now | Soon | No plans |
| Use of drugs/medications | Now | Soon | No plans |
| Pattern of sleeping | Now | Soon | No plans |
| Use of tobacco | Now | Soon | No plans |
| Handling of tension/stress | Now | Soon | No plans |
| Diet | Now | Soon | No plans |
| Use of seat belts | Now | Soon | No plans |
| Other (list) _____ | Now | Soon | No plans |
| _____ | Now | Soon | No plans |

Name_____Section_____Date_____

## Determine Your Readiness to Participate in Physical Activity

Complete the following questionnaire (reprinted from the Canadian Society for Exercise Physiology 1994) to help you determine your readiness to begin or intensify a physical activity program.

Physical Activity Readiness
Questionnaire – PAR-Q
(revised 1994)

# PAR - Q & YOU

### (A Questionnaire for People Aged 15 to 69)

Regular physical activity is fun and healthy, and increasingly more people are starting to become more active every day. Being more active is very safe for most people. However, some people should check with their doctor before they start becoming much more physically active.

If you are planning to become much more physically active than you are now, start by answering the seven questions in the box below. If you are between the ages of 15 and 69, the PAR-Q will tell you if you should check with your doctor before you start. If you are over 69 years of age, and you are not used to being very active, check with your doctor.

Common sense is your best guide when you answer these questions. Please read the questions carefully and answer each one honestly: check YES or NO.

| YES | NO | | |
|-----|-----|-----|-----|
| ☐ | ☐ | 1. | Has your doctor ever said that you have a heart condition <u>and</u> that you should only do physical activity recommended by a doctor? |
| ☐ | ☐ | 2. | Do you feel pain in your chest when you do physical activity? |
| ☐ | ☐ | 3. | In the past month, have you had chest pain when you were not doing physical activity? |
| ☐ | ☐ | 4. | Do you lose your balance because of dizziness or do you ever lose consciousness? |
| ☐ | ☐ | 5. | Do you have a bone or joint problem that could be made worse by a change in your physical activity? |
| ☐ | ☐ | 6. | Is your doctor currently prescribing drugs (for example, water pills) for your blood pressure or heart condition? |
| ☐ | ☐ | 7. | Do you know of <u>any other reason</u> why you should not do physical activity? |

## If

## you

## answered

### YES to one or more questions

Talk with your doctor by phone or in person BEFORE you start becoming much more physically active or BEFORE you have a fitness appraisal. Tell your doctor about the PAR-Q and which questions you answered YES.

- You may be able to do any activity you want—as long as you start slowly and build up gradually. Or, you may need to restrict your activities to those which are safe for you. Talk with your doctor about the kinds of activities you wish to participate in and follow his/her advice.
- Find out which community programs are safe and helpful for you.

### NO to all questions

If you answered NO honestly to <u>all</u> PAR-Q questions, you can be reasonably sure that you can:

- start becoming much more physically active—begin slowly and build up gradually. This is the safest and easiest way to go.
- take part in a fitness appraisal—this is an excellent way to determine your basic fitness so that you can plan the best way for you to live actively.

**DELAY BECOMING MUCH MORE ACTIVE:**
- if you are not feeling well because of a temporary illness such as a cold or a fever—wait until you feel better; or
- if you are or may be pregnant—talk to your doctor before you start becoming more active.

**Please note:** If your health changes so that you then answer YES to any of the above questions, tell your fitness or health professional. Ask whether you should change your physical activity plan.

<u>Informed Use of the PAR-Q:</u> The Canadian Society for Exercise Physiology, Health Canada, and their agents assume no liability for persons who undertake physical activity, and if in doubt after completing this questionnaire, consult your doctor prior to physical activity.

| **You are encouraged to copy the PAR-Q but only if you use the entire form** |
|---|

*NOTE: If the PAR-Q is being given to a person before he or she participates in a physical activity program or a fitness appraisal, this section may be used for legal or administrative purposes.*

I have read, understood and completed this questionnaire. Any questions I had were answered to my full satisfaction.

NAME _____

SIGNATURE _____     DATE _____

SIGNATURE OF PARENT _____     WITNESS _____
or GUARDIAN (for participants under the age of majority)

©Canadian Society for Exercise Physiology          *Supported by:*          Health      Santé
  Société canadienne de physiologie de l'exercice                                                  Canada     Canada

## Results and Conclusions

1. On the basis of your responses to all of the questions in this lab, list the areas of fitness and health that you need to acquire more information on and, based on what you know right now, steps you could take to improve them.

_____

_____

_____

_____

_____

2. The PAR-Q should give you an indication whether to seek medical counseling before beginning or intensifying your exercise program. Do you need to seek medical counseling before proceeding with an exercise program?

_____

_____

_____

_____

_____

3. From your findings in this lab, are you apparently healthy? _____

Do you agree with these findings? _____

Why or why not? _____

_____

_____

# Chapter 2

# Cardiorespiratory Fitness

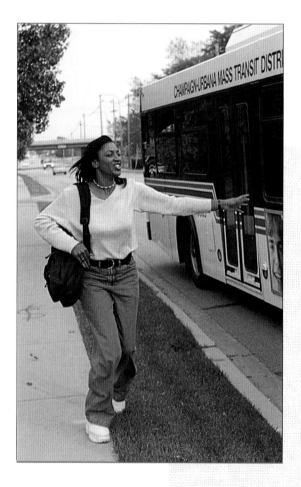

As usual, I was running late for my 8 o'clock class. Typically I catch the bus at the last minute, but I missed it, so I decided to jog over to class, about a half mile away.

By the time I got there, I could hardly breathe! I couldn't believe how out of shape I was. And I used to run on the cross-country team in high school! I haven't run for three years, but still I didn't think it'd be so hard to catch my breath. It made me think about getting back into shape, maybe starting to run again. I don't care about running competitively, like in road races or anything like that, but I *would* like to feel better the next time I have to jog when I'm late to class!

—Alicia, 18-year-old freshman

## *What do you think?*

Why did Alicia have such a hard time jogging to class and catching her breath? Would she be more fit if she walked to class every day? America is becoming a sedentary nation—how many of us would recoil in horror at the thought of walking two blocks if we could drive instead? Many people say they have no time to spend being active or exercising. They have an "all-or-nothing" attitude toward exercise—since they can't do it all, they do nothing. But how much physical activity does it really take to notice cardiorespiratory fitness gains? You might be surprised.

Cardiorespiratory endurance is certainly a key component of health-related fitness. *Cardiorespiratory* refers to the cardiac (heart) and respiratory (lung) systems. The heart and lungs provide oxygenated blood to our bodies. Aerobic activities that improve and maintain cardiorespiratory endurance such as jogging, walking, cycling, cross-country skiing, aerobic dancing, and swimming can be essential parts of a physically active lifestyle. In this chapter we'll examine how aerobic activity affects fitness and oxygen consumption, and we'll also look at the principles and components that go into designing an aerobic exercise program. In addition, we'll explore the effects of exercising in different environments (heat, cold, altitude, pollution) and consider physical activities that are alternatives to those just mentioned. We'll also take a look at the pros and cons of using different types of exercise equipment.

### AEROBIC ACTIVITY

We've all heard the term "aerobic activity," and we can easily relate it to the activities mentioned in the previous paragraph—swimming, jogging, cycling, and so on. But knowing *why* it's called *aerobic* activity will give you a better clue as to why such activity is crucial to your cardiorespiratory fitness.

*Aerobic* simply means "with oxygen." This doesn't refer to your need to breathe during an activity, but to the oxygen needed in the muscles to perform the activity. An athlete sprinting 100 meters certainly is breathing along the way, but sprinting short distances such as this is an *anaerobic* activity, because it doesn't require *additional* oxygen to be taken in by the muscles to move the body. Aerobic activities *do* require additional oxygen to be taken in to allow continued moving and functioning at the same rates and levels.

 *Aerobic* means "with oxygen." As we exercise, our muscles need a steady supply of oxygen to continue contracting and functioning.

In aerobic activity, oxygen must be present in our muscles to produce a high-energy chemical compound called *adenosine triphosphate (ATP)*. The energy for muscular contraction—that is, movement—comes from ATP; we can't continue to contract our muscles without assistance from it. Yet the body has only a small amount of stored ATP; if you are going to walk for 20 minutes, your body will constantly be producing ATP as you walk.

One way of producing ATP is through aerobic metabolism, a process occurring in the mitochondria (cellular structures that produce energy) that uses oxygen to produce this chemical compound. Regularly performing aerobic exercise for 20 to 60 minutes improves your cardiorespiratory system, which enables you to produce more ATP. The improvement results in a stronger cardiac and respiratory system and the ability to utilize oxygen more efficiently. As a result, you can continue to exercise longer and improve your maximal oxygen consumption (see page 21).

## OXYGEN CONSUMPTION

Aerobic activity is, by its very nature, directly related to cardiorespiratory fitness because it affects your oxygen consumption. When you're resting, your oxygen consumption is low because you're not exercising and you don't need much ATP. But if you walk briskly for 20 minutes, your need for ATP and your oxygen consumption ($\dot{V}O_2$) increase.

So just how is oxygen consumption determined? It is composed of the oxygen supply, the cardiac output, and the oxygen used (arterial-venous difference [$A\text{-}\dot{V}O_2$]). Cardiac output is a combination of *stroke volume* (amount of blood the heart pumps with each beat) and *heart rate* (number of beats per minute). Thus, cardiac output is the amount of blood leaving the heart per minute. The $A\text{-}\dot{V}O_2$ difference is the difference between oxygen content in *arterial blood* (higher oxygen) and oxygen content in the *venous blood* (lower oxygen). What do we mean by higher oxygen and lower oxygen? As blood leaves the heart and passes through the arteries, it is high in oxygen. Tissues that need oxygen and other nutrients use oxygen from the blood and input waste products such as carbon dioxide ($CO_2$) in the blood (see figure 2.1). The blood, now lower in oxygen, returns to the heart via the veins.

 As blood leaves the heart and passes through the arteries, it is high in oxygen. As it returns to the heart via the veins, it is lower in oxygen because much of it has been extracted along the way by tissues needing the oxygen.

Let's explain these concepts using your brisk walk of 20 minutes as an example. Before you

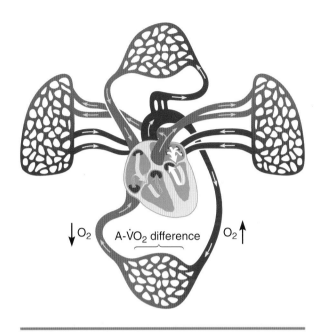

**FIGURE 2.1**  Oxygen distribution and consumption.
Adapted from Wilmore and Costill 1994.

begin walking, let's say you have been resting. Your breathing rate, heart rate, stroke volume, and use of oxygen are low. But as you start walking, your body needs more oxygen to keep muscular contractions going. You breathe more deeply and more frequently so your lungs can take in more oxygen from the air and expire more carbon dioxide. Your heart rate and stroke volume increase to supply more oxygen-rich blood to your muscles. Your leg muscles, which are contracting and thus allowing you to walk, extract and use more oxygen, which causes the arterial-venous oxygen difference to increase. All of this points ultimately to one thing: your oxygen consumption during the 20-minute walk rises (see figure 2.2).

As you look at figure 2.2, note two things:

1. When you first start walking, it takes several minutes for your breathing rate, heart rate, and oxygen consumption to reach a level stage that is referred to as *steady state* It is at this point that the activity becomes truly aerobic (aerobic metabolism supplies most of the ATP). Before you reach the

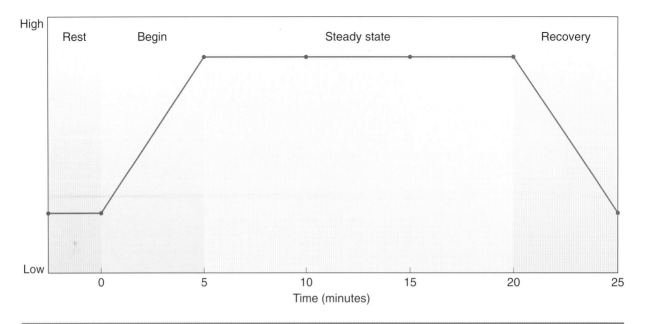

**FIGURE 2.2** Breathing rate, heart rate, cardiac output, and oxygen consumption responses to steady-state exercise.

steady state stage, most of your ATP is supplied through anaerobic metabolism.

2. After you stop walking, your breathing rate, heart rate, and oxygen consumption gradually return to resting levels. This is the *recovery phase* of the activity.

Your 20-minute walk is called "aerobic exercise" because most of the needed energy (ATP) is supplied by aerobic metabolism. However, in *any* exercise, a certain amount of energy is produced by both the aerobic and anaerobic systems. Labeling exercise as "aerobic" or "anaerobic" simply indicates the energy system that supplies *most* of the energy during the exercise.

If you maintain an aerobic exercise program for 15 weeks, for a minimum of 20 minutes each exercise session three times per week, your maximal oxygen consumption ($\dot{V}O_2$max) will increase. Regular aerobic exercise will improve your maximal oxygen consumption by improving your lung function, cardiac output, and arterial-venous oxygen difference. Many other biochemical, physiological, and anatomical changes beyond the scope of this book also occur that improve maximal oxygen consumption. One result of

these changes is that you will become more efficient at submaximal levels of exercise; exercise will become physiologically easier for you. You will be able to exercise for a longer period of time at a higher rate before becoming tired.

For instance, let's say that when you embarked on a 15-week aerobic exercise program, your submaximal exercise heart rate while walking steadily at 4 miles (6.4 kilometers) an hour was 130 beats per minute. After 15 weeks, your submaximal heart rate when walking at the same pace dropped to 120 beats per minute. Why? Your heart became stronger and your stroke volume increased. Thus you needed fewer heart beats per minute—that is, a lower heart rate—to supply the same amount of blood for the same amount of exercise. These physiological changes improve the heart's ability to conduct its activity more efficiently, the ultimate benefit being a reduced risk of coronary heart disease (this is explained in more detail in chapter 7). Think back to Alicia's brief run to class that caused her to huff and puff. As she becomes more fit, her improved cardiac function will also decrease the time needed to recover from a burst of physical activity.

## Determining Your Maximal Oxygen Consumption

One way to determine your *maximal oxygen consumption ($\dot{V}O_2max$)*—which is the best measure of your aerobic capacity and cardiorespiratory endurance—is to take a maximal exercise stress test on a treadmill or stationary cycle ergometer. During the test, you breathe into a mouthpiece attached to a metabolic measurement system that monitors oxygen and carbon dioxide. You exercise to physical exhaustion; the maximum oxygen consumption level obtained during the test is your $\dot{V}O_2max$.

Sound painful? It is. It's also difficult, time-consuming, and expensive. However, later in this chapter and in the laboratory experience that follows, you'll learn how to estimate your aerobic and cardiorespiratory fitness with tests that are more simple, less costly, and less painful.

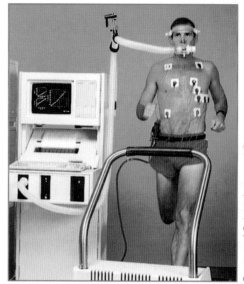

Courtesy of Quinton Instrument Co.

### HEALTHCHECK

**Does a 10 beat per minute reduction in resting heart rate really make a difference?**

Absolutely! Let's take a look at this decrease over the course of one year:

10 beats per minute × 60 minutes per hour =
600 fewer beats per hour
600 beats per hour × 24 hours per day =
14,400 fewer beats per day
14,400 beats per day × 365 days per year =
5,256,000 fewer beats per year!

## DESIGNING AN AEROBIC EXERCISE PROGRAM

By now you should have a basic understanding of what aerobic means and how it relates to cardiorespiratory fitness, which is an important component of health-related fitness. Next we'll explore how to establish and maintain an aerobic exercise program that will improve cardiorespiratory fitness. As you'll recall, the laboratory experience from chapter 1 helped you determine that you were ready to begin an exercise program. If you determined you weren't ready, then you'll need to receive medical clearance to begin an exercise program.

We'll look first at the principles of an exercise program, such as overload, specificity, individuality, and reversibility; we'll then look at a program's components, including frequency, intensity, and time; finally we'll help you put this program information in the context of an individual workout, including warm-up, exercise, and cool-down. This will give you the foundational information you'll need later on to develop your own physical activity plan.

## Principles

You should be aware of four important principles as you design an aerobic exercise program: overload, specificity, individuality, and reversibility. These principles are important for any type of exercise program, but we'll be speaking here in terms of their importance to aerobic exercise.

### Principle #1:   Overload

*To improve a physiological system, you must stress or challenge that system beyond its normal limits.*

In this case the physiological system is the aerobic system, which affects our cardiorespiratory function. Sitting on the couch won't improve our cardiorespiratory fitness! Doing aerobic exercise at a level or intensity that overloads our aerobic system *will* lead to fitness improvements.

It's important to understand that the point at which a person's aerobic system is stressed differs from person to person. Many people beginning an aerobic exercise program become discouraged when they reach their limits earlier than others. The idea isn't to "keep up with the Joneses," but to stress your *own* aerobic system as you gradually improve your fitness.

### Principle #2:   Specificity

*Your aerobic exercise program must be specifically related to your overall exercise objectives.*

If you want to improve in math, you need to study math. If you want to improve your cardiorespiratory system, you need to work your aerobic or cardiorespiratory system. It's that simple. Interestingly enough, many people who would say they are focusing on total or health-related fitness actually concentrate on only one aspect of that fitness—for instance, strength. They lift weights, which does improve their strength, but it does very little for their cardiorespiratory fitness.

### Principle #3:   Individuality

*You should evaluate your fitness level and your exercise goals on a personal level, rather than compare yourself to others.*

Each person has a unique genetic endowment, history of exercise and fitness, level of motivation, and range of responses to exercise. You need to figure out what's important to you regarding your own fitness and exercise program. As we just noted, it can be defeating to compare yourself to others who may be more fit to begin with or have exercise goals that are focused on preparing them to compete at high levels. Instead, establish and focus on your *own* goals, and recognize when you are taking the steps to achieve them. Very few of us have the genetic capacities and motivation to be an Olympic champion—or even to win a local 10K race. For most of us, it's enough to exercise regularly to improve or maintain a moderate to good level of cardiorespiratory fitness.

### Principle #4:   Reversibility

*When you stop overloading your aerobic system, your aerobic fitness level will, over time, return to its preexercise level.*

This is the principle we'd all like to avoid! But it's the unavoidable truth: it doesn't matter how hard you worked to *get* into shape—to *remain* in shape you need to remain active. When you stop training, physiological function and performance deteriorate in these areas:

- Muscle strength and power
- Muscular endurance
- Speed, agility, and flexibility
- Cardiorespiratory endurance

That's why the better aerobic goal isn't the one that will "whip you into shape" the quickest, but the one that you will most likely stick with over the long haul and that will improve your cardiorespiratory system along the way. This might be called the "tortoise-hare principle:" those who take off like the hare but don't continue will lose out to those who stick to the program, like the tortoise. If you want the health benefits of exercise and fitness, you'll need to be committed to a physically active lifestyle throughout the years.

## Components

Just as there are four important principles to be aware of in designing an aerobic exercise program, there are four components of exercise to consider. These components, appropriately enough, form the acronym *FITT:*

- **F**requency (the number of exercise sessions per week)

- **I**ntensity (the difficulty or stress levels of each exercise session)

- **T**ime (the duration of each exercise session)

- **T**ype (the type of exercise during each session)

*Frequency, intensity,* and *time* are three variables that you manipulate to establish the appropriate amounts and levels of aerobic exercise you need to improve your cardiorespiratory fitness. *Type* is simply the activity that you choose, such as jogging, cycling, swimming, and so on. As we just discussed, it's important to do enough exercise to reach a "threshold of exercise" and overload your aerobic system. We each have a zone where our exercise threshold is reached and our fitness is improved. If we don't exercise, or don't exercise enough, we don't overload the aerobic system. If we exercise *too much,* or at too great an intensity or for too long, we risk injury and burnout—which results in a loss of the health and fitness benefits that the exercise initially produced. It should be our goal, then, to exercise within the appropriate zone.

So how much exercise is enough? The American College of Sports Medicine (ACSM) guidelines for developing fitness through cardiorespiratory exercise (see table 2.1) are widely accepted. The guidelines address exercise frequency, intensity, and time, providing threshold and upper limits for all three components. The ACSM recommends that adults beginning an exercise program emphasize lower intensity and longer duration within the prescribed zones. Figure 2.3 shows the relationships that you should maintain between time and intensity to keep your aerobic exercise in the training zone. If you exercise at a higher intensity, your exercise time should decrease. If you exercise at a lower intensity, your exercise time should increase.

## Table 2.1 ACSM Exercise Guidelines

| Component | Threshold | Upper limit |
|---|---|---|
| Frequency | 3 days per week | 5 days per week |
| Intensity | 55% of maximal heart rate; 12 on the RPE scale | 90% of maximal heart rate; 16 on the RPE scale |
| Time* | 20 minutes per session | 60 minutes per session |

*Time of exercise can be achieved by accumulating multiple 10-minute sessions of exercise across the day.

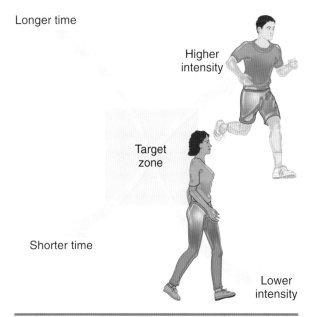

Longer time

Higher intensity

Target zone

Shorter time

Lower intensity

**FIGURE 2.3** Exercising in the target zone.

Four principles of exercise to consider are *overload, specificity, individuality,* and *reversibility.* The four *components* of an exercise program are *frequency, intensity, time,* and *type.*

### *Maximal Heart Rate*

As indicated in the ACSM exercise guidelines, you can use heart rate to guide your exercise intensity because of the heart rate's linear relationship to oxygen consumption and energy expenditure. You can measure your heart rate by taking your carotid or radial pulse (see figure 2.4). When taking either your carotid or your radial pulse, count your pulse for 15 seconds and multiply by 4 to arrive at your heart rate for 1 minute. Your estimated maximal heart rate is 220 minus your age in years. For example, if you're 20, your estimated maximal heart rate is 220 − 20, which is 200 beats per minute.

The maximal heart rate formula is based on the expected decrease in maximal heart rate due to the aging process. While the formula is pretty accurate for most people, realize that it's only an estimate. To determine your true maximal heart rate, you'd have to take a maximal stress test.

The ACSM recommends that people exercise somewhere between 55% and 90% of their maximal heart rates (see table 2.1). Based on these recommendations, the training heart rate zone for a 20-year-old (who, as we've stated, has a maximal heart rate of 200) is

110 for the lower limit (.55 × 200)

180 for the upper limit (.90 × 200)

### HEALTHCHECK

My friend plays intramural soccer twice a week, but he doesn't really exercise other than that. His games, though, are pretty intense; he's always dripping with sweat after them. I, on the other hand, jog about four times a week at a fairly easy pace. Which is the better plan for fitness?

If you're speaking of health-related fitness, your plan is better, so long as your heart rate is at least at 55% of your maximum when you jog. That's not to discount the workouts your friend is getting; but to get the full benefits of exercise, he should be supplementing his games with a few other workouts per week. And if the only exercise he gets comes from intramurals, what happens when intramurals are over?

### Perceived Exertion

Most people have a good sense of how hard they are exercising. Borg (1998) has developed a *ratings of perceived exertion scale* based on people's observations of their exercise efforts

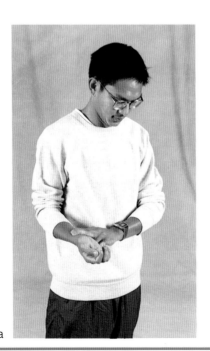

To take your pulse at the wrist, slowly slide the first two fingertips of your right hand along the edge of your left thumb toward your wrist until they rest on your arm. Feel for the pulse and count the number of beats for 15 seconds.

To take your pulse at your neck, place the first two fingertips on your neck even with your Adam's apple. Slide your fingers back until they are in the groove between your Adam's apple and the large muscle running down the front of your neck. Press *gently* to feel your pulse and count the number of beats for 15 seconds.

a

b

**FIGURE 2.4**    Taking your pulse at the *(a)* radial and *(b)* carotid arteries.

## If All Else Fails, Use Common Sense

If you're 20 years old, your maximal heart rate is most likely right around 200, based on the 220 − your age formula. According to the ACSM exercise guidelines (see table 2.1), you should be exercising at a heart rate of 55% to 90% of your maximal rate, which works out to 110 to 180 beats per minute.

Let's say you think you're in relatively decent shape; you've been exercising fairly regularly and feel pretty fit. So you decide to start exercising at a 150 heart rate (75% of your maximal rate), thinking that this will be somewhat difficult but not overwhelmingly so.

Now let's say your response to exercising at that heart rate is either, "Hey! That was too easy," or "Hey! Who stole the [puff, puff] oxygen mask?" Yet your heart rate was right in the middle of where you thought it should be. What do you do?

Adjust to a rate that's more comfortable. Your maximal heart rate is only estimated; it can lead to an incorrect training heart rate zone. A very unfit person can improve cardiorespiratory fitness by exercising at less than 55% maximal heart rate, while a very fit person may be able to exercise at 90% maximal heart rate. Research shows that when people exercise at an intensity level that they choose or prefer, it is usually a level that improves their fitness. This doesn't discount using a training heart rate zone (especially for beginners), but it does emphasize the importance of listening to your body.

(see figure 2.5). You simply rate your exercise intensity based on your perceptions. (To fully understand the RPE scale and its administration, it is necessary for all users to read *Borg's Perceived Exertion and Pain Scales*.) The intensity recommended by the ACSM is 12 (threshold) to 16 (upper limit). In your lab experiences for this chapter you will become familiar with heart rate and ratings of perceived exertion steps for setting an exercise intensity zone.

## The Complete Program

Understanding the principles and components of an exercise program will get you two-thirds of the way home toward designing your program. The final leg involves putting those principles to practice—that is, designing the actual workout! Wilmore and Costill (1999) list the following as parts of a complete program:

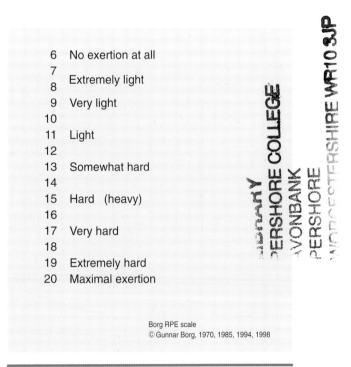

**FIGURE 2.5** The Borg RPE scale for perceived exertion.
Reprinted from Borg 1998.

- Warm-up and stretching
- Cardiorespiratory endurance exercise
- Cool-down and stretching
- Flexibility activities
- Strength activities

A basic workout consists of the first three items on the list, with flexibility incorporated into your warm-up and cool-down. Flexibility and strength activities help develop the musculoskeletal components of health-related fitness; in chapter 3 we'll explore how to develop and maintain flexibility and strength programs. However, in the following sections we will address the first three parts of the "complete program:" warm-up and stretching, cardiorespiratory endurance, and cool-down and stretching.

- **Warm-up and stretching.** Your warm-up and stretching should last about 5 to 10 minutes and should include several minutes of low-intensity physical activity of the same mode that you will be performing during your cardiorespiratory phase. Your warm-up will increase your body temperature, heart rate, and breathing rate. These changes will help your heart, lungs, blood vessels (arteries and veins), and muscles to function efficiently during the more rigorous cardiorespiratory phase. A good warm-up will also decrease your chance of muscle or joint injury and reduce the amount of muscle and joint soreness that you will experience as you begin an exercise program. Always warm up *before* stretching to reduce the risk of injury from stretching "cold" muscles.
- **Cardiorespiratory endurance exercise.** A wide variety of activities will improve your cardiorespiratory endurance. Wilmore and Costill (1999) note that the most often prescribed types of exercise include
  - walking,
  - jogging,
  - running,
  - hiking,
  - cycling,
  - rowing, and
  - swimming.

However, if none of these suits your fancy, you can improve your cardiorespiratory endurance through numerous other activities, including aerobic dance, bench stepping, and most racket sports (Wilmore and Costill 1999). What's most important is that you select an activity that you enjoy and that you are more likely to stick with. Don't choose an activity that you think is "good for you" but that you're not motivated to do.

- **Cool-down and stretching.** Immediately after finishing your cardiorespiratory exercise, you should begin your cool-down phase, lasting 5 to 10 minutes and consisting of the same activities and stretching that you performed in your warm-up. The cool-down is essentially your warm-up repeated. The cool-down time is an especially good time to stretch because your muscles are warm. Many people are more flexible after aerobic exercise and can greatly improve their flexibility during the cool-down phase. Cooling down helps lower the risk of joint or muscle injury, prevents the pooling of blood in the arms or legs, and returns the body to resting conditions.

**KEY POINT**

A complete workout program consists of warm-up and stretching, cardiorespiratory endurance exercise, cool-down and stretching, flexibility exercises, and strength training.

---

**HEALTHCHECK**

**Why do people develop cramps in their legs or sides ("side stitches") while exercising?**

These cramps can be caused by a number of factors:

- failure to hydrate yourself well before activity;
- failure to warm up or stretch properly;
- lack of sufficient vitamins and minerals in your diet; and
- trying to do too much in your workouts instead of gradually increasing time and intensity.

If you get these cramps while exercising, stop and slowly stretch the muscle to its greatest length—don't bounce!

## If the Shoe Fits . . .

In a recent evaluation of running shoes, *Consumer Reports* magazine offered the following suggestions to keep in mind when shopping for new athletic shoes:

▮ You're more likely to get sound help and advice at an athletic footwear store than at other types of stores.

▮ When looking for running shoes, bring in your old shoes to help you analyze your gait and places of most wear, and buy new shoes that match your gait.

▮ When trying on shoes, wear the socks you'll exercise in.

▮ Shop late in the day, when your feet are at their largest.

▮ Jog or walk around the store in the potential shoes if possible.

▮ Inexpensive shoes are usually fine for walking but are usually not acceptable for jogging. Be prepared to spend at least $50 for good running shoes. Buying discontinued shoe models can save you money.

As a runner you should replace your shoes every 500 miles (about 800 kilometers); this translates to about every eight months if you're running 15 miles (about 24 kilometers) per week. Walking and hiking shoes should also be replaced every 500 to 600 miles (every year if you walk about 9 to 12 miles per week; every two years if you hike 5 miles per week). Aerobic shoes should be replaced after every 100 hours of activity (every eight months if you take an hour-long class three times per week).

## EXERCISING IN DIFFERENT ENVIRONMENTS

As you're designing your exercise program, you'll want to consider one other factor: the environment you'll be exercising in. It can affect both your exercise performance and your health. Here we'll look at the effects of exercising in heat, cold, altitude, and air pollution and give you tips to minimize health risks in each environment.

## Heat

Exercise with caution in hot environments, because heat stresses the body and makes it difficult to control body temperature within a normal range (thermoregulation). The body's inability to dissipate heat can ultimately lead to *hyperthermia*, a state in which the body's temperature has risen to a dangerous level. Early symptoms of hyperthermia "include clumsiness, stumbling, excessive sweating (or the cessation of sweating), headache, nausea, dizziness, apathy, and any gradual impairment of consciousness" (ACSM 1987). Older people are more susceptible to heat illnesses than young adults. And a person who has had one heat-related incident is more likely to succumb again than is a person who has not had a heat-related incident. Anyone having a hyperthermic response to exercise should seek immediate medical attention.

The full effect of heat is not confined to the ambient temperature. Radiant heat (direct sunlight exposure), humidity (moisture in the air), heat conduction (physical contact between your body and another surface), and heat convection (air movement across the body) interact with the ambient temperature to bring about the full effect of heat. See figure 2.6 to learn more about the interaction between ambient temperature and humidity.

In extremely humid environments, the body is unable to dissipate heat (which is typically dissipated through sweating). This inability to regu-

## HEALTHCHECK

I ran a 10K race last summer in 70-degree weather with only about 40% humidity—which doesn't appear within the "caution" range in the heat and humidity index [see figure 2.6]. Yet I felt dizzy and disoriented toward the end and sweated profusely for several hours. I was shaky all day. Why?

The ambient temperature and humidity index provides only a general guide to when you might encounter heat-related problems. Individual tolerances for heat and humidity will vary. In addition, the index in figure 2.6 doesn't take into account the effect of radiant heat. You'll need to be well hydrated before your next race in similar weather conditions, to keep hydrated, and to listen to your body—slow down or stop if dizziness, nausea, or related symptoms appear. If any symptoms do appear, you should seek immediate medical assistance.

| | Temperature | | | | | | | | |
|---|---|---|---|---|---|---|---|---|---|
| % relative humidity | 60 | 65 | 70 | 75 | 80 | 85 | 90 | 95 | 100 |
| 0 | | | | | | | | | |
| 10 | 59 | 62 | 64 | 67 | 69 | 72 | 74 | 77 | 79 |
| 20 | 59 | 62 | 65 | 68 | 70 | 73 | 76 | 79 | 82 |
| 30 | 59 | 62 | 65 | 68 | 72 | 75 | 78 | 81 | 84 |
| 40 | 59 | 63 | 66 | 69 | 73 | 76 | 79 | 83 | 86 |
| 50 | 59 | 63 | 67 | 70 | 74 | 76 | 81 | 85 | 88 |
| 60 | 60 | 63 | 67 | 71 | 75 | 79 | 83 | 87 | 91 |
| 70 | 60 | 64 | 68 | 72 | 76 | 81 | 85 | 88 | 93 |
| 80 | 60 | 64 | 69 | 73 | 78 | 82 | 86 | 91 | 95 |
| 90 | 60 | 65 | 69 | 74 | 79 | 84 | 88 | 93 | 98 |
| 100 | 60 | 65 | 70 | 75 | 80 | 85 | 90 | 95 | 100 |
| | Caution | | | | Extreme caution | | | | |

*Note.* Use as a conservative guide, because the radiant heat load is not considered.

**FIGURE 2.6** Interaction between ambient temperature and humidity.

From *On the Ball* by B.A. Franklin, N.B. Oldridge, K.G. Stoedefalke, and W.F. Loechel, 1990. (Madison, WI: Brown & Benchmark), 15, 49. Reprinted with permission from McGraw-Hill.

late the body's temperature can lead to heat exhaustion, heat stroke, and ultimately death. When the body can't dissipate heat, heat exhaustion results, then heat stroke. This is why it's so important to stop activity if you experience any symptoms of heat exhaustion. But you can take steps to limit your risks of encountering these dangers.

The most important step you can take is to ingest fluids both before and during your physical activity. Many sports drinks replace electrolytes and minerals lost during physical activity. But the most important loss to replace is water.

You can also limit your risks by exercising

- early or late in the day, when the heat and humidity may not be quite as high as at midday;
- indoors in a cooler environment, rather than outdoors;
- near a fan or in the shade; and
- while wearing clothing that will not hold your body heat and moisture in (clothing should be porous, light-colored, and loose-fitting and

## POINT OF INTEREST

### Water or Sports Drinks?

Sports drinks have long been available for use before, during, and after exercise. These drinks are various mixtures of water, carbohydrate, electrolytes, and minerals that replace fluids and energy potential lost during exercise. There's some debate as to the ideal mixture for sports drinks: those with too little carbohydrate won't provide enough energy benefit, and those with too much carbohydrate produce an uncomfortable feeling of fullness and stay longer in the stomach. But the bigger issue is when to use sports drinks to replenish lost fluids and when to use water.

Wilmore and Costill (1999) make four recommendations regarding the use of sports drinks and water:

- The most important fluid to drink is water. The hotter or more humid the climate, the more water is needed.

- For most exercise sessions of less than an hour (unless it's very hot or humid), you don't need to replace fluids *during* exercise. Do drink adequate amounts both before and after exercise, however. If you exercise longer than an hour, especially in hot or humid weather, you can benefit from sports drinks or water during exercise.

- A sports drink with 4 to 8 grams of carbohydrate per 100 milliliters (approximately 3 to 4 ounces, or half a cup) of water is a good mix for most people. This mix will provide an energy boost and won't remain too long in the stomach, thus slowing the delivery of fluids to the body.

- Drink 100 to 150 milliliters (3 to 4 ounces) for every 10 to 15 minutes of exercise. This rate will reduce the risk of dehydration and hyperthermia while providing energy during the exercise.

If you will be using a sports drink during exercise, check out its taste first. Each of these drinks has a distinctive taste—and if you choose one that you don't like, you probably won't drink it when you most need it!

One final note: Sports drinks (and any other beverage high in citric acid and sugar) can, when consumed frequently, erode teeth and promote tooth decay. If you use a sports drink, avoid holding or swishing the drink in your mouth, and consider using a straw to drink it.

should "wick" away moisture to the surface of the material so that evaporation can occur).

## Cold

At the other extreme, risk-wise, is exercising in cold weather. One of the risks is becoming hypothermic. *Hypothermia* refers to the body's inability to maintain heat; as this occurs, the body's temperature can drop to dangerous levels. Severity of hypothermia is defined by these body core temperatures, in Fahrenheit:

- Mild hypothermia: 97 to 95 degrees
- Moderate hypothermia: 95 to 90 degrees
- Severe hypothermia: below 90 degrees

Early hypothermia symptoms include shivering, euphoria, and the appearance of being disoriented (much like intoxication). Moderate and severe hypothermia symptoms are similar, but more severe. As with heat, paying attention to cold weather conditions can minimize risks. Just

as humidity and other factors exacerbate the effects of heat, wind and wetness exacerbate the effects of cold (see figure 2.7). Use extreme caution when exercising outdoors in cold weather, especially when wetness and wind are factored into the equation. When exercising in the cold, maintain body heat by layering clothing that can be easily removed as your core temperature increases. It is especially important to wear appropriate clothing in environments that are cold *and* wet.

## Altitude

The higher the altitude, the more the lack of oxygen pressure in the air affects aerobic performance. When you exercise at higher altitudes (i.e., 6,000 feet [about 1,800 meters] or above), you'll have to work harder to achieve the same performance because your aerobic system will be taxed that much harder. Many great African distance runners from Africa and elsewhere train

| Actual thermometer reading (°F) | | | | | | | | | | | | |
|---|---|---|---|---|---|---|---|---|---|---|---|---|
| | 50 | 40 | 30 | 20 | 10 | 0 | -10 | -20 | -30 | -40 | -50 | -60 |
| Wind speed (mph) | Equivalent temperature (°F) | | | | | | | | | | | |
| Calm | 50 | 40 | 30 | 20 | 10 | 0 | −10 | −20 | −30 | −40 | −50 | −60 |
| 5 | 48 | 37 | 27 | 16 | 6 | −5 | −15 | −26 | −36 | −47 | −57 | −68 |
| 10 | 40 | 28 | 16 | 4 | −9 | −21 | −33 | −46 | −58 | −70 | −83 | −95 |
| 15 | 36 | 22 | 9 | −5 | −18 | −36 | −45 | −58 | −72 | −85 | −99 | −112 |
| 20 | 32 | 18 | 4 | −10 | −25 | −39 | −53 | −67 | −82 | −96 | −110 | −124 |
| 25 | 30 | 16 | 0 | −15 | −29 | −44 | −59 | −74 | −88 | −104 | −118 | −133 |
| 30 | 28 | 13 | −2 | −18 | −33 | −48 | −63 | −79 | −94 | −109 | −125 | −140 |
| 35 | 27 | 11 | −4 | −20 | −35 | −49 | −67 | −82 | −98 | −113 | −129 | −145 |
| 40 | 26 | 10 | −6 | −21 | −37 | −53 | −69 | −85 | −100 | −116 | −132 | −148 |

Little danger (for properly clothed person)   Increasing danger   Great danger

Danger from freezing of exposed flesh

**FIGURE 2.7** Wind chill index.

Reprinted from Sharkey 1997.

at higher altitudes; the *hypoxic* (reduced oxygen level) environment they encounter can potentially improve their performances as it helps develop their aerobic systems.

However, assuming you're not training to be a world class runner, what's important for you to realize is that exercising at higher altitudes will impair your performance. This is especially true for travelers (campers, hikers, skiers, and so on) who don't live in higher altitudes. If you're new to high altitudes and you exercise in such an environment, you'll notice that you'll become exhausted more quickly. Symptoms of having altitude-related problems include headache, difficulty sleeping or breathing, rapid heartbeat, and dizziness. Severe levels of these symptoms can be life-threatening.

The key is to adjust gradually to higher altitudes. Initial activity should be shorter and less intense than what you would perform at lower altitudes. If you're in better shape, you'll probably be able to adjust more quickly than those who are just beginning an exercise program. But realize that full acclimatization usually takes several weeks or months. At higher altitudes, you'll probably never be able to demonstrate the same levels of fitness that you attain at lower altitudes. And you'll note that you won't have to work as hard to achieve your heart training zone.

## Air Pollution

If you live in a large city, you might be concerned about the effects of air pollution on your physical activities. Pollution, smog, carbon monoxide, and the like do have irritating effects on the airways leading to the lungs, and they can ultimately impact your ability to exercise.

You can take a few simple steps to help minimize the impact of air pollution on your exercise. First, if possible, exercise indoors, where the air is filtered. Second, if you must exercise outdoors, do so early in the morning, before motor vehicle pollution has its greatest effect. Try to work out in areas with less traffic. And pay attention to smog alerts—move your workouts indoors when these occur.

**KEY POINT**

Make the proper adjustments to your exercise plans when exercising in heat, cold, altitude, and air pollution. This includes adjusting the frequency, intensity, time, and type of exercise.

## ALTERNATE PHYSICAL ACTIVITIES

So far in this chapter we've laid the groundwork for understanding cardiorespiratory fitness and the ways in which you can attain that fitness, improve your health, and lower your risk for a variety of diseases by designing an aerobic exercise program. But the truth is, most Americans don't adhere to such a program and don't experience the health and fitness benefits that come with being physically active. Does that mean that the majority of you, then, will never actually experience those benefits? Not necessarily.

First, there's a distinction between *health* benefits and *fitness* benefits. Second, you can experience health benefits through a variety of alternate activities—that is, activities that are linked more to lifestyle than to adherence to an exercise program. We'll discuss those alternate activities in a moment, but first let's revisit the distinction between fitness and health.

In chapter 1 we defined health as the presence of sufficient energy and vitality to carry out daily tasks and recreational activities without undue fatigue. Consider health as the broad foundational rock upon which we want to build. Fitness is something that we are continuously chiseling out of that foundational rock of health. Its components, remember, are cardiorespiratory fitness, body composition, and musculoskeletal fitness (flexibility, strength, muscular endurance).

In other words, we can experience the benefits of health without necessarily adhering to a strenuous exercise program. The U.S. Centers for Disease Control and Prevention and the ACSM developed a summary statement titled "Physical Activity and the Public Health" in which they suggest that alternate activities can have a significant health benefit (Pate et al. 1995). And while the ACSM and the Centers for Disease Control and Prevention recommend that adults be moderately active for at least 30 minutes on most or all days of the week, studies have shown that three 10-minute sessions of moderate activity throughout the day have nearly the same effect on health as one 30-minute workout at the same effort.

So while we certainly recommend that you exercise within the ACSM guidelines shown in table 2.1, we emphasize that you can attain health benefits and improve your quality of life by engaging in physical activities that are below 55% of your

## POINT OF INTEREST

### Exercise Equipment, Infomercials, and You

Turn on your TV and you'll see an abundance of infomercials selling all sorts of exercise equipment. Equipment to improve cardiorespiratory fitness is especially "hot." Prices—and claims made regarding the equipment's value—vary widely.

Now go to your newspaper and look in the classifieds. You'll see a long section of ads for "barely used, like new!" equipment—the same exercise equipment that is sold on the infomercials.

In 1997, consumers spent about $5.3 billion on home exercise equipment. Unfortunately, more than one third of equipment owners say they once used their equipment but have stopped. That probably says more about people's long-term motivation to exercise regularly than it does about the value of the equipment. But it does make you think twice about buying exercise equipment.

The greatest piece of exercise equipment isn't worth a penny if you just use it to gather dust. On the other hand, a relatively inexpensive and rudimentary piece of equipment may be worth its weight in gold if you use it regularly and gain good workouts from it.

The bottom line lies with *you,* not the equipment. You can get a great workout using no equipment at all. You can also get a great workout using exercise equipment.

If you are interested in purchasing equipment, first be honest with yourself: Will you use it over the long haul? Are you truly more motivated to exercise when using equipment? If so, be a smart shopper. Try the equipment out—and several similar pieces of equipment, if you can—before purchasing. Can you return the equipment if you try it at home and don't like it?

The equipment itself—stair steppers, cycles, treadmills, rowing machines, air gliders, cross-country skiing machines, and so on—can be convenient, safe, and worthwhile. These devices can add satisfaction to all of your workouts, they can be used as an occasional alternative to your regular exercise routine, and they can even be a motivating force for those who prefer working out indoors or who like to squeeze a workout in while watching the news (or another infomercial!) on TV.

So long as the focus is on the exercise, not the TV.

Three 10-minute workouts of moderate activity have nearly the same effect on health as one 30-minute workout at the same effort. But if you're not one to plan workouts, realize that you can attain health benefits just by living an active lifestyle—so long as your "unstructured" activity is at least equivalent to any "structured" workout that you might plan.

maximal heart rate. These physical activities are more accurately described as lifestyle choices rather than formal exercise. Examples include

parking your car farther away from your destination and walking; raking leaves, gardening, and doing other yard work; using stairs instead of elevators or escalators; dancing; housework; and so on.

The Metropolitan Life Insurance Company (1995) developed an "Exercise and Activity Pyramid" that depicts four levels of lifestyle physical activity behaviors, with suggestions for either maintaining or increasing activity, depending on your level (see figure 2.8). Review the pyramid and identify steps you can take to improve your lifestyle behaviors related to physical activity.

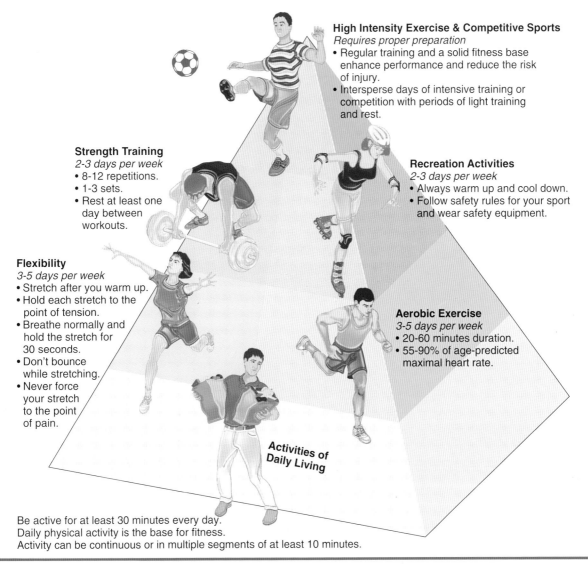

**High Intensity Exercise & Competitive Sports**
*Requires proper preparation*
- Regular training and a solid fitness base enhance performance and reduce the risk of injury.
- Intersperse days of intensive training or competition with periods of light training and rest.

**Strength Training**
*2-3 days per week*
- 8-12 repetitions.
- 1-3 sets.
- Rest at least one day between workouts.

**Recreation Activities**
*2-3 days per week*
- Always warm up and cool down.
- Follow safety rules for your sport and wear safety equipment.

**Flexibility**
*3-5 days per week*
- Stretch after you warm up.
- Hold each stretch to the point of tension.
- Breathe normally and hold the stretch for 30 seconds.
- Don't bounce while stretching.
- Never force your stretch to the point of pain.

**Aerobic Exercise**
*3-5 days per week*
- 20-60 minutes duration.
- 55-90% of age-predicted maximal heart rate.

**Activities of Daily Living**

Be active for at least 30 minutes every day.
Daily physical activity is the base for fitness.
Activity can be continuous or in multiple segments of at least 10 minutes.

**FIGURE 2.8** The exercise and physical activity pyramid.

Adapted from "Exercise and Activity Pyramid," Metropolitan Life Insurance Company 1995.

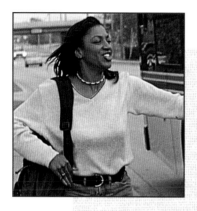

# Health Concepts

As you'll recall, Alicia was surprised at how out of shape she was when she had to jog to class. She assumed that since she had run in high school, she'd still be in decent cardiorespiratory shape. But her half-mile jog told her a much different story.

The good news is that Alicia can greatly improve her oxygen consumption through regular physical activity. Regular aerobic exercise improves maximal oxygen consumption by improving lung function, cardiac output, and arterial-venous oxygen difference.

The key word there is *regular*. As we noted in the preceding chapter, fitness has a dynamic relationship with physical activity. The phrase "use it or lose it" is very apropos here.

And that's why designing an aerobic exercise program is so important. It's hard enough to exercise regularly even when we plan to. When we *don't* plan exercise into our day, we're virtually assuring ourselves that we won't exercise regularly—and thus will never attain higher levels of cardiorespiratory fitness!

## SUMMARY

▌ *Aerobic* means "with oxygen;" *anaerobic* means "without oxygen." In aerobic activity, oxygen must be present in our muscles to produce a high-energy chemical compound called *adenosine triphosphate (ATP)*. The energy for muscular contraction—that is, movement—comes from ATP. Small amounts of ATP are stored in our body; as we exercise, we produce more ATP through aerobic metabolism.

▌ Cardiac output is the amount of blood leaving the heart per minute, determined by the *stroke volume* (amount of blood pumped by the heart with each beat) and *heart rate* (number of beats per minute).

▌ The arterial-venous oxygen difference is the difference in oxygen content between arterial blood and venous blood. The blood is richer in oxygen when it is pumped through the arteries than when it returns through the veins. Tissues that need oxygen and other nutrients extract oxygen from the blood and input waste products such as carbon dioxide in the blood. Oxygen consumption is composed of available oxygen in the blood, cardiac output, and the oxygen used (as determined through the arterial-venous oxygen difference).

▌ Four important principles to consider in designing an aerobic exercise program are *overload, specificity, individuality,* and *reversibility.* Four components of an exercise program are *frequency, intensity, time,* and *type.*

▌ You should aim to exercise at between 55% and 90% of your *maximal heart rate,* which can be estimated by subtracting your age from 220. You should sandwich your cardiorespiratory exercise with 5 to 10 minutes of warm-up and cool-down activities, including stretching. Take specific precautions when exercising in heat, cold, altitude, and air pollution.

▮ You can experience the health benefits of physical activity without necessarily adhering to a strenuous exercise program. Three 10-minute workouts of moderate intensity have nearly the same health benefits as one 30-minute workout at the same effort. Participating in physical activities that are below 55% of your maximal heart rate, such as taking the stairs or gardening, are lifestyle choices that can also give you health benefits and improve your quality of life.

*Cardiorespiratory fitness is the cornerstone of health-related fitness. Next we'll explore the effects of physical activity on another important facet of health-related fitness: muscular fitness.*

## KEY TERMS

| | |
|---|---|
| adenosine triphosphate (ATP) | hyperthermia |
| aerobic | hypothermia |
| anaerobic | maximal oxygen consumption ($\dot{V}O_2$max) |
| cardiorespiratory | steady state |

# 2

# Determining Heart Rate Training Zone, Workout Intensity, Aerobic Capacity, and Physical Activity Level

### THE PURPOSES OF THIS LAB EXPERIENCE ARE TO

▌ determine your heart rate training zone,

▌ estimate the intensity of your workouts through the ratings of perceived exertion,

▌ estimate and evaluate your aerobic capacity, and

▌ estimate your physical activity level.

### Determine Your Heart Rate Training Zone

There are several ways to determine your heart rate training zone; the easiest way is by using your maximum heart rate. Your maximal heart rate is estimated by subtracting your age from 220.

To establish your heart rate training zone, you need to determine the lower and upper ends of the zone. The lower end should be at 55% of your maximal heart rate; the upper end should be at 90%. Determine this zone by completing the following:

(220 − your age) × .55 = _____ (lower end of zone)

(220 − your age) × .90 = _____ (upper end of zone)

You can also use the ratings of perceived exertion to determine your heart rate training zone. Do so by referring to figure 2.5 and by completing the following steps.

1. Warm up.

2. Engage in aerobic activity (e.g., walk, jog, cycle, stair climb).

3. When you perceive that the exercise is of moderate intensity (12 on the 20-point scale), check your heart rate and compare it to 55% of your maximal heart rate.

4. Continue to exercise until you perceive the effort to be very hard (16 on the 20-point scale). Now compare your heart rate to 90% of your maximal heart rate.

You'll likely find different results when using your maximal heart rate and the ratings of perceived exertion to determine your heart rate training zone. That's why we estimate a *zone* instead of a specific target heart rate.

## Estimate Workout Intensity

Use the ratings of perceived exertion in figure 2.5 to estimate your workout intensity. On the 20-point scale, your exertion should be between 12 (moderate) and 16 (hard) if you are to gain aerobic and health benefits.

## Estimate and Evaluate Your Aerobic Capacity

We'll use two ways to estimate your aerobic capacity: the Rockport Walking Test and a nonexercise method.

### Rockport Walking Test

1. Walk 1 mile as quickly as you can.
2. Record your time for the mile.
3. Record your heart rate immediately following the walk by taking your 15-second pulse count and multiplying by 4 to calculate the beats per minute. Then complete the following formula (from Kline et al. 1987) to estimate your aerobic capacity.

> Estimated $\dot{V}O_2$max (ml/kg/min) = 132.853
> - (0.0769 × body weight [pounds])
> - (0.3877 × age [years])
> + (6.3150 × gender [female = 0; male = 1])
> - (3.2649 × 1-mile walk time [in minutes and hundredths])
> - (0.1565 × 1-minute heart rate at end of mile [beats per minute])

For example, consider a 20-year-old male who weighs 230 pounds, walked a mile in 15:32, and had a heart rate of 203 beats per minute after the walking test:

> Estimated $\dot{V}O_2$max = 132.853      132.853
> - (0.0769 × 230)      - 17.687
> - (0.3877 × 20)      - 7.754
> + (6.3150 × 1)      + 6.3150
> - (3.2649 × [15 + 32/60])      - 50.71
> - (0.1565 × 203)      - 31.77
>      = 31.25 ml/kg/min

On the basis of the validity (R = .88) and standard error of estimate (5.0 ml/kg/min), you can be about 68% sure that your true $\dot{V}O_2$max is ± 5.0 ml/kg/min of your calculated value. For example, if your predicted $\dot{V}O_2$max is 40 ml/kg/min, there is a 68% likelihood that your actual value is between 35 and 45.

### Nonexercise Estimation of Your Aerobic Capacity

Jackson et al. (1990) developed a method to estimate your aerobic capacity by using the Physical Activity Rating (PAR) Scale and your weight and height. First, find the number (0 to 7) that best describes your level of physical activity as outlined in the following PAR Scale.

*I don't participate regularly in programmed recreation, sports, or heavy physical activity.*

0—I avoid walking or exertion (e.g., I use an elevator instead of stairs; I drive when possible instead of walking).

1—I walk for pleasure, routinely use stairs, occasionally exercise hard enough to perspire or breathe heavily.

*I participate regularly in recreation or work requiring modest physical activity (such as golf, horseback riding, calisthenics, gymnastics, table tennis, bowling, weight lifting, yard work).*

2—This activity takes 10 to 60 minutes per week.

3—This activity takes more than 60 minutes per week.

*I participate regularly in heavy physical exercise (such as running or jogging, swimming, cycling, rowing, skipping rope, or engaging in vigorous aerobic activity such as playing tennis, basketball, or racquetball).*

4—I run less than 1 mile per week or spend less than 30 minutes per week in comparable activity.

5—I run 1 to 5 miles per week or spend 30 to 60 minutes per week in comparable physical activity.

6—I run 6 to 10 miles per week or spend 1 to 3 hours per week in comparable physical activity.

7—I run over 10 miles per week or spend over 3 hours per week in comparable physical activity.

**Now plug your PAR number into the following equation.**

Estimated $\dot{V}O_2$max (ml/kg/min) = 56.363

+ (1.921 × PAR)

− (0.381 × age in years)

− (0.754 × [weight in pounds / 2.2]) / (height in inches × 0.0254)$^2$

+ (10.987 × gender [female = 0; male = 1])

The standard error for this equation is 5.70 ml/kg/min.

For example, consider a 23-year-old female who weighs 130 pounds, is 5 feet 4 inches tall, and has a PAR of 2:

| Estimated $\dot{V}O_2$max = 56.363 | 56.363 |
|---|---|
| + (1.921 × 2) | + 3.842 |
| − (0.381 × 23) | − 8.763 |
| − (0.754 × [130 / 2.2]) / (64 × 0.0254)$^2$ | − 16.860 |
| + (10.987 × 0) | + 0 |
| | = 34.58 ml/kg/min |

## Evaluate Your Aerobic Capacity

Now that you've estimated your $\dot{V}O_2$max, use the following chart (adapted from Howley and Franks 1992) to evaluate your fitness level (ml/kg/min).

| Age | $\dot{V}O_2$max (ml/kg/min) Female | Male |
|---|---|---|
| **GOOD** | | |
| 15-34 | > 40 | > 45 |
| 35-54 | > 35 | > 40 |
| 55-70 | > 30 | > 35 |
| **ADEQUATE FOR MOST ACTIVITIES** | | |
| 15-34 | 35 | 40 |
| 35-54 | 30 | 35 |
| 55-70 | 25 | 30 |
| **BORDERLINE** | | |
| 15-34 | 30 | 35 |
| 35-54 | 25 | 30 |
| 55-70 | 20 | 25 |
| **NEEDS TO IMPROVE AEROBIC CAPACITY** | | |
| 15-34 | < 25 | < 30 |
| 35-54 | < 20 | < 25 |
| 55-70 | < 15 | < 20 |

## Estimate Your Physical Activity Level

Review the following Physical Activity Questionnaire (based in part on questions from the U.S. Centers for Disease Control and Prevention 1996) and circle the level that best describes your physical activity level. If you are at Level 4 or higher, you are probably engaging in enough physical activity to enjoy its health benefits.

| Physical activity | Description | Examples |
|---|---|---|
| Level 1 "Sedentary" | Essentially no physical activity above minimum demands of daily living | • Watching TV<br>• Working at desk<br>• Riding in car<br>• Eating |
| Level 2 "Minimally active" | Activity during normal daily routine to limber body and provide light muscle contraction<br>• Total of 15-30 minutes per day<br>• Daily<br>• Very light to fairly light perceived exertion | • Walking<br>• Occasional stair climbing<br>• Light gardening<br>• Light home repairs |
| Level 3 "Mildly active" | Activity to limber body and provide moderate muscle contraction to large muscle groups<br>• Total of 30-60 minutes per day<br>• Daily<br>• Fairly light to somewhat hard perceived exertion | • Walking<br>• Calisthenics<br>• Heavy gardening<br>• Major home repairs |
| Level 4 "Moderately active" | One or more dynamic activities with large muscle groups<br>• 15 minutes or more per session<br>• 1-3 sessions per week<br>• Exercise maintains heart rate in target zone | • Running/jogging<br>• Lap swimming<br>• Bicycling<br>• Fast walking<br>• Calisthenics/dancing<br>• Aerobics classes<br>• Stair climbing<br>• Nonaerobic sports* |
| Level 5 "Vigorously active" | One or more dynamic activities with large muscle groups<br>• 20 minutes or more per session<br>• 3 or more sessions per week<br>• 65% or greater maximal heart rate or somewhat hard to hard perceived exertion | Same exercises as in Level 4, including:<br>• Bench classes<br>• Aerobic sports** |
| Level 6 "Very vigorous" | One or more dynamic activities with large muscle groups<br>• 30 minutes or more per session<br>• 4 or more sessions per week<br>• 65% or greater maximal heart rate or somewhat hard to hard perceived exertion | Same exercises as in Levels 4 and 5, including:<br>• Cross-training<br>• Fitness activities<br>• Bench classes and running<br>• Lap swimming and bicycling |
| Level 7 "Competitive" | One or more dynamic activities with large muscle groups<br>• 40-60 minutes per session<br>• 5-6 sessions per week<br>• 65% or greater maximal heart rate or somewhat hard to hard perceived exertion | Same exercises as in Levels 4 through 6, including:<br>• Competitive athletic training (triathlon training,10K training, marathon training) |

*For example, tennis, basketball, baseball, downhill skiing
**For example, roller skating, cross-country skiing, soccer

# Chapter 3

# Muscular Fitness

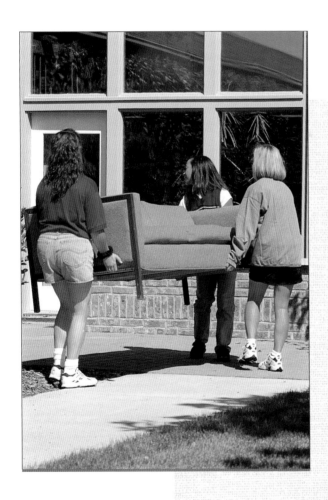

Dawn and I helped Heather move into her new apartment yesterday. This morning I woke up all stiff and sore, but Dawn said she didn't feel it at all. She said it was probably because she works out at the student fitness center. She lifts weights and stretches three or four times a week. She has decent muscle tone, but she certainly doesn't look like the weight lifters I've seen in magazines. I'm not interested in becoming a bodybuilder, but I would like to "carry my own weight," so to speak, so that the next time I help someone move I don't get so stiff and sore! Plus, I'll probably play coed volleyball next semester, and I'm thinking a little additional strength wouldn't hurt. But if I do lift weights and become stronger, does that mean I'll become less flexible, too? I don't want to get too big and bulky.

—Melissa, 21-year-old senior

*W*hat *do you think?*

Strength and flexibility are two components of musculoskeletal fitness that are commonly misunderstood. Athletes tend to value strength because it can help them perform better, and men in general also value strength because it's usually seen as a desired trait for men. But what about women? If women lift weights, will they, as Melissa fears, become "big and bulky," masculine and unattractive? Are the benefits of becoming stronger simply superficial, or are there additional fitness and health benefits?

Similarly, the value of being flexible is often clouded with controversy. If you're not an athlete who *needs* to become more flexible to perform better, are there any reasons to work at increasing your ranges of motion? Do stretching exercises really help prevent injuries and enhance performance? Are there actual *health benefits* to becoming more flexible?

In reading this chapter, you'll be able to separate fact from fiction regarding strength and flexibility. You'll learn the benefits and principles of building strength and learn how to increase strength and muscular endurance through basic and advanced techniques. You'll be exposed to a series of weight-lifting exercises working the muscles throughout the body. And you'll encounter similar types of information about flexibility: its benefits and the factors that affect it; different types of stretching; and a series of stretching exercises designed to increase range of motion in the body's major muscle joints. Along the way you'll also gain some insight into two of the muddier areas of strength and flexibility: the issue of women, weight lifting, and bulk, and the controversy surrounding stretching and injury prevention.

## STRENGTH

*Strength* is defined as the ability of a muscle to produce force. It is largely determined by how much muscle a person has, and can be measured in terms of how much we can lift, push, or pull in a single, all-out effort. This effort can be as-sessed by using barbells or weight machines or by using computer-assisted systems that accurately measure force production.

Another factor that influences strength is the proportion of fast-twitch muscle fibers. The body is composed of three types of muscle fibers: fast-twitch red, fast-twitch white, and slow-twitch red. Fast-twitch fibers produce more force than slow-twitch fibers. If two people have the same muscle mass but one has a greater percentage of fast-twitch fibers, the one with more fast-twitch fibers will be able to generate more force. The percentage of fast-twitch and slow-twitch fibers doesn't affect health, but it does affect performance. People with more fast-twitch fibers tend to have more power and speed; people with more slow-twitch fibers tend to have more endurance. The proportion of fast-twitch and slow-twitch fibers is determined by genetics, and is altered only slightly by factors such as training or aging.

*Muscular endurance* refers to a muscle's ability to produce force over and over again. Generally when we speak of *muscular* endurance we are thinking of exercise that we can sustain for a few seconds to a few minutes; when we speak of endurance in general we are usually thinking of exercise that we can sustain for many minutes or hours. This endurance is determined by both muscular fitness and cardiorespiratory fitness, which we discussed in chapter 2.

*Power* refers to the amount of work performed in a given amount of time. "Work" is the product of force and the distance through which that force is applied. People who are stronger are usually more powerful because they can produce more force. As with muscular endurance, the amount and quality of muscle largely determine power. Both power and strength are influenced by other factors, including training and qualities of the central nervous system.

 *Strength* refers to a muscle's ability to produce force; *muscular endurance* refers to a muscle's ability to keep on producing force; and *power* refers to a muscle's ability to produce force quickly.

For example, our ability to exert strength and power is normally monitored, as it were, by the central nervous system. This system has a degree of inhibition that keeps our muscles from actually producing as much force as they are capable of producing; this reduces the risk of a muscle tearing itself off a bone. In extraordinary circumstances this inhibition is decreased. Women (or men) don't normally go around lifting cars off the ground, but when a car is partially over a child, they might find the strength to do so.

That, of course, is the extreme example. The more normal way of decreasing muscular inhibition is to train the muscles consistently for months.

You need minimal levels of strength to perform such mundane tasks as turning a steering wheel, carrying a load of laundry, and shelving groceries. But you'll benefit by having greater-than-minimal levels of strength. Strength, in fact, has many benefits.

## Benefits of Strength

Strength can improve physical performance. Strength will help you get greater enjoyment from recreational sport and from leisure activities such as camping and canoeing, hiking and climbing, or mountain biking. You don't need to be overly strong to enjoy these activities, but moderate strength will help you take part in them with less fatigue and more enjoyment. If you're in shape, you'll go farther and feel better.

Being stronger can also help protect you from injuries. Many activities, such as recreational sports, present some risk of injury. Other recreation or leisure pursuits can also lead to injuries. Consider the examples in the previous paragraph. Camping involves lifting and carrying. There are backpacks with tents and supplies of water, food, and wood for the fire. Having adequate strength (and practicing good lifting habits) can help minimize the risk of injury by making tasks less stressful on your body.

When you increase your muscle mass, you increase your resting metabolic rate—more muscle mass burns more calories, even at rest. From a weight control point of view, your muscles will be working for you 24 hours a day. And, of course, it takes energy to build muscle. As you burn calories to *become* stronger, you're burning more calories because you *are* stronger.

As you age, you lose bone mineral density and muscle mass. By building muscular strength you can prevent, or at least postpone and minimize, these losses. It's hard for most college students to imagine what it will be like when they're 70 years old and retired. Will you be stooped and weak, or standing tall, feeling fit, and enjoying an active life? Now is the time to build and maintain a healthy level of strength.

There are other advantages to working out regularly to improve your strength. You may experience an improved sense of well-being through the physical effects of improving strength, and the more subtle psychological effects: when you go into the weight room with a reasonable goal, and you achieve that goal, you'll naturally feel good. And finally, for many people, looking good equals feeling good. Many years ago, exercise physiologists used to judge the effectiveness of a program by observing changes in parameters such as strength and power, or aerobic endurance when people were participating in an aerobic fitness program. One fitness program director figured it out—he realized that people were interested in looking good and feeling good, not in having a lower resting heart rate or a higher-max lift in the bench press. Stick with your program and you'll be looking good and feeling good!

 When you improve your strength you can improve your physical performance, protect yourself from injuries, increase your resting metabolic rate, prevent or minimize bone mineral density loss, and help yourself look and feel good.

## Principles of Building Strength

To safely build and maintain strength for fitness, you need to first understand and apply basic training principles. You'll remember that in chapter 2 we discussed four important principles—overload, specificity, individuality, and reversibility—in relation to improving cardiorespiratory fitness. You can also apply these four principles to a strength-training program.

### Principle #1: Overload

*To increase strength, we must tax our muscles beyond their accustomed loads.*

We develop strength by creating tension within our muscles. The more tension we create (the more force we produce), the more strength we'll build. So, the load we place upon our muscles must be significant enough to cause physiological adaptations. When we train our muscles systematically, our muscles will respond by becoming larger; this is called *hypertrophy*. Weight lifting is the most common recreational way to bring about hypertrophy; but construction work and

other jobs that rely on heavy physical labor also create tension and build strength. You use the overload principle to reach strength goals; once you've reached them, you work to maintain what you've gained.

### Principle #2: Specificity

*Your strength-training program must be specifically related to your overall exercise objectives.*

Only the muscles we work can gain strength. Within an individual muscle, only the fibers that you activate during a training session or activity can get stronger. Simply put, your body responds very specifically to your exercise or activity. In terms of building strength, this means that if you use push-ups to build chest muscles, those muscles will become stronger and you'll *specifically* increase your ability to perform push-ups. You'll also *generally* increase your ability to perform other activities that call for muscular endurance in your chest muscles, but you'll most notice your muscular endurance gains when performing the push-ups that brought you those gains.

 Our bodies respond very specifically to exercise. Only the muscle fibers that we activate during a training session can increase in strength.

### Principle #3: Individuality

*You should evaluate your fitness level and your exercise goals on a personal level rather than compare yourself to others.*

If you lift weights regularly, typically you'll become stronger. But as mentioned in chapter 2, each person has a unique genetic endowment, history of exercise and fitness, level of motivation, and range of responses to exercise. Some people respond very quickly to a strength-training program, while others don't experience gains until they've trained regularly for weeks or months. On the same note, some people must work very hard to see progress while others seem to hardly break a sweat and still get stronger. Some people like to perform the same routine at each exercise session, and others have to vary their workouts and really shake things up to stay interested and see the benefits they want. The most important idea behind individuality is that everyone will benefit from a strength-training program; realize as you begin your program that your body's response to training and your individual workout needs will be different from someone else's.

### Principle #4: Reversibility

*When you stop overloading your muscles, your strength and muscular fitness will, over time, return to their preexercise levels.*

You've heard the expression "use it or lose it." The results of any training program, including strength training, are not permanent. You have to keep overloading your muscles to maintain the benefits. Reversibility doesn't mean that if you miss a week in the gym you'll shrink back to your original size. But if you stop exercising completely for a long period of time, you lose

- muscle strength and power;
- muscular endurance;
- speed, agility, and flexibility; and
- cardiorespiratory endurance.

With reversibility, you gradually experience a shrinking of the muscles; this is called *atrophy.* Atrophy is most obvious when a cast comes off after a person has broken an arm or leg. The injured limb is noticeably smaller after the immobilization, when there was little load, let alone overload.

## Types of Muscle Action

Weight lifting and other strength-training programs depend ultimately on the types of muscle action used in the activity. There are two basic ways to train your muscles: through *isometric exercise* and *isotonic exercise.*

In isometric exercise, your muscles stay at the same length. They don't shorten (contract), but they do produce force. If you hold a weight with your arm straight down and then raise the weight until your arm is bent at a 90-degree angle, and then stop the motion, you're no longer contracting your biceps; your muscles are no longer shortening. They are, however, still exerting

### Strength Differences in Men and Women

Women can increase strength and muscle mass, but the average woman won't become as big or strong as the average man because men's testosterone levels, which kick in at puberty, enable them to build a larger muscle mass. After puberty, both men and women can increase strength and muscle mass, but even if a woman makes the same relative improvement (percentage increase) as a man, her absolute improvement (pounds or kilograms of muscle) will be less. Of course, there is a wide range of "trainability" in both men and women, meaning that some people—regardless of gender—can make greater improvements than others. However, very few women can develop large muscles. In addition, their muscle mass will be less evident than that of a man because women tend to have more body fat (see chapter 4).

The bottom line is that both men and women can develop and maintain strength at a level that benefits their health and well-being.

force to hold the weight in place. This is an *isometric muscle action.*

With *isotonic muscle action,* your muscles are contracting or lengthening. When you contract a muscle, the action is *concentric;* when you lengthen a muscle, the action is *eccentric.* In both cases the muscle action applies force as the muscle goes through its movements. For example, when you perform a biceps curl, your biceps contract as you bring the weight from your waist to your shoulders. This is a *concentric muscle action.* As you lower the weight, your biceps lengthen; this is an *eccentric muscle action.*

Another form of isotonic exercise is *isokinetics,* which means "the same rate of shortening." Isokinetics is used mainly in rehabilitation and research, and involves the use of sophisticated, computer-assisted devices that control the rate of movement and measure the force that is produced. Through *isokinetic muscle action* we can facilitate rehabilitation by moving a joint at a constant rate and through the same range of motion.

## BUILDING STRENGTH AND MUSCULAR ENDURANCE

As you begin to create a program to build your muscular endurance and strength, you should be aware of several factors that affect your training. Most important is the *training routine.* We'll describe the components of a training routine and define training techniques that will help you reach health and fitness goals.

As you enter into your routine, one of the first questions you might have is how quickly you'll progress. We'll explain the factors that affect how rapidly you improve, and we'll also look at cross training as it pertains to building strength and muscular endurance.

### Training Routine

A training routine is based upon knowing the appropriate type of exercise, intensity, frequency, and duration. Use the acronym FITT to remember the components of a training routine:

- **F**requency (how many times you exercise per week)
- **I**ntensity (how hard you exercise; in this case how heavy a weight you lift)
- **T**ime (the duration of each workout; in this case how many exercises and how many sets and repetitions of each exercise)
- **T**ype (what type of exercise you perform)

There are numerous routines or systems to choose from; within reason, it doesn't matter exactly which system you choose, so long as you incorporate wise training principles. To understand wise training principles, we first need to define some weight-lifting terms.

 You can vary your training routine so long as you stick to wise training principles.

A *repetition* or "rep" is one complete movement, such as bringing a dumbbell from your waist to your shoulder and then lowering it back to its starting position. A *set* is a series of repetitions—for example, you might do one set of 8 reps, or three sets of 8 reps. A *one-repetition maximum (1-RM)* is the heaviest weight that you can successfully lift one time while maintaining proper form. A 1-RM is a measure of your strength. An 8-RM or 12-RM is a measure of your muscular endurance.

This doesn't mean that when you perform a set of 8 reps you must go to "muscle failure" at the end of the set—that is, be unable to perform another rep. Do remember the overload principle, however; submit your muscles to an overload in order to gain strength. For example, determine your 12-RM for a certain exercise, and then lift that weight 10 times. This will feel hard, but you should feel as though you could lift the weight one or two more times at the end of the set.

A basic routine is to choose 8 to 10 exercises that work the major muscle groups and perform

**HEALTHCHECK**

**Can using anabolic steroids make me stronger?**

Steroids *can* improve strength—but they come with high risks. Using steroids increases the risk of coronary artery disease and can cause many other serious health problems. Steroids are banned in organized sport and can't be obtained legally for the purpose of more rapid strength gain. They have no place in anyone's personal fitness program.

one set of 8 to 12 reps for each exercise. Do this workout three times per week with a day off in between each workout. You'll build strength by following such a routine.

You might increase your strength gains by performing three sets of 6 to 10 reps for each exercise, but you'll spend more time and energy in doing so. There's probably a greater risk of injury with a more intense workout such as this, and the workout will take two to three times as long.

A more intense workout may also result in muscle soreness. Even performing a series of one-set exercises can cause soreness when you begin a program. Soreness is caused by damage to the older, more susceptible muscle fibers; if you exercise (especially with intensity) in a way you haven't done recently, you'll damage these fibers. But subsequent bouts of similar exercise won't produce the same damage and resulting soreness, because you'll have fewer old fibers to damage. The key is to start slowly—don't see how much you can do in the first day. Building strength comes through consistent effort, not occasional all-out effort.

As you begin your program, you may feel stiff and sore 24 to 48 hours after lifting. This is referred to as DOMS—*delayed onset muscle soreness.* Delayed onset muscle soreness is an inflammatory response that causes swelling around the muscles as the older fibers are damaged; this swelling causes the soreness. The soreness usually dissipates within a few days, and no permanent muscle damage occurs. The soreness isn't harmful, and it's okay to exercise when you're sore, though it will be uncomfortable. In fact,

**Ten Signs of Overtraining**

According to Baechle and Groves (1998), signs of overtraining include
1. extreme muscle soreness the day after training;
2. a gradual *increase* in muscle soreness from one training session to the next;
3. weight loss (if no attempt to lose weight is being made);
4. an inability to finish a training session that you'd normally be able to finish;
5. an increase of 8 to 10 beats per minute in your resting heart rate (taken every day at the same time and in the same conditions);
6. an increase in minor illnesses such as colds, headaches, and so on;
7. a loss in appetite;
8. swollen lymph nodes in the neck, groin, or armpits;
9. constipation or diarrhea; and
10. an unexplained drop in physical performance.

usually the soreness will subside somewhat during the exercise. And once you've established your routine, the soreness should be minimal.

## Training Techniques

Just as there are numerous training routines to choose from, there are also a number of training techniques you can employ to build strength and muscular endurance. Following are brief descriptions of some of these techniques; for more detail on training techniques, see *Designing Resistance Training Programs* (Fleck and Kraemer 1997) and *Essentials of Strength Training and Conditioning* (National Strength and Conditioning Association 1994).

• **Vary the order of your lifts.** The common practice is to work the large muscle groups before working the small muscle groups (e.g., the chest muscles before the biceps and triceps). The reasoning here is that if you work the smaller muscles first, then they'll be too fatigued to do their supporting work as you move to the larger muscle groups. However, as you advance in your program, you might want to consider a technique that many experienced weight lifters at least occasionally employ: targeting the smaller muscles first—performing a series of different exercises all designed to work, say, the triceps. Just understand that other lifts that call on the triceps for support (such as the bench press, which primarily works the chest muscles) will suffer that day.

• **Isolate the muscles you're exercising.** Many lifts call on numerous muscles working together to lift the weight. The bench press, for example, uses the chest muscles, the front of the shoulders, and the triceps, while bench stepping uses the quadriceps, hamstrings, and gluteals. Some exercises, however, isolate muscles, ensuring that only an individual muscle or set of muscles is doing the work. For instance, the triceps extension isolates the triceps, and the leg flexion isolates the hamstrings and gluteals.

• **Split your routine.** Our basic exercise prescription has you perform the same exercises each workout day. As you advance, however, you might consider another technique that many experienced lifters use: splitting the routine. On one workout day, for example, you might perform exercises for your thighs, abdominals, and chest; on the next workout day, you'd exercise your calves, arms, and back. This allows you to work out four days a week with each body part receiving a 48-hour break between workouts.

*Note:* Although it's possible to work out six or even seven days a week with this schedule, it's not advisable. Just as a specific muscle needs time to recover, so does your body in general. Even serious athletes take days off. Plus, if you build rest days into your weekly schedule, you'll have a day to catch up if for some reason you weren't able to work out on the day you had planned.

• **Use a partner to assist in some lifts.** While at first this technique may seem contrary to making strength gains, many experienced lifters use a partner to help with the concentric (positive) action. Muscle fibers are able to produce more force in an eccentric (negative) action. With a little help on the concentric action, you can increase the training stimulus on your muscles. You shouldn't try this, though, unless you're an advanced weight lifter; this technique, with the greater weight lifted during the eccentric actions, can cause DOMS and brings with it a greater risk of injury.

• **Use periodization as you progress.** *Periodization* refers to the planned progression of workouts over time. This progression doesn't just mean more reps, more sets, and more weight; rather, it refers to cycles of workouts. As you progress, you might increase some elements of your workout while decreasing other elements. For example, you might perform more reps while using slightly less weight than usual. Or, if you were going to move from doing one set of 12 reps of an exercise to doing three sets, you might cut back on both the number of reps per set and the weight until you were used to the increased number of sets.

### HEALTHCHECK

**If you want to improve your muscular endurance for activities such as jogging, cycling, or playing tennis, are you better off by performing fewer reps with high weights or more reps with low weights?**

You'll improve muscular endurance by performing a greater number of repetitions with lower weights. Muscular strength is improved through performance of fewer repetitions at higher weights.

The shortest cycle you might consider is one week. You might lift on four days and split your routine, as we suggested, by alternating between body parts. You might use more reps and lighter weights on the first session for each body part, and fewer reps and heavier weights on the second session. Periodization slightly changes the stress on the muscles, reducing the risk of injury. As you change the stimulus through periodization, you increase the likelihood of adaptation. That is, when you stress a muscle with high resistance, it should respond (adapt) by becoming stronger and being able to generate more tension. During another workout you might increase your reps, and your muscles should respond by increasing muscular endurance. Over several months, the emphasis gradually shifts from high volume with low intensity (to develop mass), to moderate volume with relatively high intensity (to develop muscular endurance), to low volume with high intensity (to develop strength), and finally—at least for athletes—to low volume with high-intensity and high-speed lifting (to develop power). So, through periodization, you first develop muscle mass, then muscular endurance, then strength, and finally power.

By changing the emphases in the cycles of your workouts, you can develop muscle mass, then muscular endurance, then strength, and finally power.

## Determining Your 1-RM

As we saw earlier, a 1-RM is the heaviest weight you can successfully lift one time while maintaining proper form. To determine your 1-RM, you should be rested and ready. After a few warm-ups with a light weight, try a weight that you believe is close to your maximum on that exercise. If you succeed, rest 2 to 3 minutes and try something heavier. When you find a weight you can't lift with proper form, either rest and try that weight one more time, or try a weight slightly lighter (but heavier than the greatest weight you've achieved in that session). Don't make more than five or six attempts in a testing session, or fatigue may affect the outcome. Likewise, don't test for more than two or three 1-RMs (in different lifts) in any one session.

Now that you know how to determine your 1-RM, you might wonder "Why do I need to know?" One point to remember: While determining your 1-RM does give you an indication of your strength, if you're training for health and basic fitness, it's not essential that you determine your 1-RM. Many athletes monitor their strength training by testing their 1-RMs at regular intervals, and some then base their training weights in each exercise on percentages of this maximum; however, you can increase your strength without ever checking your 1-RM.

All right, you now understand that your 1-RM is an indicator of strength. How do you know what weight to use in your workouts? We've previously recommended using a weight that allows you to perform 8 to 12 reps. Sets involving more reps (12 to 15) produce gains in muscular endurance. One to three sets of 8 to 12 reps produce gains in muscle mass and strength. You can accomplish lifting for overall fitness with one to three sets of 8 to 12 reps—enough reps to stimulate muscle development and muscular endurance. The key is to use enough weight to stimulate strength gain. You can determine this weight for each exercise in three ways.

1. The first way to determine your 12-RM is to plan to do three sets of 10 reps with this weight.

## Training for Power

Power is the product of force and speed. To be powerful you must have great strength and be able to produce force quickly. The principle of specificity tells us that if we want to become more powerful, we must train not just to make separate gains in strength and in speed, but to gain in our ability to produce great force quickly.

Just as you can modify any strength exercise into a muscular endurance exercise by performing more reps, so you can modify an exercise to develop power by performing it faster. *Plyometrics* is a form of exercise used to develop power. Plyometrics involves jumping, hopping, and bounding movements for the lower body and swinging, quick-action push-offs, and catching and throwing weighted objects for the upper body. The basic idea of plyometrics is to "store" energy in the muscles and then immediately release the energy in the opposite direction.

For example, in jumping, the object is to land and immediately release in the opposite direction (i.e., upward). As you jump, your quadriceps (the large muscles in the front of your thighs) stretch like a rubber band. As you land, they recoil, and as you jump again, some of the force is due to the elastic recoil.

This has two effects. The immediate effect is that you should be able to jump higher because you're combining the elastic recoil with your muscles' own force production. The training effect is that your body will, over time, learn to produce force faster on the rebound—which increases your power to perform those movements. See the exercise descriptions of half knee bends and knee push-ups on pages 60 and 65, respectively, for specific examples of how to adapt strength-training exercises into power-training exercises. Check out the second edition of *Jumping Into Plyometrics* (Chu 1998) for more information on this training method.

---

Finding your 12-RM isn't quite as easy as determining your 1-RM. Let's say you're interested in determining your 12-RM for the bench press. You first try 50 pounds and find you can lift it 20 times. You rest, then try 60 pounds, which you lift 14 times. You rest again, try 65 pounds, and get only 10 reps. But could you have done more reps if you weren't tired from your previous attempts?

2. The second way to determine a weight for your three sets of 10 reps is through trial and error. Pick a weight and see if you can perform three sets of 10 reps. If the first two sets are challenging and the last set is downright difficult (or you couldn't finish all 10 reps), then you've done a good job of guessing the weight you should start with. If you can't finish even 10 reps of the first set, you'll know you have to decrease the weight to accomplish three sets. And if you feel as though you could do about 50 more reps after the first set, then obviously you need to add a little weight to test for the next two. A drawback to this method is that if you pick a weight that is too heavy for the first set, even if your next pick is a good one you may be too tired to complete the final two sets. Nevertheless, after trying this

method on different days, you'll soon learn what weight you can handle for the reps and sets you're planning.

3. The first two methods overlook one important concept: after your first exercise of the day, you'll be tired for every other exercise. Maybe you *can* do three sets of 10 reps with 60 pounds for the bench press . . . when you're fresh. But if you usually perform the bench press *after* the military press, you may be able to perform only 10 sets of 50 pounds. To avoid this problem, the third method applies the trial-and-error technique across your entire workout. The first exercise in your order of exercises will be the first one for which you will, for certain, learn which weight is most appropriate. Then, for each subsequent exercise, you'll be able to determine what weight you can handle after having performed the previous exercises, just as you would for your normal routine. We'll take you through this method in the lab exercises for this chapter.

Regardless of the method you choose to determine the appropriate resistance, be patient—it will take you some time. Be prepared to discover that once you've finally determined the best weight for each exercise, you'll have developed enough strength to increase the weight on some of your exercises! There are two important things to remember here. First, if you increase weight in one exercise, it may affect how much you can lift or the reps you can finish in subsequent exercises. Second, even if you don't have exactly the "right" weight, lifting the bar will make you stronger! Don't get too tied up in calculating your 1-RM and 12-RM—get in there and start lifting!

You've probably noticed that we haven't told you exactly how many reps to perform each day, and you might think that "8 to 12" is a little vague. But what you do—and what you *can* do—each day is determined not just by your 12-RM and some magic exercise prescription, but also by how you feel, by what you've been doing during the day, by the time of day, and by various environmental conditions. If 10 reps seems too tough one day, settle for 8. If you're feeling great and 12 seems easy, go ahead and do 12 today (and remember that it's fine to do your usual 10 the next time!).

## Progression

Three factors will affect how quickly you progress as you engage in a weight-lifting program:

1. Your genetic ability. People have varying genetic abilities to increase strength.

2. Your starting point. If you haven't been active, your initial progress will be faster than the progress of someone who has been exercising regularly.

3. Your commitment. Gaining and maintaining higher levels of strength take a steady commitment.

That commitment of time and energy will result in a greater level of health and fitness. And that commitment is often fueled by the appreciable gains in strength noticed soon after you begin a program. In many cases, beginning lifters find that they have made appreciable strength gains after only one or two weeks of training. The motivation is sometimes harder to come by once you've made some initial gains and have leveled off, or "plateaued." But typically plateaus can be followed by more gains in strength. It's during these times of leveling off that many weight lifters employ some of the training techniques described previously, such as periodization, partner-assisted lifts, and so on.

 Your initial gains will be followed by a "plateau" period. But by using various training techniques—and maintaining your workouts—you can make further strength gains.

## Cross Training

People originally spoke of *cross training* in connection with athletes who, in training for one

**HEALTHCHECK**

**What are the pros and cons of using free weights versus machines to build strength?**

Many athletes are convinced that using free weights is the best way to build the most strength. Certainly, free weights can be used effectively to develop explosive power. Free weights also require (and help develop) balance and coordination. Machine weights and free weights can both be used to build strength, and unless you're a power athlete, any differences probably aren't meaningful to you. The big advantage of machines lies in their relative safety. Especially if you're a beginner, free weights have a greater potential to cause injury because they require skill, balance, and coordination (and because they can fall on you!).

someone who runs, cycles, and lifts weights is "cross training." Two advantages of cross training are that you reduce risk of overuse injury and that you may avoid the boredom that comes from training in the same way each day.

Seen in this more general context, cross training has application in weight lifting. For instance, you can perform strength training by using different equipment such as free weights, Nautilus equipment, and a Universal Gym. You can benefit through each of these systems, and you get to see improvement in many more individual exercises.

By taking the idea of cross training a bit further, you can use many different exercises to strengthen the same muscle. For example, the bench press is the primary exercise for strengthening the pectoralis major—the chest muscle responsible for bringing your arms forward or pushing an object away from your body. You can also raise the bench to a 35-degree angle and perform an "inclined" press to work these muscles in a slightly different way. Or you can perform push-ups, with your hands close together and then farther apart for different effects.

sport, "crossed over" and used training from another sport to improve performance in the first sport. Now when most people speak of cross training, they are simply referring to one person doing multiple types of training: for instance,

### Safety Tips

▌ Warm up with exercises, jogging, light lifting, and stretching.
▌ Don't hold your breath or hyperventilate. Breathe rhythmically with your lifting.
▌ Protect your back by holding weights close to your body and by not arching your back (weight belts can help you prevent this from happening).
▌ Keep your hands dry.
▌ Check for secured collars and pins on free weights or machines.
▌ Avoid deep squats, to prevent knee injuries.
▌ Use a slow, balanced lifting cadence with a full range of motion for each exercise. Don't jerk the weights to get in one more rep.
▌ Use a spotter when working out with free weights.
▌ You don't have to work to muscle "failure" in every set to achieve benefits—it's better to think you could have done one more rep than to hurt yourself trying.
▌ Use proper technique to decrease the risk of injury. You're most likely to slip into poor lifting techniques when you're tired or distracted.

## STRENGTH EXERCISES

You can perform the following exercises by using machines or free weights. Select the body areas or muscle groups that you want to work and choose exercises for these areas. It's to your advantage to learn from an experienced instructor in the club or gym how to perform the exercises you choose; however, the pictures and descriptions accompanying the exercises will point you in the right direction.

The 17 exercises are categorized by legs; upper back, shoulder, and chest; lower back and abdomen; and arms. Refer to figure 3.1 to see which muscles are being worked with the various exercises.

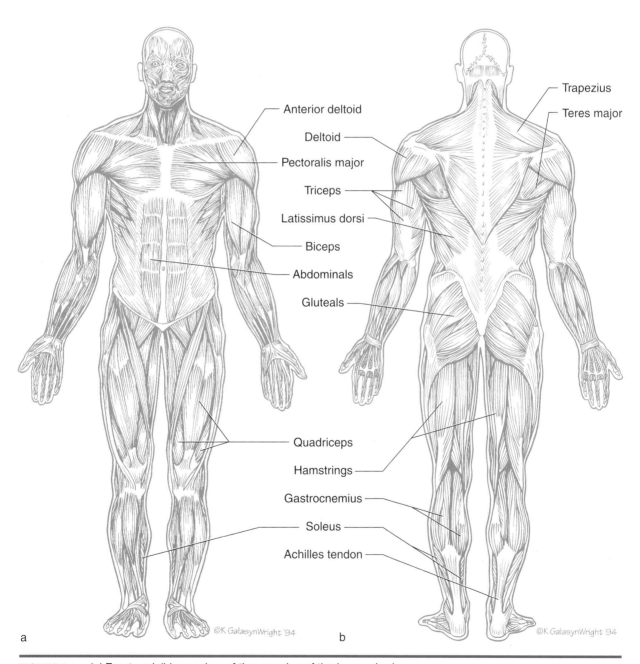

a    b

**FIGURE 3.1** *(a)* Front and *(b)* rear view of the muscles of the human body.

## Leg Exercises

The first six lower body exercises work the quadriceps, hamstrings, gluteals, and calves. The muscles worked are noted within each exercise description. How will greater leg strength benefit you? Having increased leg strength and muscular endurance means that daily tasks are less demanding on your body; for example running up a flight of stairs won't leave you out of breath with sore legs.

### LEG PRESS

Muscles worked: Quadriceps, hamstrings, gluteals

Place your feet on the pedals with your knees flexed at about a 90-degree angle and grasp the seat handles. Press your feet forward until your legs are almost straight, but don't lock your knees. Return to the starting position and repeat.

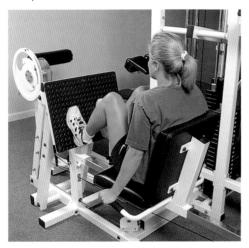 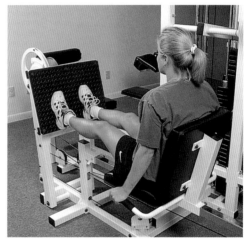

### LEG EXTENSION

Muscles worked: Quadriceps

Sit on the bench with the tops of your feet resting under the padded bar and grasp the seat handles. Slowly extend your legs (don't lock your knees) to lift the weight. Return to the starting position and repeat. Don't let your lower legs or feet rotate during the exercise.

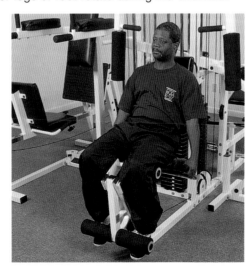 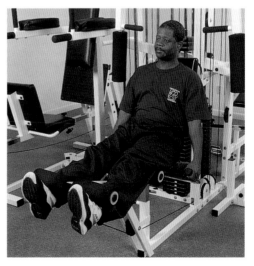

## Waiting to Exhale

To breathe or not to breathe, that is the question. Many weight lifters hold their breath while lifting a heavy weight or performing the last few reps of a set, because it's easier to complete the lift. This breath-holding technique is known as the *Valsalva maneuver.* Tightening the muscles around a lungful of air stabilizes the trunk and provides a sturdy platform from which to lift. However, the technique can have two harmful effects. First, it can increase your blood pressure, because as your heart tries to pump blood through the body, the chest muscles are contracting and constricting the vessels, so the pressure rises. Second, these constricting blood vessels also restrict the flow of blood returning to the heart. So after a few moments of high blood pressure, your blood pressure drops. In extreme cases this can lead to light-headedness, fainting, or even an irregular heartbeat.

The bottom line is that using the Valsalva maneuver may help you squeeze out a few more reps, but it places stress on your heart and cardiovascular system. So, to answer the original question: You should breathe throughout the exercise. Most people exhale as they lift and inhale as they return the weight to the starting position, but the main point is to breathe with each rep.

## LEG FLEXION

Muscles worked: Hamstrings, gluteals

Lie facedown on the bench with your heels under the padded bar, keeping your knees slightly flexed. Flex your legs to lift the weight. Return to the starting position and repeat. Be careful not to overarch your back while lifting.

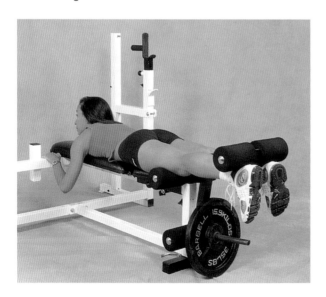 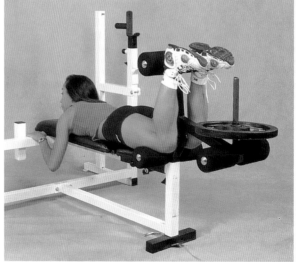

## BENCH STEPPING

Muscles worked: Quadriceps, hamstrings, gluteals, calves (gastrocnemius and soleus)

Using a four-step motion, step up and down on a bench as fast as possible for 30 seconds (up with right foot, up with left foot, down with right foot, down with left foot). Then switch the lead leg and repeat. You can also do bench stepping with a loaded pack or wrist weights, or while holding dumbbells to increase resistance. Don't use ankle weights, and make sure the bench isn't too high—the bench height should be at or below knee level.

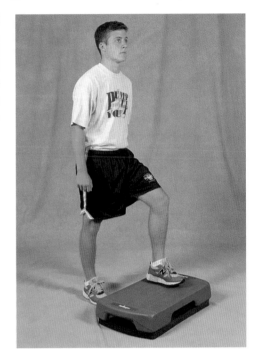

## HALF KNEE BENDS

Muscles worked: Quadriceps, hamstrings, gluteals

With your feet apart and hands on your hips, squat until your thighs are parallel to the ground. Return to the starting position and repeat. Start by performing 10 to 15 repetitions. You'll soon build up to 30 or more, although your reps should be fewer when you add resistance. Try a 2-inch (5-centimeter) block under the heels to aid balance. For variety, use a backpack or hold dumbbells. This exercise is a good one to adapt for power or for plyometric training (see page 54). To develop power, remove the 2-inch block, and instead of just returning to the original standing position after your squat, jump as high as you can. Don't stop when you land—squat and jump again and again as rapidly as possible. You'll probably find a set of 10 quite demanding! For variety, hold your hands at waist height with your palms facing downward and bring your knees up to your hands at the height of your jump.

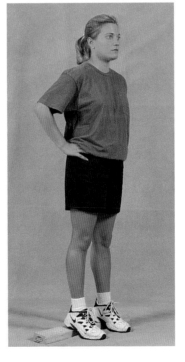
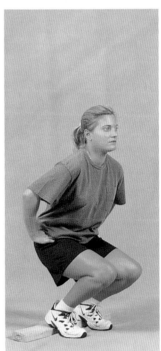

## HEEL RAISES

Muscles worked: Calves (gastrocnemius, soleus)

Stand erect with your hands at your sides or hips, your feet close together. Rise up on your toes 20 to 40 times. You can also try heel raises with the front of your feet on a 2-inch platform, or with a loaded pack, or while holding dumbbells to add resistance. Keep your knees slightly flexed and your ankles straight throughout the exercise.

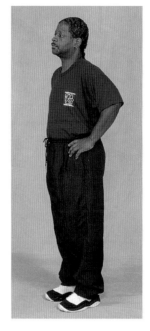
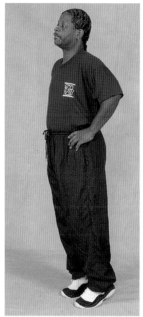

## Upper Back, Shoulder, and Chest Exercises

The next seven exercises work the various muscles of your upper back, shoulders, and chest. The particular muscles worked are noted with each exercise. Developing your upper body strength and endurance will also make everyday tasks seem easier. Carrying your books or groceries will be less fatiguing, and you may also be less prone to injuries. Upper body strength is especially important in many sport and recreational activities.

## PULL-DOWNS

Muscles worked: Latissimus dorsi, pectoralis major, biceps

Kneel on one or both knees or sit on a bench, and grasp the handles. Pull the bar down until it rests on the back of your neck and your upper arms are about parallel with the floor. Slowly return to the starting position and repeat.

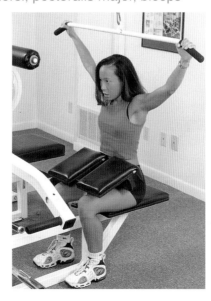
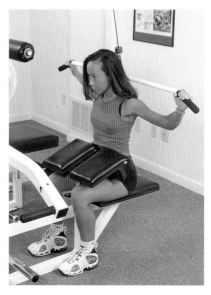

## MODIFIED CHIN-UPS

Muscles worked: Latissimus dorsi, trapezius, teres major, biceps

Stand with the bar at about chest height. Using an underhand grasp, hang from the bar with your body straight and your feet on the ground in front of the bar—not directly under it. Pull up until your chin is above the bar. Return to the starting position and repeat, doing as many as possible. To perform a more difficult version of the chin-up, stand straight up at a higher bar and pull yourself up instead of letting your feet touch the floor. You can also grip the bar with an overhand grip to form another variation.

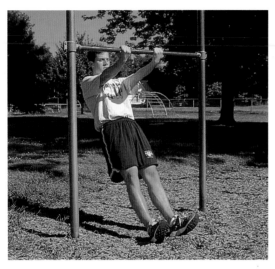 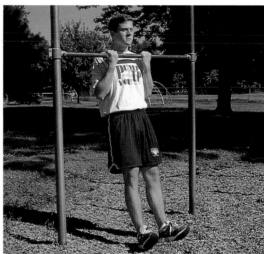

## BENT ROWING

Muscles worked: Latissimus dorsi, teres major, biceps, lower back

Stand in a bent-over position with your back flat and slightly above parallel with the floor. Spread your feet shoulder-width apart, with your knees slightly bent. Grasp a barbell with an overhand grip; your hands should be slightly farther than shoulder-width apart. Pull the bar to your chest, then lower it to the starting position and repeat, keeping your upper body stationary.

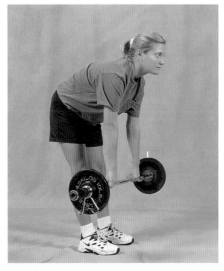 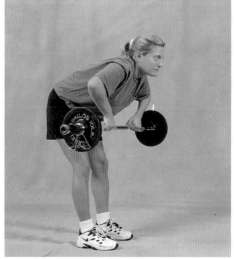

## MILITARY PRESS

Muscles worked: Deltoids, triceps

Stand erect with your feet comfortably apart and grasp a barbell with an overhand grip. Raise the bar to your upper chest, then press the bar overhead until your elbows are fully extended. Return to the starting position and repeat.

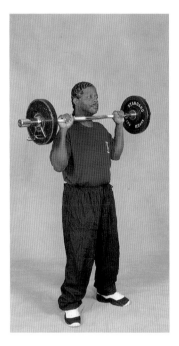 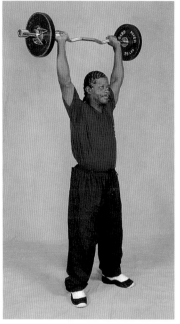

## BENCH PRESS

Muscles worked: Pectoralis major, anterior deltoid, triceps

Lie flat on your back with your feet planted firmly on the floor to either side of the bench. Grasp the bar with your hands a little farther than shoulder-width apart, with your arms extended. Slowly lower the bar to your chest, then press it back up to the starting position. When you're performing this exercise with free weights, a partner should spot you at all times. Don't arch your back when lifting; if you're prone to lower back pain, you can perform this exercise with your feet on the bench.

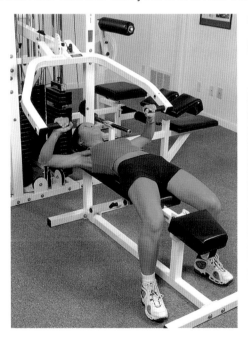 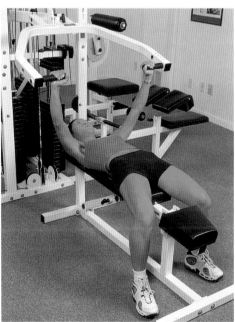

## Cheaters Sometimes Prosper

The adage "Cheaters never prosper" is not wholly accurate in weight lifting. "Cheating"—that is, not using strict form—has its good and bad points. Lifters normally cheat when they are struggling to lift a weight. They end up using other (and usually stronger) muscles to help complete the reps. For example, in the military press, instead of using only the shoulder muscles to push the weight upward, you can "cheat" by bending your knees at the start and then straightening your legs to gain a little momentum. Then, near the end of the upward movement, you might arch your back slightly, gaining further advantage by using chest and leg muscles and by dropping below the bar rather than pushing it fully above you.

*Disadvantages of cheating:* You're not training only the muscles that the lift was designed to train. You're accomplishing the lift by calling on other muscles to assist you. And, if you distort your form (usually by arching your back) *too* much, you risk injury.

*Advantages of cheating:* You're using your leg, back, and chest muscles in a coordinated movement. You strengthen more muscle groups and learn to recruit various muscles to perform a coordinated action.

You can also cheat by not going through the full range of motion. For example, if the weight is too heavy, you might not lower the bar or the dumbbells all the way in the bench press. Or in bent rowing, you might not be able to lift the weight all the way to your chest. In this case you won't gain strength throughout the full range of motion. However, *occasionally* using a weight that you can't handle through the full range of motion can help you improve your strength at the ranges where you want or need to be the strongest. For example, if you're "stuck" at 40 pounds in the bent row, you could benefit by going to 50 pounds and completing 80% of the range of motion.

## PUSH-UPS

Muscles worked: Pectoralis major, anterior deltoid, triceps

Lie facedown with your hands on the floor a little more than shoulder-width apart. Push up, keeping your back straight; lower your body until your chest almost touches the floor, then repeat. Do as many as possible.

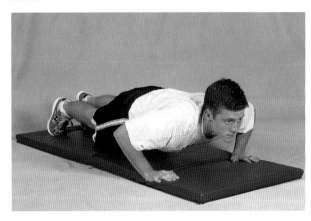
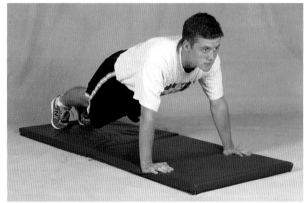

## KNEE PUSH-UPS

Muscles worked: Pectoralis major, anterior deltoid, triceps

Knee push-ups are a little easier than regular push-ups. With your hands a little more than shoulder-width apart and your knees bent, push up, keeping your back straight; lower your body until your chest almost touches the floor, then repeat. Do as many as possible. This exercise is another one that can be easily modified to become a power exercise for the upper body. As you push up, extend your arms quickly and forcefully so your hands are pushed off the floor. Be careful not to smack your chin on the floor as you catch yourself at the end of each repetition. Continue pushing up as rapidly as possible without pausing in the down position. Start with 5 or 10 repetitions at first and gradually work your way up. For variety (and to ensure that you keep extending your arms hard enough to push your hands off of the floor), clap your hands together each time you push up.

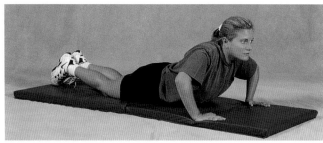
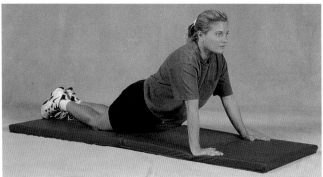

## Lower Back and Abdominal Exercises

From a function point of view, strengthening the lower back and abdominal muscles provides a solid "platform" so that as you run, cycle, work at a desk, lift weights, or throw, you are working with a sturdy base. This translates into better performance, less fatigue, and hopefully a reduced risk of injury. In addition, strengthening these muscles improves posture and puts less strain on the back; and from an aesthetic perspective, good posture is attractive! Perform these two exercises regularly— preventing low back pain (which is discussed in more detail in chapter 8) is much easier than recuperating from it.

## CRUNCHES

Muscles worked: Abdominals

Lie on your back with your arms crossed on your chest, or hands behind your neck, and your knees bent. Curl up to a semi-sitting position. Return to the starting position and repeat 10 to 15 times. If you place your hands behind your neck, don't pull on your head while curling up—let your abs do the work! For variation, you can do crunches very fast, do them on an inclined board, or do them holding a weight on your chest. You can also do them very *slowly,* holding in the contracted position and lowering slowly to the floor.
*Note:* Here are a few variations of crunches you can perform:

- Do crunches or curl-ups with your feet up on a chair or bed. This isolates the abdominal muscles and doesn't allow you to "cheat" by using your hip flexors.

- Hook your feet under a desk or have someone hold your feet as you perform crunches. This allows you to do more crunches and to bring your body through a complete range of motion.

- Perform crunches with your knees bent and your hands behind your head. Lock your hands behind your head, curl up, and attempt to touch your right elbow to your left knee, and on your next time up touch your left elbow to your right knee; continue to alternate in this fashion. In the beginning, you may not be able to curl all the way up without bouncing or throwing your arms forward to gain momentum. If this is the case, start with your hands at your sides rather than behind your head, and curl up by trying to slide your hands forward toward your feet.

- Do a series of crunches with one foot flat on the floor and the other crossed so the ankle rests on the knee of the opposite leg. Lock your hands behind your head. Curl up as far as possible and try to touch your elbow to the opposite knee. Repeat on both sides.

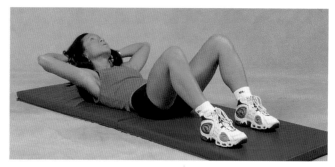

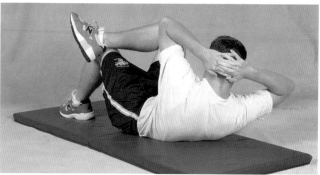

## LEG LIFTS

Muscles worked: Lower back

Lie facedown on the floor or mat. With a partner holding your trunk down, raise your legs 5 to 10 times. Your knees should only be a few inches off the ground—don't lift your legs too high or you could hyperextend your back.

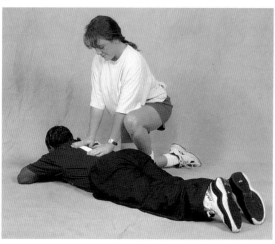 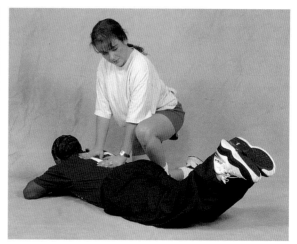

## Arm Exercises

The next two exercises work either the biceps or triceps muscles. Upper body strength doesn't occur naturally—you have to work at it. But the benefits are worth it; your chores will seem easier, you'll be able to lift and carry heavier objects, and you'll get tired out less easily. We may live in an automated world, but chances are you still have to carry books, lunch trays, laundry, and groceries!

## BICEPS CURLS

Muscles worked: Biceps

Stand with your feet comfortably apart and knees slightly flexed. Hold the bar in front of your thighs with an underhand grip, your hands about shoulder-width apart; your arms should be straight. Flex your elbows and lift the bar to your chest, keeping your elbows close to your sides. Don't lean backward or bounce the bar with your leg motion. Return to the starting position and repeat. You can also perform this exercise with dumbbells.

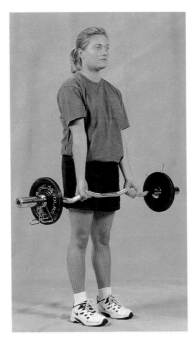 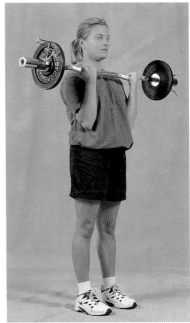

## TRICEPS EXTENSION

Muscles worked: Triceps

Sit on a bench with your back straight. Grasp the bar with your hands about 2 inches (5 centimeters) apart, using an overhand grip. Bring the bar to full arm extension above your head. Lower the bar behind your head, keeping your elbows stationary.

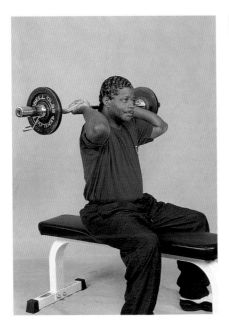 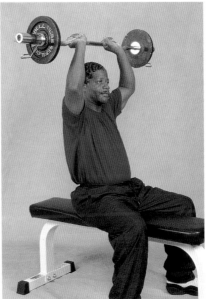

## Do You Have to Go to a Gym to Get Stronger?

We've provided some specific exercises that you can do in a typical gym or health club, or at home using your own equipment. We've also included some additional exercises, like crunches and push-ups, that develop strength and power without the need for a club membership or special equipment. So no, you don't necessarily have to go the gym to participate in an organized and effective strength-training program.

In chapter 2 we discussed the small daily changes, such as taking the stairs or parking farther from your destination, that you can make to contribute to your cardiovascular health. You may be wondering the same thing about muscular fitness: How can I adjust my lifestyle to develop an adequate level of strength? Certain lifestyles require—and develop—strength and muscular endurance. For example, a typical manual laborer can be quite strong without participating in an organized strength-training program. Imagine "real-life" exercises that mimic each of the exercises described earlier. The question becomes, Do you lead this kind of lifestyle? If you hike regularly with a backpack, canoe frequently, climb trees, chop wood, and so on, you probably don't need to head to the weight room to develop strength in at least some areas of your body.

If you don't have a physically challenging job or regularly perform activities that require a reasonable amount of strength, you can try to adjust your lifestyle to make it more physically demanding. For example, take the stairs two at a time, carry your own groceries, scrub your own floor, hammer your own nails, or hike (instead of driving) to a scenic view. A physical hobby, such as gardening, can also have its benefits. Digging holes, pulling and chopping weeds, stooping, carrying pots and bags of mulch, mowing, and pruning can all help develop your strength.

## Sample Programs

You may begin with one set of each exercise; then increase to three sets (while dropping back the resistance for each exercise by about 10%) after you have become accustomed to the exercises, are over the expected muscle soreness, and know what weight you can handle.

Following are two sample programs and a training log to help you get started:

- A three-times-a-week program that works the major muscle groups throughout the body (see table 3.1)

- A four-times-a-week program that alternates between upper body and lower body on alternate days (see table 3.2)

- A training log to help you track your workouts and your progress (see table 3.3 on page 70)

## FLEXIBILITY

*Flexibility* refers to the range of motion that you can achieve at any joint through any particular movement. Flexibility is joint-specific, meaning that having flexibility in your hip doesn't

## Table 3.1 Sample Strength Training Program—Same Workout Three Times per Week

| Exercise | Sets | Reps | Muscle groups |
|---|---|---|---|
| Bench press | 3 | 10 | Chest, triceps |
| Bent row | 3 | 10 | Upper back, lower back, biceps |
| Military press | 3 | 10 | Upper chest/back (deltoids), triceps |
| Pull-downs | 3 | 10 | Latissimus dorsi, biceps |
| Half knee bends | 3 | 10 | Quadriceps, hamstrings, gluteals |
| Heel raises | 3 | 10 | Calves (gastrocnemius, soleus) |
| Sit-ups | 3 | 15 | Abdominals |

## Table 3.2 Sample Strength Training Program—Split Routine

**Monday-Thursday focuses on upper body**

| Exercise | Sets | Reps | Muscle groups |
|---|---|---|---|
| Bench press | 3 | 10 | Chest, triceps |
| Bent row | 3 | 10 | Upper back, lower back, biceps |
| Military press | 3 | 10 | Upper chest/back (deltoids), triceps |
| Pull-downs | 3 | 10 | Latissimus dorsi, biceps |
| Biceps curls | 3 | 10 | Biceps |
| Triceps extension | 3 | 10 | Triceps |
| Sit-ups | 3-5 | 15 | Abdominals (or intersperse abdominal exercises between the other exercises above) |

**Tuesday-Friday focuses on lower body**

| Exercise | Sets | Reps | Muscle groups |
|---|---|---|---|
| Squats | 3 | 10 | Quadriceps, hamstrings, gluteals |
| Heel raises | 3 | 10 | Calves (gastrocnemius, soleus) |
| Leg flexion | 3 | 10 | Hamstrings, gluteals |
| Leg extension | 3 | 10 | Quadriceps |
| Half knee bends | 3 | 10 | Perform as plyometrics to develop power in quadriceps, hamstrings, and gluteals |
| Sit-ups | 3-5 | 15 | Abdominals (or intersperse abdominal exercises between the other exercises above) |

mean you'll be flexible in your shoulders. Flexibility can also be specific from one side of the body to the other: right-handed tennis players, for example, might be more flexible in the right shoulder than in the left because they're moving the right shoulder through wider ranges of motion.

There are different types of flexibility. *Passive flexibility* is the range of motion you can attain when someone pushes or pulls on you (without causing pain or injury, of course!). *Active flexibility* is the range of motion that you can achieve by actively contracting your muscles. Regardless of the type of flexibility, being flexible has many benefits.

Flexibility is very specific: you may be flexible in some joints and not very flexible in others.

## Table 3.3 Sample Training Log

| Exercise | Date | | |
|---|---|---|---|
| | **6-12-99** | **6-14-99** | **6-16-99** |
| Bench press | 3/10/60* | 3/10/60 | 3/12/60 |
| Bent row | 3/10/45 | 3/10/45 | 3/10/45 |
| Military press | 3/10/50 | 3/10/50 | 3/10/50 |
| Pull-downs | 3/10/80 | 3/10/80 | 3/10/80 |
| Squats | 3/10/120 | 3/10/120 | 3/10/120 |
| Heel raises | 3/10/120 | ★ | 1/10/100 |
| Sit-ups | 3/15 | 3/15 | 3/20 |

Comments:
* Sets/reps/weight (pounds).
★Calf was cramping so didn't finish doing heel raises.

| Exercise | Date | | | | |
|---|---|---|---|---|---|
| | _____ | _____ | _____ | _____ | _____ |
| _____ | _____ | _____ | _____ | _____ | _____ |
| _____ | _____ | _____ | _____ | _____ | _____ |
| _____ | _____ | _____ | _____ | _____ | _____ |
| _____ | _____ | _____ | _____ | _____ | _____ |
| _____ | _____ | _____ | _____ | _____ | _____ |
| _____ | _____ | _____ | _____ | _____ | _____ |
| _____ | _____ | _____ | _____ | _____ | _____ |
| _____ | _____ | _____ | _____ | _____ | _____ |
| _____ | _____ | _____ | _____ | _____ | _____ |
| _____ | _____ | _____ | _____ | _____ | _____ |
| _____ | _____ | _____ | _____ | _____ | _____ |
| _____ | _____ | _____ | _____ | _____ | _____ |
| _____ | _____ | _____ | _____ | _____ | _____ |
| _____ | _____ | _____ | _____ | _____ | _____ |
| _____ | _____ | _____ | _____ | _____ | _____ |

## Benefits of Flexibility

Earlier, we stated that some degree of strength was necessary for everyday activities—for everything from putting away the groceries to mowing the lawn. Similarly, some degree of flexibility is necessary to perform everyday activities. It's impossible to put a 10-pound bag of flour up on the shelf if you can't raise your arms above your shoulders. In addition, flexibility can enhance performance in some activities, and it may even help reduce the risk of injuries. Let's address these two benefits.

Certainly, extreme flexibility is required for a high jumper who arches backward over the bar, a diver or a gymnast who is performing a move, or a swimmer who is reaching with both the feet and the arms. Athletes must be able to move their limbs through large ranges of motion and often be able to produce force at these ranges.

On the other hand, *extreme* range of motion isn't necessary in many sport activities. How flexible must runners be? They don't raise their knees very high or extend their hips very far, so they really don't need tremendous flexibility. For them, as for many athletes, the importance of flexibility in performance is that they are able to produce force (i.e., that they can use their strength) throughout the necessary working range of motion. Even recreational athletes who aren't concerned about extreme flexibility will find that developing and maintaining a reasonable degree of flexibility enhances their performance and enjoyment. Flexibility is important for you whether you're training for a triathlon every day or walking every day and playing softball on the weekends.

While it's easy to understand the role flexibility can play in physical performance, its role in preventing injuries is a little more elusive. Quite simply, this potential benefit is harder to pin down because it's not ethical to design a research study in which the plan is to injure participants! Therefore we rely heavily on anecdotal evidence. (According to the American College of Sports Medicine, "while there is a lack of randomized, controlled, clinical trials defining the benefit of flexibility exercise in the prevention and treatment of musculoskeletal injuries, observational studies support stretching in both of these applications.") Everyone knows someone who was "tight as a drum," or who never stretched, or who forgot to do a warm-up one day, and then got injured. We believe that inadequate flexibility or an inadequate warm-up led to the injury. However, many people become injured despite being flexible and performing a warm-up, and other people aren't very flexible and don't warm up—and yet they escape injury!

Nevertheless, flexibility is an important aspect of fitness. It enhances performance and enjoyment of many activities, and it may contribute to a reduced risk of injury. Certainly, as you age, it's imperative that you strive to maintain range of motion at all the joints.

## Factors That Affect Flexibility

Joint flexibility ranges dramatically from one person to the next. Differences in flexibility can be attributed to factors you *can* change, such as physical activity patterns, and to factors you *can't* change, such as genetic predisposition, gender, and age.

As with most things, there is of course a genetic component. Some people just will never be able to bend the way a gymnast or an acrobat can. What about gender? It is commonly assumed that women are more flexible than men. Certainly, girls perform better than boys on a sit-and-reach test that is designed to assess hip flexibility. However, there really doesn't appear to be a strong or consistent difference in flexibility between men and women. And what about aging? Again, there is a common assumption that flexibility declines as a person ages, after reaching adulthood. Flexibility does seem to be highest during the middle teen years and to decline slightly after that. Aging often results in changes within the muscle-tendon unit that directly lead to an increased rigidity of the tendons. However, there is compelling evidence that age-related loss in flexibility can be reduced by regular physical activity, including stretching exercises.

So, what can you do to improve flexibility or, as you get older, to maintain flexibility? First, we must consider what actually limits range of motion at a joint. To begin with, there is the structure of the joint, the way the bones articulate. Ligaments, which attach bone to bone, also restrict motion; but this provides structural support, preventing unwanted movement. We don't want to increase range of motion by reducing joint stability. That leaves the muscles and connective tissue (the tendons that attach muscles to bone). Most efforts to increase range of motion target the muscles. The goal is twofold: first, to increase the normal length of the muscle and second, to reduce the tension in the muscle when you aren't using it to perform exercise. When you perform stretching exercises, the idea is that the muscle will remain slightly lengthened even after you have stopped actually stretching it. Stretching may also reduce the level of tension (force production in a muscle). Other methods of causing muscles to relax include specific relaxation techniques or meditation, massage, and warm baths.

As you read at the beginning of this chapter, Melissa was concerned that weight lifting might cause her to become big, bulky, and less flexible. It used to be that people mistakenly believed that having large muscles meant having poor flexibility. But that's not true. Having *tight* muscles—muscles that are producing force and tension—does limit your range of motion. So the answer to Melissa is that weight lifting won't reduce flexibility, but stretching exercises can improve it.

## HEALTHCHECK

### How far should you take a stretch?

To the point of discomfort but not beyond. Going beyond risks injury. If your muscles begin to quiver or you feel pain, you're going too far. Keep in mind the adage "Train, don't strain."

## Types of Stretching

Three different ways to improve flexibility through stretching are *static stretching*, *ballistic stretching*, and *proprioceptive neuromuscular facilitation*.

*Static stretching* involves stretching either actively (i.e., with no assistance) or passively (i.e., with assistance) and holding the stretch for anywhere from 3 to 60 seconds. While you probably obtain optimal benefits by holding the stretch for about 30 seconds, you can also benefit by stretching for 6 to 10 seconds, easing off, and then repeating the stretch three times.

You can increase flexibility by holding a stretch for 30 seconds or by stretching for 6 to 10 seconds, easing off, and repeating the stretch three times.

*Ballistic stretching* involves dynamic movements—for example, bouncing movements to stretch a particular muscle. With the bouncing motion, you stimulate receptors in the muscles being stretched; these receptors, known as muscle spindles, sense the rapid stretching and stimulate a reflex response that tries to contract the muscles to prevent overstretching. While ballistic stretching may have its place with experienced athletes who understand its limits and dangers, for most people it is not a good way to stretch. Muscles are stretched by your momentum and shortened by their own force production—often resulting in muscle pulls or tears.

*Proprioceptive neuromuscular facilitation* is a type of stretching that takes advantage of the body's reflex responses to enhance muscle relaxation and joint range of motion. Proprioceptive neuromuscular facilitation techniques are usually performed with a partner; they include contract-relax, hold-relax, and slow reversal-hold-relax. These techniques involve contracting and relaxing both the agonist and antagonist muscles: for example, to stretch the hamstrings (hip extensors) and increase the range of motion during hip flexion, lie on your back with your knee extended and your ankle flexed to 90 degrees and have your partner push your leg toward your chest until you feel slight discomfort in the hamstrings. You then push against your partner's resistance by contracting your hamstrings isometrically. After pushing hard for 10 seconds, the hamstrings should relax. Then, your leg is lowered and the quadriceps, which are the agonist muscles in this example, are contracted concentrically while your partner resists your effort. When you contract your hip flexors concentrically, moving your leg toward your chest, your body relaxes the opposite hamstrings. This type of contract-relax stretching can be used to stretch any muscle in the body.

## STRETCHING EXERCISES

Use the following stretches as part of your warm-up before lifting weights or taking part in any physical activity. You'll make the greatest improvements in your flexibility if you also stretch *after* exercise. If you don't have time to perform all these stretches before an activity, choose the ones that will benefit you most. For instance, if you're focusing on upper body lifts one day, perform the upper body stretches. If you're warming up prior to a run, use lower body stretches to increase flexibility in your legs and potentially reduce the risk of injury.

Within any preexercise activity, you have the choice of performing either the warming exercises or the stretching exercises first. The preferred method is to lightly warm up and then stretch to reduce the risk of tearing a "cold" muscle. Another good reason to warm up (e.g., by jogging, cycling, or lifting very light weights) *first* is that warm muscles are less viscous and can be stretched further. On the other hand, if you have tight muscles, you may want to stretch them first. For example, jogging with tight hamstrings might worsen the tightness, so you would want to stretch them before doing the warming activities.

After your workout, perform a cool-down to gradually bring your body back to its resting state. After your cool-down, your muscles will still be warm, and this is a good time to stretch. In fact, many people believe that this is the best time to improve flexibility.

The following 15 stretches are categorized by neck; shoulders, chest, and upper back; arms; trunk and lower back; and legs and hips. Let's work our way from top to bottom. Except for the head tilt, which is done slowly, all of these stretches require that you slowly stretch a muscle and take your joint to the limit of its *pain-free* range of motion and then hold the stretch for about 10 seconds. You can do each stretch twice or even three times.

## Neck Stretch

### HEAD TILT

Areas stretched: Neck flexors and extensors, upper back

You may not think of the neck as a joint, but it is a complicated joint that requires a good range of motion. Tilt your head slowly to each side and to the front by tucking your chin on your chest, then your left ear on your left shoulder, then your right ear on your right shoulder—now you're back where you started. Do several slow tilts in all directions.

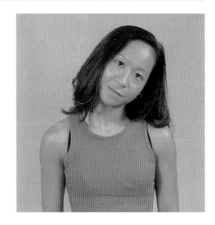

## Shoulders, Chest, and Upper Back Stretches

### ARM CIRCLES

Area stretched: Shoulder muscles and ligaments

Stand with your feet shoulder-width apart and hold your arms straight out to the sides with your palms facing up. Gently move your arms in small and then gradually larger circles in one direction, then reverse directions. Do several circles in each direction.

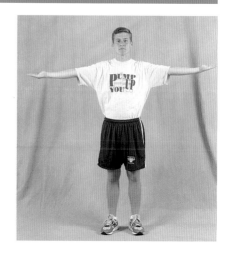

### ACROSS-THE-BODY

Areas stretched: Shoulders, upper back

With your right hand, grasp your left elbow and pull it slowly across your chest toward your right shoulder. You'll feel the stretch along the outside of your left shoulder. Hold, and then repeat with the other arm.

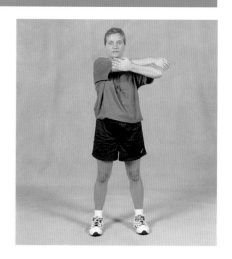

### REACH-BACK

Areas stretched: Chest, shoulders

Grasp your hands behind your back and slowly lift your arms upward. If you're not able to grasp your hands, simply reach back and then up as far as possible. Hold when you reach the limit of your range of motion.

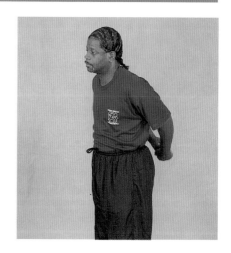

## CHAIR STRETCH

Area stretched: Chest

Kneel in front of a chair or other low supporting object. Place both forearms on top of the chair and gradually let your head and chest sink toward the floor.

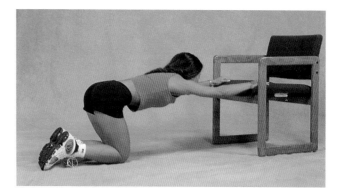

## ARM EXTENSIONS

Area stretched: Upper back

Stand with your feet shoulder-width apart and knees slightly flexed. Clasp your hands straight out in front of your body and rotate your wrists to press your palms forward. Keep your pelvis tucked in and let your upper back round slightly to perform the stretch.

You can also devise all sorts of exercises using a 3- to 4-foot (around 1 meter) broomstick. For example, cup each end of the stick in the palm of your hand and alternately push one hand or the other as far behind you as possible, taking different paths to get there (e.g., start with the stick horizontal at eye level and push one hand back so that it stays at eye level, or start with the stick at a 45-degree angle and push back over your shoulder).

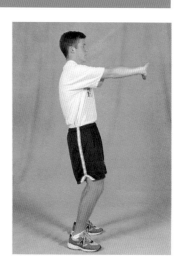

## Arm Stretches

## BICEPS STRETCH

Area stretched: Biceps (upper arms)

Stand with your back to a door frame or wall with your feet shoulder-width apart and your knees slightly flexed. Place one hand against the door frame or wall and slowly turn your arm so your biceps face upward, until you feel the stretch. Hold, and then repeat with the other arm.

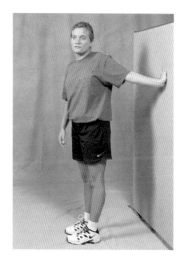

## TRICEPS STRETCH

Area stretched: Triceps (upper arms)

Bring both arms overhead and hold your left elbow with your right hand. Bend your left arm at the elbow and let your left hand rest against your right shoulder. Pull with your right hand to slowly move the left elbow behind your head toward your right shoulder until you feel the stretch. Hold, and then repeat with the other arm.

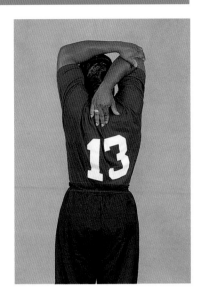

## Trunk and Lower Back Stretches

Trunk and back flexibility is important in sport. However, these exercises must be performed carefully and with an understanding of the risks involved, especially for individuals with low back pain. Additional back exercises are described in detail in chapter 8.

## SIDE STRETCH

Areas stretched: Trunk, pelvic region

Stand erect with your feet shoulder-width apart and knees slightly flexed. Extend one arm overhead and place the other hand on your hip. Slowly bend to the side. Hold, and then repeat on the opposite side.

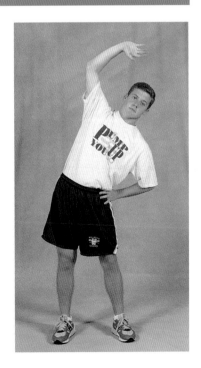

## SITTING TRUNK ROTATION

Areas stretched: Trunk, lower back, hips

Sit on the floor with your legs straight in front of you, arms straight with palms on the floor behind you. Bend your right leg, cross it over your left knee, and place the sole of your right foot on the floor. Now, bring your left hand off the floor and push against the outside of your right thigh with your left elbow, just above your right knee. Slowly rotate your upper body toward your right hand and arm. You should feel the stretch in your back, hips, and buttocks. Hold, and repeat on the opposite side.

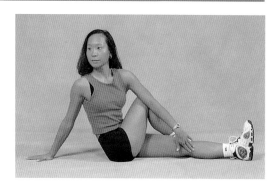

# Leg and Hip Stretches

## QUAD STRETCH

Areas stretched: Quadriceps, hip flexors, knee ligaments

Quadriceps are rarely a tight muscle group because they are in a stretched state when you sit in a chair. However, you can also use this quad stretch to focus on the hip flexors, which really need to be stretched because they are in a shortened state when you sit in a chair.

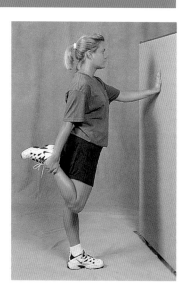

Using a wall or stationary object for balance, bend your right leg at the knee, grasp your right foot, and hold it behind you. Pull up gently on your foot so that your knee remains stationary. You should feel the stretch along the front of your thigh. To place emphasis on the hip flexor, pull your foot gently up and away from your buttocks, causing your right knee to move back slightly. You'll feel the stretch higher in the front of your right thigh. Hold, and repeat with the other leg. Keep your body upright when you do this exercise. Remember, for this and all other stretches, the point is not to see how far you can pull your foot; the point is to stretch the target muscle, in this case the hip flexors. You gain nothing by bending forward at the waist while pulling up on your foot.

## FRONT LUNGE

Areas stretched: Hip, quadriceps

Another way to focus on the hip flexors and quadriceps is to perform a slow "lunge." Take a giant step forward with your left foot and then bend your left knee so that your hips drop toward the ground. You'll feel the stretch high up on the front of your right thigh. Hold, then repeat with the opposite leg.

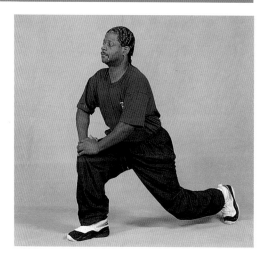

## BUTTERFLY STRETCH

Areas stretched: Hip adductors, groin, inner thigh

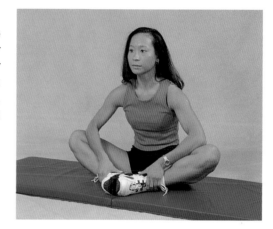

Sit on the floor and bring your feet in close to you so that the soles are touching. Rest your elbows or forearms on your thighs and push your legs downward. For variety, use your legs to resist the movement when you first begin to push them toward the floor, then relax and push them down for the stretch. You can also lean forward while pushing down to try to touch your head to your feet or the floor.

## MODIFIED HURDLER STRETCH

Areas stretched: Hamstrings, lower back

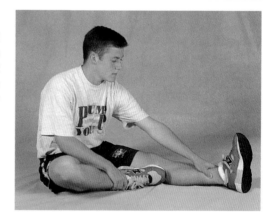

Sit with your legs straight in front of you. Bend your right leg and bring the sole of your right foot to rest gently against the inside of your left knee. Slowly bend forward at the hips, and make certain to keep the toes of your left foot pointing up. You should feel the stretch in the back of your left leg and in your lower back. Hold, and repeat with the other leg.

## WALL STRETCH

Areas stretched: Calves, Achilles tendon

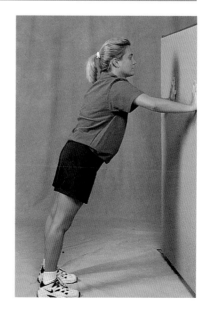

Stand with your feet slightly apart and your legs straight, about 2 feet (about 0.6 meters) away from a wall or stationary object. Lean forward and place your hands against the wall. Slowly bend your elbows so that your body moves closer to the wall. Keep your back straight and your heels on the ground. You'll feel the stretch in your calves.

For variation, you can alternately allow your right and left heels to rise off the ground slightly. Avoid arching your back. And remember the purpose is to stretch. You won't gain anything by moving way back and then having to extend your arms completely or pike at the waist.

Other muscles that cross the ankles can be gently stretched by actively or passively performing ankle rotations. Also, try to invert and evert the ankle. You invert the ankle when, for example, you twist your foot to look at the sole and evert your ankle when you twist your foot so you can see the outside edge.

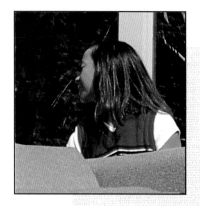

# Health Concepts

As related at the beginning of the chapter, Melissa wanted to start lifting weights but was concerned that doing so would make her big and bulky. She also wanted to know if she needed to stretch in order to not become less flexible as she became stronger.

She can rest assured that lifting weights will increase her strength but won't produce bulky, masculine muscles. Women can increase strength and muscle mass, but the average woman won't become as big or strong as the average man because men's testosterone levels enable them to build a larger muscle mass. And stretching can both help increase flexibility and reduce the risk of injury. Both strength and flexibility are important components of fitness, and they can be developed together.

## SUMMARY

▌ *Strength* is the ability of a muscle to produce force. *Muscular endurance* is the ability of a muscle to produce force over and over again. *Power* is the ability of a muscle to produce force quickly.

▌ Three important principles in building strength are *overload, specificity,* and *individuality.* We build strength by putting tension on our muscles. We increase strength by taxing our muscles beyond their accustomed loads. Muscle development is specific—that is, only the muscle fibers that are activated can gain strength. Our bodies respond very specifically to exercise.

▌ Muscle soreness often occurs 24 to 48 hours after a strength-training workout. This is called DOMS—delayed onset muscle soreness. The soreness usually dissipates within a few days and isn't harmful.

▌ Strength-training techniques include varying the order of your lifts, isolating the muscles you're exercising, splitting your routine (upper body one day, lower body the next), using a partner to assist in lifts, and using periodization in your training. Your progress in building strength is affected by your genetic ability, your starting point, and your commitment.

▌ Flexibility is joint-specific; you can be flexible in some joints and not so flexible in others. It is also side-specific; you can have greater range of motion in joints on one side of your body than on the other.

▌ Flexibility can enhance performance and may reduce the likelihood of injury. It is affected by many factors, including age, gender, activity, and stretching.

▌ Three ways to stretch include static stretching, ballistic stretching, and proprioceptive neuromuscular facilitation. Proprioceptive neuromuscular facilitation normally involves another person; ballistic stretching is not recommended because it can lead to injury. Static stretching is the best way for most people to stretch on their own.

*Strength and flexibility affect our fitness and ability to perform everyday tasks as well as physical activity. Next we'll look at another issue that both affects and is affected by physical activity—obesity.*

## KEY TERMS

| | |
|---|---|
| atrophy | muscular endurance |
| ballistic stretching | one-repetition maximum (1-RM) |
| concentric muscle action | periodization |
| cross training | plyometrics |
| delayed onset muscle soreness (DOMS) | power |
| eccentric muscle action | proprioceptive neuromuscular facilitation |
| flexibility | repetition (rep) |
| hypertrophy | set |
| isokinetic muscle action | static stretching |
| isometric muscle action | strength |
| isotonic muscle action | Valsalva maneuver |

# 3

# Selecting Weight-Lifting Exercises, Calculating Your 1-RM and 12-RM, Assessing Strength and Muscular Endurance, and Determining the Effect of Stretching on Range of Motion

### THE PURPOSES OF THIS LAB EXPERIENCE ARE TO

▌ familiarize yourself with different exercises that you can use to strengthen various muscle groups,

▌ calculate your 1-RM and 12-RM,

▌ determine your level of muscular strength and endurance,

▌ understand the effect of prior exercise on measures of muscular strength and endurance,

▌ assess your muscular fitness, and

▌ determine the effect of stretching exercises on hip joint range of motion.

## Familiarize Yourself With Various Exercises

This "take-away" assignment doesn't necessarily require any weight lifting on your part. However, you have the option of testing yourself, if the facility you choose allows you to do so. After you've identified what muscles you think each exercise targets, *do* the exercise with a light weight and see for yourself which muscle groups are affected!

Go to the university weight room, the athletics facility (if available to you), or a local health club—any place where people are performing weight-lifting exercises at exercise stations or on pieces of equipment. Obtain permission to observe, but don't ask for any assistance from the staff yet. For each machine or station, watch a person perform the exercise, and then identify as best you can what muscle group is being used (you don't have to give the proper name of the muscle if you don't know it, just its location). Many exercises use primarily one muscle group but also involve others to some degree. Can you identify other muscle groups involved? If you're observing at a facility with less than 12 stations, complete the chart that follows for however many stations are available.

As you identify the prime movers for each exercise, highlight them on the muscle map provided in figure 3.1 on page 57. After completing your investigation, look at the muscle map. Is it completely highlighted? Did the stations in the rotation target all the major muscle groups (or body parts)? Which were left out?

Now, ask a knowledgeable employee for 5 minutes of his or her time. For each station in the rotation, have the person tell you the main muscle group involved. Compare this information with the answers that you provided in the chart. How did you do? Make any corrections with a red pen before you turn in your report. Ask the employee who helped you to sign the form.

If you can, go through the rotation yourself. If you haven't been lifting regularly, be sure to use very light weights to avoid injury and soreness.

Name of the weight-lifting facility _____

| Exercise station | Brief description of the action | Primary (P) and secondary (S) muscles |
|---|---|---|
| 1 | | P |
| | | S |
| 2 | | P |
| | | S |
| 3 | | P |
| | | S |
| 4 | | P |
| | | S |
| 5 | | P |
| | | S |
| 6 | | P |
| | | S |
| 7 | | P |
| | | S |
| 8 | | P |
| | | S |
| 9 | | P |
| | | S |
| 10 | | P |
| | | S |
| 11 | | P |
| | | S |
| 12 | | P |
| | | S |

To the fitness specialist who helped this student perform this observation, thank you for your time and for sharing your expertise. Please sign here, acknowledging the student's participation.

Fitness specialist _____

## Determine Your 1-RM and 12-RM

For this portion of the lab, you'll measure your chest muscle (pectoralis) strength and muscular endurance. Specifically, you'll determine your 1-RM for the bench press and the number of reps you can perform at 80% of your 1-RM. You'll see the effect of prior exercise on strength by determining your bench press 1-RM immediately after an exhaustive set of bench press reps using 80% of your 1-RM. Finally, you'll also measure your arm flexor muscle endurance by determining the 12-RM for arm curls.

Your lab instructor may substitute other chest and biceps exercises or may use completely different exercises depending on the availability of equipment. Read through the lab completely before coming to class and beginning to collect data.

There are several things you can do to avoid injuries, in this lab and any other time you're in the weight room. First, pay attention to what's going on around you. Second, use proper form. And third, use a spotter. Especially when you're trying for a 1-RM or nearing exhaustion in a test of muscular endurance, it's important to concentrate on maintaining your form and correct breathing. Perform all lifts in a controlled fashion. For all lifts, refrain from performing the Valsalva maneuver. Even though we've said this, you'll soon find that performing the Valsalva maneuver and holding your breath does permit a higher 1-RM or number of reps in an endurance test. While we are not recommending you do this, we realize it's almost impossible not to—just be sure not to overdo it, and certainly let the instructor know if you're feeling light-headed after lifting (in which case, sit down before you fall down!).

You can expect muscle soreness after this lab experience. That's not an injury. It will go away in a few days.

### Determine Your Chest Muscle Strength

After a short warm-up, including stretching for the pectoral muscles, your lab instructor will demonstrate proper technique. You'll be lying on the bench with both knees bent or one or both feet up on the bench close to your buttocks—this should keep your back from arching. With the help of a spotter, grasp the bar with your hands slightly more than shoulder-width apart. Lower the bar in a controlled fashion to your chest, pause, and then push it upward (see page 84). Perform 5 to 10 presses with a light weight (try 1/4 of your body weight if you're a woman, 1/3 of your body weight if you're a man). From here, it's a process of trial and error. Try to perform 1 rep with a heavier weight, rest 3 to 5 minutes, try an even heavier weight, and so on until you can't perform the lift. Once you can't lift the weight, either rest and try again one more time, or try a weight slightly lighter (but still heavier than the greatest weight you've already lifted). A reasonable 1-RM is just over 1/2 body weight for women and close to body weight for men. This should help you select appropriate weights to start out with. You want to achieve your 1-RM on the fourth or fifth attempt. Note that if you have five successful lifts and one or two failures, this process can take almost 30 minutes. Record each successful attempt as well as each failure.

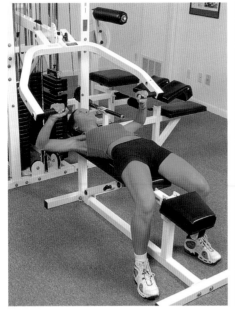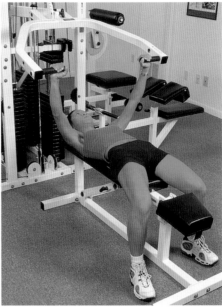

### SAMPLE RESULTS

**Student A:**

√ 8 × 50 pounds (warm-up)

√ 80 pounds

X 100 pounds

√ 90 pounds

√ 95 pounds

X 97.5 pounds

1- RM = 95 pounds

**Student B:**

√ 10 × 70 pounds (warm-up)

√ 110 pounds

√ 125 pounds

√ 135 pounds

√ 140 pounds

X 145 pounds

X 142.5 pounds

1- RM = 140 pounds

Your results:

_____

_____

_____

_____

## Determine Your Chest Muscle Endurance

Five to ten minutes after determining your 1-RM, load the bar with 80% of your 1-RM. Perform as many reps as possible with this weight.

1-RM _____ 80% 1-RM _____ Weight used _____ Number of reps _____

### Effect of Prior Exercise on Your Chest Muscle Strength

Five minutes after the muscular endurance test, repeat the determination of your 1-RM.

**Your results:**

_____

_____

_____

_____


### Determine Your 12-RM for the Biceps Curl

The first set can serve as the warm-up. You may find that after three or four attempts you're willing to estimate a value. See data for student B below for an example. To perform a biceps curl, stand with your feet comfortably apart and knees slightly flexed. Hold the bar in front of your thighs with an

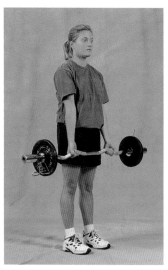 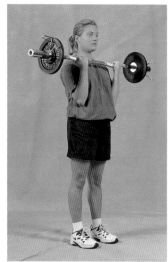

underhand grip, hands about shoulder-width apart; your arms should be straight. Flex your elbows and lift the bar to your chest, keeping your elbows close to your sides. Don't lean backward or bounce the bar with your leg motion.

---

**SAMPLE RESULTS**

| **Student A:** | **Student B:** |
| --- | --- |
| √ 12 × 50 pounds—not too hard | √ 12 × 40 pounds—really easy |
| √ 12 × 80 pounds—hard | √ 12 × 60 pounds—not too hard |
| √ 12 × 85 pounds—barely finished | √ 12 × 75 pounds—hard |
| 12-RM = 85 pounds | X 12 × 85 pounds—couldn't do 12 reps |
| | Estimate: 12-RM = 83 pounds (you may estimate that the 12-RM is 85 pounds, when you're rested) |

## Questions:

1. Is there a relationship between strength (bench press 1-RM) and muscular endurance (bench press reps using 80% of 1-RM)?

   To answer this question, plot the class data for muscular endurance (number of bench press reps using 80% 1-RM) on the y-axis against strength (bench press 1-RM) on the x-axis. Note that this is a measure of relative muscular endurance where the resistance used is "relative to" (or determined by) your strength.

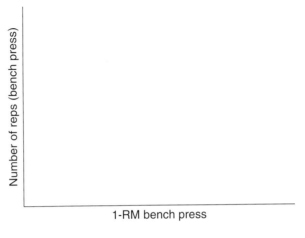

   *Answer:*

   _____

   _____

2. Is there a relationship between strength (bench press 1-RM) and muscular endurance (arm curl 12-RM)?

   To answer this question, plot the class data for muscular endurance (arm curl 12-RM) on the y-axis against strength (bench press 1-RM) on the x-axis. Note that this time we've used an absolute measure of muscular endurance.

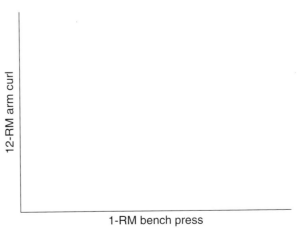

   *Answer:*

   _____

   _____

## Assess Your Muscular Fitness

You've practiced resistance training and developing your own program in this chapter. Now you can do some simple evaluations of your muscular fitness. You'll be doing three tests from the FITNESSGRAM, developed by the Cooper Institute for Aerobics Research (1992), and adapted for our purposes from Morrow et al. (1995).

### Curl-Up Test

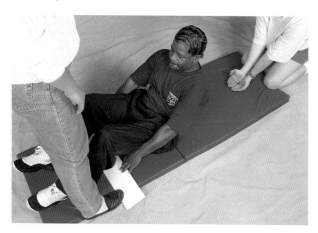

**Purpose:** To measure abdominal strength and endurance.

**Objective:** The individual performs as many curl-ups as possible to a maximum of 75.

**Equipment:** Gym mats, cardboard strips (30 inches by 4.5 inches [about 75 by 11.5 centimeters]), tape player and audiotape (for controlling cadence).

**Instructions:** Perform this test in groups of three. One person performs the curl-ups, the second supports the head of the performer, and the third secures the strip so it doesn't move. The person being tested lies in a supine position on the mat with knees bent at about 140 degrees, legs apart, arms straight and parallel to the trunk with the palms resting on the mat. The fingers are extended and the head is in the partner's hand, which is resting on the mat. The cardboard strip is placed under the knees with the performer's fingers touching the nearer edge. The third person stands on the strip so it doesn't move during the test. The performer curls up so that the fingers slide to the other side of the strip. The performer does as many curl-ups as possible while maintaining a cadence of one curl-up every 3 seconds, but stops at a maximum of 75.

**Scoring:** Record the number of curl-ups to a maximum of 75.

|  | *Males* | *Females* |
|---|---|---|
| Health goal | 24 curl-ups | 18 curl-ups |
| Fitness goal | 47 curl-ups | 35 curl-ups |

### Trunk Lift Test

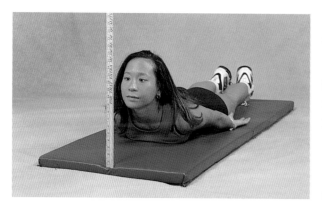

**Purpose:** To measure trunk extensor strength and flexibility.

**Objective:** The person lifts the upper body from the ground using the muscles of the back and holds the position to allow an accurate measurement from chin to the ground.

**Equipment:** Gym mats, yardstick or ruler.

**Instructions:** The person being tested lies face-down on a mat. The toes are pointed and the hands are placed alongside the body. The person lifts the upper body up, at a slow and controlled pace, to a maximum of 12 inches (31 centimeters). The performer holds the position until another person takes a measurement from the floor to the chin. Two trials should be done for this test.

Scoring: Record the highest score of the two trials, up to a maximum of 12 inches.

|  | *Males* | *Females* |
|---|---|---|
| Health goal | 9 inches (23 centimeters) | 9 inches (23 centimeters) |
| Fitness goal | 12 inches (31 centimeters) | 12 inches (31 centimeters) |

## Push-Ups Test

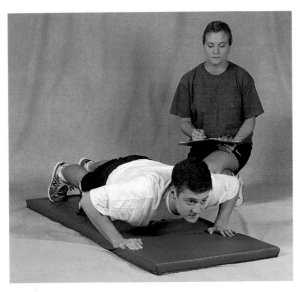

Purpose: To measure upper body strength and endurance.

Objective: The individual completes as many push-ups as possible.

Equipment: Tape player and audiotape to control the cadence of one push-up every 3 seconds.

Instructions: Working in pairs, one person counts while the other is tested. The person being tested lies facedown on the ground with the hands under the shoulders; fingers stretched; legs straight, parallel, and slightly apart; and the toes tucked under the feet. At a start command the person pushes up with the arms until they are straight. The legs and back should be kept straight throughout the test. The person lowers the body using the arms until the arms bend to a 90-degree angle and the upper arms are parallel to the floor. This action is repeated as many times as possible following the cadence of one repetition every 3 seconds. The test is continued until the person can't maintain the pace or demonstrates poor form.

Scoring: Record the number of push-ups performed.

|  | *Males* | *Females* |
|---|---|---|
| Health goal | 18 push-ups | 7 push-ups |
| Fitness goal | 35 push-ups | 15 push-ups |

## Determine the Effect of Stretching Exercises

The purpose of this experience is to help you evaluate the effect that different types of stretching exercises have on the range of motion (ROM) of your hip joint.

The first step is for everyone in the class to perform the sit-and-reach test to determine the initial range of motion. Work in groups of three or four—one person is being tested, and the others read the score, record it, and make sure the person being tested uses the correct technique. To perform the sit-and-reach test, you can use either a professionally made sit-and-reach flexibility tester or simply place a yardstick on top of a box that's approximately 12 inches tall. Warm up with a few minutes of activity and stretching to avoid injury. Start the test by sitting straight-legged on the floor with your feet flat against the box. Place one hand on top of the other, and, keeping your feet flat on the box and

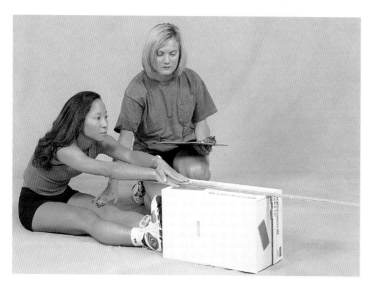

your legs straight, slowly slide your hands along the top of the box and reach forward as far as possible. Record the distance reached, and use the best of three tries as the final score.

Your instructor will now rank everyone from highest to lowest on the sit-and-reach test and divide you into three groups. Those ranked 1, 4, 7, etc. will form group 1; those ranked 2, 5, 8, etc. will form group 2; and those ranked 3, 6, 9, etc. will form group 3. Enter each person's first sit-and-reach score in the ROM1 column using the format of the following table:

Group 1

| Name | ROM1 | ROM2 | Change |
| --- | --- | --- | --- |
|  |  |  |  |
| Mean |  |  |  |

Group 2

| Name | ROM1 | ROM2 | Change |
| --- | --- | --- | --- |
|  |  |  |  |
| Mean |  |  |  |

Group 3

| Name | ROM1 | ROM2 | Change |
| --- | --- | --- | --- |
|  |  |  |  |
| Mean |  |  |  |

Everyone in group 1 now performs a static stretch of the hip extensors, and everyone in group 2 performs a proprioceptive neuromuscular facilitation technique stretch. Group 3 will be the control group and does not perform any stretch. Within three minutes of performing the stretch (or about 20 minutes after the last person in group 3 performed the sit-and-reach test), determine the ROM through the sit-and-reach test one more time. Enter the score for each group member in the ROM2 column of the table.

Calculate the change in ROM for each person and enter this number in the change column. Then calculate each group's average change. Compare the groups' mean change values: Does stretching improve ROM? Is one stretching technique better than the other in improving ROM? Note that we had one group do nothing so we could be reasonably sure that any changes to ROM after performing a stretch were actually due to the stretch and not, for example, just a practice effect (if ROM improves as much in the control as in the stretching groups, you would conclude that you could just save your energy and not stretch!).

One problem with this experiment is that you don't know if the people in group 1, for example, just respond better to stretching than the others if their average change turns out to be the greatest. Although you've tried to make the groups similar by placing each successive person (by initial ROM score) in an alternate group , we still can't be sure that some factor other than our stretching will also affect the results. To rule this out, every person can perform each technique (static stretch, proprioceptive neuromuscular stretch, and no stretch). With every person acting as his or her own control group, you can get a good comparison of how effective each technique is.

# Part II

# Physical Activity and Weight Control

Obesity is one of the greatest threats to good health and a high quality of life; issues related to obesity and weight control greatly impact health. In chapter 4 you'll learn about obesity and the health problems associated with it. You'll also explore the techniques used to measure and evaluate percent body fat, and you'll determine a healthy weight for yourself. In chapter 5, you'll learn about food nutrients, the dietary status of Americans, the components of a good diet, and the steps to establish a good diet and restrict calories of little nutritional value. In chapter 6, you'll examine the basic principles of weight loss through healthful nutrition and physical activity, and you'll learn about the importance of resting metabolic rate and lean body mass. You'll also explore "caloric balance" and other issues related to weight control. Through part II, you should be able to understand the issues involved in obesity and weight control and establish a healthful diet to help control your weight and body composition.

# Chapter 4

# Obesity

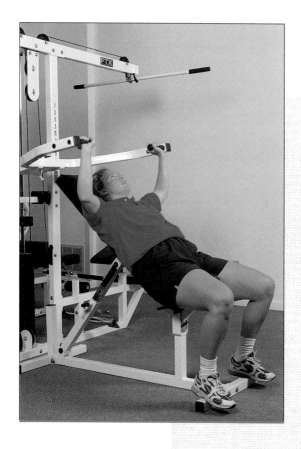

I've been on a regular program of walking and lifting weights for the past year now. I've been really consistent—more so than ever before. So I figured I was in pretty decent shape. I've gained a few pounds but I'm also stronger from lifting weights. I think most of the added pounds are muscle.

But at my yearly physical a few weeks ago, the nurse said I'm overweight according to the height/ weight charts (I'm 5 feet 7 inches and weigh about 160 pounds). She even says I may be bordering on obesity! That sounds ridiculous—but it scares me. Am I supposed to look like some model who disappears when she turns sideways? I have tons of energy and feel great. Since I feel so good, I figure my weight can't be too unhealthy. I wish I could figure out what's a healthy weight for me.

—Kate, 20-year-old junior

*What do you think?*

Should Kate be trying to look like a Parisian model—or is her weight where it should be? Are the standard height/weight charts an accurate guide to determining obesity? How does weight affect health? America has long had a distorted view of what healthy body weight is, thanks in part to Madison Avenue's long love affair with bone-thin models. But if Madison Avenue is wrong, who's right? If you say that neither extreme of the weight continuum is healthy, you're on the right track.

In this chapter you'll learn what obesity is, how it differs from overweight, and how it affects the body. We'll examine ways to determine your level of body fat. And we'll explore that most mysterious of questions: What's a desirable (healthy) weight for you? There is a way to determine that desirable weight—and we'll show you how.

## DRAWING THE LINE BETWEEN OVERWEIGHT AND OBESITY

The terms "overweight" and "obesity" conjure up immediate images, but an understanding of the terms is often subjective and murky. Where does overweight stop and obesity begin? The terms are related, but they do involve distinct differences. We say people are *overweight* when their weight exceeds an arbitrary figure according to their height and frame size (most suggest that anyone who is 20% over this figure could be called overweight). Of course, their weight includes not only fat, but also bones, muscle, and vital organs.

We say people are *obese* when their percent of body fat exceeds a certain level. A person's percent of body fat is a much truer measure of relative health than is weight. For men, we define *obesity* as 25% body fat or greater; for women, 30% or greater. Later in this chapter we'll show you how to determine your body fat level. But for now, understand that obese levels of body fat increase the risk of contracting diseases that impair the quality of life and that are often fatal.

**KEY POINT**

Although *overweight* and *obesity* are highly related and often used interchangeably, there is a difference. *Overweight* indicates too much body weight for a given height and frame. *Obesity* refers to an overfat level that brings with it increased risks of serious and often fatal diseases. A person can be overweight without being obese.

We'll explore what those risks of disease are a little later in this chapter. But first let's look at how obesity develops. The popular conception is that people who are obese are that way simply because they eat more than nonobese people. If that's true, then what about your 50-year-old Uncle Ed, the beanpole who has always eaten more than any two people in your family? Uncle Ed never met a pizza or a hot fudge sundae he didn't like. Why isn't he obese?

### Where Those Pounds Come From

Three factors help determine whether a person becomes obese: genetics, energy balance, and lifestyle.

#### Genetics

Heredity has much to say about who becomes overly fat. In fact, about 25% of body fat is related to a genetic component, according to studies of twins and parental associations for both humans and animals (Bouchard et al. 1988).

Children of obese parents have a greater chance of becoming obese themselves than do children of parents who are not obese. (It's likely, therefore, that Uncle Ed's parents didn't carry a lot of extra weight, either!)

---

### HEALTHCHECK

**If your parents are normal weight, can you assume you don't have to worry about becoming obese?**

No. Heredity increases the *probability* that you will have a body composition similar to that of either or both of your parents, but it's not a given.

---

### Energy Balance

A person's energy balance also plays an important role in determining obesity. A *positive energy balance* simply means that you consume more calories than you expend. This is the only way you can gain weight. A *negative energy balance* means you consume fewer calories than you expend—which is, of course, the only way to lose weight.

Supermarket tabloids would like us to think otherwise, judging by their headlines: "Alien Reveals Weight Loss Secrets to New Jersey Woman!," "New Rutabaga Diet Melts Pounds Away!" For all the miracle diets on the market, weight gain and loss boil down to this rather dull concept:

TAKE IN MORE CALORIES THAN YOU EXPEND, AND YOU GAIN WEIGHT. EXPEND MORE CALORIES THAN YOU TAKE IN, AND YOU LOSE WEIGHT.

You can eat five pizzas a day (not that we recommend it!) and not gain weight, so long as you expend the same amount of calories that those pizzas add up to. And your Uncle Ed? Somehow he's been expending all those calories he's been consuming. It could be just a hyperactive metabolism, or perhaps he leads a lifestyle that is quite physically active.

A long-term *positive energy balance*—which means that you consume more calories than you expend—leads to obesity. A positive energy balance is affected by your genetics and by how physically active you are.

### Lifestyle

Many Americans have sedentary occupations and lifestyles, involving little or no physical activity. College students, with their busy schedules, are hardly immune from being inactive. Such a lifestyle lowers the rate of caloric expenditure, which tilts the scales toward a positive energy balance. To get a rough idea of whether this is true for you, take this quick quiz. In your free time, you are most likely to

A. sit in front of a TV;

B. graze on nachos, potato chips, or *[insert your favorite junk food here]*;

C. *think* about exercising;

D. A, B, and C;

E. do something physically active: in-line skating, jogging, bike riding, tennis, or the like.

If you answered "D," you have plenty of company. About 100 million adults don't get enough physical activity to gain health benefits. If you answered "E," congratulations! You're doing something quite healthy. As you know from the previous chapters, an active lifestyle is a key to gaining and maintaining health.

Now that you know the factors that affect obesity, let's look at different *types* of obesity.

## Apples and Pears

Obesity can be described by type *(android* and *gynoid obesity)* and trend *(creeping obesity)*.

*Android obesity* occurs when a person has much more fat on the upper body than lower body, resulting in an apple-shaped form. The American Heart Association (1994) reports that such people have higher risks of cardiovascular disease than do those who have *gynoid obesity*, in which the distribution of fat is much greater below the waist (pear-shaped; see figure 4.1). Why people with android obesity have increased risk of cardiovascular disease is complex and not perfectly understood; for our purposes, it is important to simply recognize the increased risk.

---

### HEALTHCHECK

**Think of the adult men and women you know. Which gender do you associate with android obesity, and which with gynoid obesity?**

Males tend to store more fat around their midsections—android obesity. Females tend to store fat around the hips and thighs—gynoid obesity.

---

*Creeping obesity* refers to a gradual and consistent weight gain over the years. If you're like most people, you'll gain about 1.5 pounds (about 0.7 kilograms) of *fat* per year. At your 25-year college reunion, that means you'll be packing nearly 40 more pounds (about 18 kilograms) over your current weight! No wonder we need name tags at reunions. Rather than looking trim and healthy at 50 years old, like your Uncle Ed, you may end up gaining weight at a rate similar to that for the person in figure 4.2. This weight gain results from a combination of factors, all of which lead back to energy balance. As you age, your metabolic rate naturally decreases. On top of that, as people age they often become more sedentary because of lack of time for physical activity and a number of other factors. If you continue to consume the same amount of food (or more), the pounds start to add up.

Even if you don't put on weight at the rate others do, it's not hard to see that overweight and obesity are serious problems in our society. Just how prevalent is obesity in America? Let's take a look.

**FIGURE 4.1** *(a)* Android and *(b)* gynoid obesity.

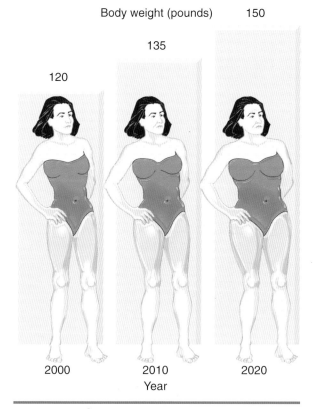

Body weight (pounds)

120    135    150

2000    2010    2020
Year

**FIGURE 4.2** Creeping obesity.

## How America Weighs In

As we have mentioned, obesity is strongly linked to being overweight—and the percentages of various American adult populations who are overweight have risen sharply since 1960. Across the board, the percentage of people in this country considered overweight—that is, 20% or more above their desirable weight—increased from 25% in 1980 to 33% in 1991. And obesity among children has also dramatically increased. Today, approximately 11% of children ages 6 through 17 are considered overweight. This is up from 5% in the 1960s and 1970s. The percentage of children who are described as "superobese" has increased the most.

Figure 4.3 shows the percentages of men and women, grouped according to age, who are overweight. Again the percentages increase over the years, although men do show a slight decline in their later years. However, even with this slight decline, almost twice the percentage of older men are still overweight in comparison to men aged 20 to 34.

### THE REAL SKINNY ON FAT

Obesity causes many health problems, ranging from cardiovascular disease to diabetes to high blood pressure to some cancers. These and related problems have been well documented by the American Heart Association, the American Cancer Society, the American Diabetes Association, the American Medical Association, the

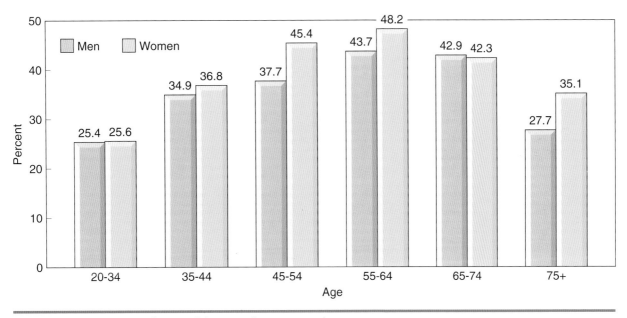

**FIGURE 4.3** Prevalence of overweight according to sex and age.

Data from Centers for Disease Control and Prevention (CDCP), National Center for Health Statistics.

## Overweight and Obesity: Risky Business

People who are overweight are twice as likely to have high blood pressure, and one and a half times as likely to have high cholesterol, compared with normal-weight people.

According to Nieman (1995), people who are obese run the following risks in comparison to normal-weight people:

- Higher levels of depression and anxiety
- Lower levels of self-esteem, income, and career advancement
- Less likelihood of marriage and of achieving academic potential
- Higher risks for colon, breast, prostate, gallbladder, ovarian, and uterine cancer
- Three times the chance of getting diabetes or cardiovascular disease
- Up to twice the chance of premature death

United States Public Health Service, and many other organizations. (See "Overweight and Obesity: Risky Business," from Nieman 1995) Persons who are obese also tend to have higher levels of depression and anxiety and lower levels of self-esteem. Some of these health risks are enormously high when compared with the risks for people who are not obese. For example, the person who is obese has up to three times the chance of contracting cardiovascular disease and diabetes. The all-cause mortality rate is up to twice as great for persons who are obese. The list goes on and on.

While people who are obese do have greater health risks than those who are not obese, they can turn those health risks around by losing weight. For example, when people who are obese and have high cholesterol lose weight, their cholesterol levels decrease and their risk of cardiovascular disease goes down. In recognition of this, the *Healthy People 2000: National Health Promotion and Disease Prevention Objectives* (1990) established a goal of reducing the prevalence of obesity in the adult population to no more than 20%.

Closer to home, what this means for you is quite simple: if you are overweight or obese, attempt to lose the extra weight, either on your own or with professional help. And if you are just slightly overweight now, remember that the average weight gain is 1.5 pounds of fat (about .7 kilograms) per year. Physical activity and good nutrition will keep that extra fat away and help you maintain a healthy weight.

Up to this point we've talked about being overweight or obese and about the unhealthy consequences. We defined obesity as a body fat percent of 25% or more for men and 30% or more for women. Now we'll get to the core of the matter and tell you what you need to know about how to actually assess your percent body fat.

## FIGURING OUT YOUR BODY COMPOSITION

*Body composition* refers to what our bodies are made of: muscle and bone, organs and fat, and other matter, such as connective tissue. Or, from another perspective, our bodies are composed of *lean tissue* and *fat tissue* (see figure 4.4). We have discussed the health risks of carrying too much fat; don't infer from that, however, that the goal is to rid your body of *all* fat. As will be described in chapter 6, our bodies need a certain amount of fat to provide insulation, store energy, and assist in the normal functioning of the body. Too little fat affects the hormonal balance in women and can cause excessive bone loss, bone fractures, loss of muscle mass, and other sometimes life-threatening physiological problems.

Many people use the standard height/weight charts to assess whether they are overweight or not. These charts categorize weights for various heights according to body frame: light, medium, and heavy. But this doesn't tell us anything about a person's body composition: two people who are each 6 feet 2 inches and 250 pounds could be vastly different in their percent fat. (Envision one of these being a professional football player and the other a professional couch potato.)

Similarly, classifying body types as ectomorphic (slender and angular), mesomorphic (husky and muscular), or endomorphic (plump and fat) has little real value. Two people with similar ectomorphic builds might have markedly differing percent body fat; a person with a mesomorphic build might have a lower percent body fat than a person with an ectomorphic build.

We've told you ways that *don't* work well in assessing body composition. What does work?

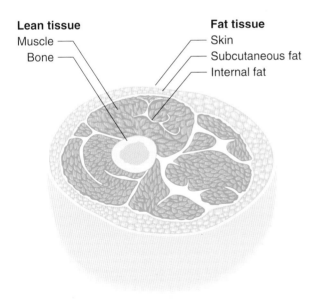

**Lean tissue**
Muscle
Bone

**Fat tissue**
Skin
Subcutaneous fat
Internal fat

**FIGURE 4.4** Lean tissue (skeletal muscle, organs, and bones and connective tissue) and fat tissue (subcutaneous fat and visceral fat).

**HEALTHCHECK**

**What is the advantage of using body composition characteristics rather than total weight when assessing relative risk that a person will develop cardiovascular disease?**

Total body weight includes lean and fat weight. When you assess body composition, you can evaluate the fat weight component—which is the component that increases the risk of cardiovascular disease.

## Lab Methods for Determining Body Composition

Actually, the most accurate way to determine someone's percent body fat is through dissection. You could simply dissect a body and place individual parts into the proper piles: fat or lean. However, relatively few subjects sign up for this method.

Dissection aside, here is a brief overview of methods used in a laboratory setting to determine a person's percent body fat.

• **Underwater weighing.** This involves measuring body density and converting that to percent body fat. *Body density* is the body's weight divided by its volume. The volume is discovered through *hydrostatic* (underwater) *weighing*; the difference between a person's scale weight and weight under water, when corrected for the density of the water, equals the body's volume, including lung volume and intestinal gas.

Confused? Think of it in terms of Archimedes' principle of buoyancy: Archimedes wanted to see if the king's crown was pure gold or if it was just overlaid with gold. He placed the king's crown, and then a same-weight silver crown, in equal containers of water. Archimedes knew that gold is more dense than silver. He also knew that if two objects weighed the same, the more dense object would not displace as much water. So if the king's crown was pure gold, it would not displace as much water as the silver crown. (Archimedes found, in fact, that the crown was only overlaid with gold.) In much the same way, a pound of lean tissue takes up less space (has less volume) than a pound of fat. The less water someone displaces, the less volume the person has.

• *Bioelectric impedance.* This method was developed in the 1980s. It estimates percent body fat by measuring the resistance to a very small electrical current flowing from the right wrist to the right ankle. Electrical current passes more easily through lean tissue than through fat tissue. The amount of resistance the current meets (i.e., the time it takes to travel through the body) reflects the amount of fat.

• **Other lab methods.** Other methods include using ultrasound, x-rays, and magnetic resonance imaging. But these techniques are hardly accessible to the average person who wants to learn how to assess percent body fat. There are, however, techniques you can actually put to use.

## Real-World Methods for Determining Body Composition

The following methods don't require advanced degrees or sophisticated equipment, or involve dissection.

• *Body mass index (BMI).* This method estimates obesity by dividing body weight (in kilograms) by the square of the body height (in meters). The lower a person's BMI, the lower the chance of developing cardiovascular disease. Body mass index is useful in large-scale surveys; for individual evaluations of body composition, skinfold measurements and circumference measurements (discussed next) are more appropriate. To calculate your BMI, and to see desirable ranges of BMI, see the BMI table on page 106 in the lab.

Note, however, that BMIs can be misleading in exactly the same way height/weight charts can be. For example, a 5-foot 10-inch football player who weighs 210 pounds is considered to be at grade 2 level obesity. The player, however, may have a very low body fat percent and actually be in very good health. Another 5-foot 10-inch male who weighs 170 pounds is considered to have an acceptable BMI; however, this person might have an abundance of body fat that puts him at much greater risk than the football player. In addition, someone who is 6 feet 4 inches and who weighs 110 pounds has a very low BMI and would be considered to have a low risk of cardiovascular disease. This person's low weight may in fact put him at high risk for other health-threatening conditions. So consider BMI values in the proper perspective—don't

## ⬤ OF INTEREST

**POINT**

### The Real Cost of Overweight

The health care cost of obesity approaches $100 billion per year in the U.S., but Paffenbarger and Olsen (1996) tell us of another cost of being overweight: *leanness*. Aside from the health hazards of being overweight, leanness has also become a marker of superior social or cultural status, as well as a quality essential to achieving such status. The social pressures to be thin in this country are enormous. Icons of male and particularly female beauty are almost impossibly gaunt. And there's even ample evidence to suggest a link between body weight and financial success. One study of business school graduates found that men who were at least 20% above their "desirable" weights made $4,000 less per year than their leaner colleagues, and the earnings gap widened over the years (Harvard Medical School 1994).

place all your "weight," so to speak, on your BMI alone.

- **Skinfold measurements.** You can estimate body fat by taking *skinfold measurements*, which quantify subcutaneous fat (the fat that lies just below the skin) at various sites on the body. These sites differ for men and women because the sexes store fat differently. Measurements are taken with calipers (see the photos in Lab 4 on pages 109 and 110), and the results are used in equations that are age-, race-, and gender-specific. The results have a margin of error of ± 3% for men and ± 4% for women. See the tables on pages 111 and 112 in the lab for the sites measured and the corresponding estimates of percent fat.

- **Circumference measurements.** You can also use circumference measurements to estimate percent fat (see the photos in Lab 4 on page 107). These measurements are best used with people who appear obese, because it may be difficult to get accurate skinfold measurements from them. Skinfold measurements are more accurate for people who are not obese, though, because two people who have the same circumference measurements may differ considerably in fat content.

You can use the *waist circumference/hip circumference ratio* to help detect android obesity and its inherent cardiovascular disease risk. Calculate the ratio by dividing the circumference of the waist by the circumference of the hips. The higher the ratio, the greater the risk. People with gynoid obesity have a lower waist/hip ratio than those with android obesity.

For example, let's say your Uncle Ed has a 31-inch waist and 36-inch hips. That means his waist/hip ratio is 31 divided by 36, or 0.86. The American Heart Association (1994) suggests that desirable waist/hip ratios are less than 1.00 for men and less than 0.80 for women. (You probably already figured Uncle Ed was in a safe range.)

Enough about Uncle Ed; his weight and body composition are fine. The much more important question: How are *your* weight and body composition?

## WHAT SHOULD *YOU* WEIGH?

By knowing your percent body fat and weight, and choosing a healthy percent body fat goal, you can establish your *desirable body weight.* Notice we didn't say *ideal* weight. No one can accurately set an exact, ideal weight for anyone. Instead, we'll concentrate on determining a healthy *range* of weight and fat. See table 4.1 for healthy ranges of body fat for men and women.

Here's an example of establishing a desirable body weight. Remember Kate, who regularly walks and lifts weights? She is 5 feet 7 inches, 160 pounds. She wanted to know if she was too heavy. When the nurse told her she was overweight, she decided to investigate. She had her skinfold measurements taken, and her body fat was estimated to be 25%. She and her doctor decided that though 25% is in the healthy range (see table 4.1), 20% might be better for her.

So how much weight does Kate have to lose to get to her 20% body fat goal? Here's how to figure it out:

1. **Determine her fat weight** by multiplying her body weight by her percent body fat.

   160 pounds $\times$ .25 = 40 pounds of fat weight

2. **Find her fat-free weight** by subtracting her fat weight from her total weight.

   160 pounds − 40 pounds of fat weight = 120 pounds of fat-free weight

3. **Figure her goal for fat-free mass** by subtracting her goal for her body fat from 100%.

   100% − 20% body fat = 80% fat-free mass

4. **Find her body weight goal** by dividing her current fat-free mass by her new fat-free mass goal.

   120 pounds divided by .80 = 150 pounds

5. **Determine her fat loss goal** by subtracting her body weight goal from her current weight.

   160 pounds − 150 pounds = 10 pounds fat loss

| Table 4.1  Body Fat Ranges | | |
| --- | --- | --- |
| Type | Males | Females |
| Essential fat | >5% | > 8% |
| Desirable for good performance | 5%-13% | 12%-22% |
| Desirable for good health | 10%-25% | 18%-30% |
| Overfatness (obesity) | >25% | > 30% |

Remember, this formula does not find the absolute perfect weight for you; it helps you determine what you need to lose, given your goal of percent body fat. There's a healthy *range* of weight and fat, not an *ideal* weight. Let's pursue our example one step further. It takes a negative caloric balance of approximately 3,500 calories to lose 1 pound (0.45 kilograms) of fat. A safe weight loss goal is 1 to 2 pounds per week. Therefore, Kate must create a 35,000 (3,500 calories × 10 pounds) negative caloric balance in order to lose 10 pounds. This translates into 3,500 to 7,000 calories per week (500 to 1,000 per day) for 5 to 10 weeks to achieve her weight goal safely.

You need to know what your percent body fat is to calculate your *desirable body weight*. Base your desirable weight on achieving a healthy body composition—10% to 25% body fat for most men, and 18% to 30% for most women.

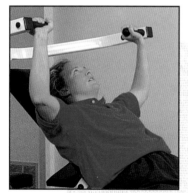

## Health Concepts

Remember Kate's questions about her weight? She learned that her body fat is within a healthy range for her, but she decided to lose weight to get into the lower end of that range. With simple calculations she determined that a 10-pound weight loss would put her where she wanted to be.

It's a good thing Kate is thinking about these issues now, because obesity is a serious health problem that tends to worsen with age. The average weight gain for adults is 1.5 pounds (about 0.7 kilograms) of fat per year. Obesity impairs the quality of life and increases the chance of contracting many serious diseases, including cardiovascular disease and cancer. People who have a positive energy balance—consuming more calories than they expend—tend to become overweight and risk becoming obese. Genetics and lifestyle also affect obesity.

# SUMMARY

▮ The term *overweight* is used when a person's weight exceeds an arbitrary figure, according to that person's height and frame size, by 20%. *Obesity* refers to a person's percent of body fat. Obesity is defined as 25% body fat or greater for men and 30% or greater for women. Genetics has much to say about who becomes overly fat.

▮ *Android obesity* occurs when a person has much more fat on the upper body; *gynoid obesity* occurs when a person has much more fat on the lower body. People who have android obesity are likelier candidates for cardiovascular disease than are those with gynoid obesity.

▮ Obesity is associated with higher levels of depression and anxiety; lower levels of self-esteem, income, and career advancement; higher risks for diabetes, cardiovascular disease, and a number of cancers; and premature death.

▮ Body fat levels can be assessed through various means, including underwater weighing, bioelectric impedance, BMI, skinfold measurements, and circumference measurements. Having an accurate estimate of your percent body fat, and knowing what ranges of body fat are healthy, you can determine your desirable weight.

*In this chapter we've explored the health risks of obesity; in the next chapter we take a look at the basics of sound nutrition and how nutrition affects physical activity.*

## KEY TERMS

android obesity

bioelectric impedance

body composition

body density

body mass index (BMI)

creeping obesity

desirable body weight

gynoid obesity

hydrostatic weighing

negative energy balance

obesity

overweight

positive energy balance

skinfold measurements

waist circumference/hip circumference ratio

# 4

# Determining Body Composition and Desired Weight Range

**THE PURPOSES OF THIS LAB EXPERIENCE ARE TO**

▌ determine your BMI,

▌ assess your cardiovascular disease risk using the waist/hip ratio from circumference measurements,

▌ estimate your percent body fat using skinfolds, and

▌ determine a desirable and healthy weight for you.

## Determine Your Body Mass Index

Use the table on the back of this page (adapted from Morrow et al. 1995) to determine your BMI.

What is your BMI? _____

What is your level of obesity? (Check color codes.)

_____

_____

_____

## Body Mass Index

**Height in inches**

| Wt. (lb) | 48 | 49 | 50 | 51 | 52 | 53 | 54 | 55 | 56 | 57 | 58 | 59 | 60 | 61 | 62 | 63 | 64 | 65 | 66 | 67 | 68 | 69 | 70 | 71 | 72 | 73 | 74 | 75 | 76 | 77 | 78 | Wt. (kg) |
|---|---|---|---|---|---|---|---|---|---|---|---|---|---|---|---|---|---|---|---|---|---|---|---|---|---|---|---|---|---|---|---|---|
| 100 | 30.6 | 29.3 | 28.2 | 27.1 | 26.1 | 25.1 | 24.2 | 23.3 | 22.5 | 21.7 | 20.9 | 20.2 | 19.6 | 18.9 | 18.3 | 17.8 | 17.2 | 16.7 | 16.2 | 15.7 | 15.2 | 14.8 | 14.4 | 14.0 | 13.6 | 13.2 | 12.9 | 12.5 | 12.2 | 11.9 | 11.6 | 45.5 |
| 105 | 32.1 | 30.8 | 29.6 | 28.4 | 27.4 | 26.3 | 25.4 | 24.5 | 23.6 | 22.8 | 22.0 | 21.3 | 20.5 | 19.9 | 19.2 | 18.6 | 18.1 | 17.5 | 17.0 | 16.5 | 16.0 | 15.5 | 15.1 | 14.7 | 14.3 | 13.9 | 13.5 | 13.2 | 12.8 | 12.5 | 12.2 | 47.7 |
| 110 | 33.6 | 32.3 | 31.0 | 29.8 | 28.7 | 27.6 | 26.6 | 25.6 | 24.7 | 23.9 | 23.0 | 22.3 | 21.5 | 20.8 | 20.2 | 19.5 | 18.9 | 18.3 | 17.8 | 17.3 | 16.8 | 16.3 | 15.8 | 15.4 | 14.9 | 14.5 | 14.2 | 13.8 | 13.4 | 13.1 | 12.7 | 50.0 |
| 115 | 35.2 | 33.7 | 32.4 | 31.2 | 30.0 | 28.8 | 27.8 | 26.8 | 25.8 | 24.9 | 24.1 | 23.3 | 22.5 | 21.8 | 21.1 | 20.4 | 19.8 | 19.2 | 18.6 | 18.0 | 17.5 | 17.0 | 16.5 | 16.1 | 15.6 | 15.2 | 14.8 | 14.4 | 14.0 | 13.7 | 13.3 | 52.3 |
| 120 | 36.7 | 35.2 | 33.8 | 32.5 | 31.3 | 30.1 | 29.0 | 27.9 | 27.0 | 26.0 | 25.1 | 24.3 | 23.5 | 22.7 | 22.0 | 21.3 | 20.6 | 20.0 | 19.4 | 18.8 | 18.3 | 17.8 | 17.3 | 16.8 | 16.3 | 15.9 | 15.4 | 15.0 | 14.6 | 14.3 | 13.9 | 54.5 |
| 125 | 38.2 | 36.7 | 35.2 | 33.9 | 32.6 | 31.4 | 30.2 | 29.1 | 28.1 | 27.1 | 26.2 | 25.3 | 24.5 | 23.7 | 22.9 | 22.2 | 21.5 | 20.8 | 20.2 | 19.6 | 19.0 | 18.5 | 18.0 | 17.5 | 17.0 | 16.5 | 16.1 | 15.7 | 15.2 | 14.9 | 14.5 | 56.8 |
| 130 | 39.8 | 38.1 | 36.6 | 35.2 | 33.9 | 32.6 | 31.4 | 30.3 | 29.2 | 28.2 | 27.2 | 26.3 | 25.4 | 24.6 | 23.8 | 23.1 | 22.4 | 21.7 | 21.0 | 20.4 | 19.8 | 19.2 | 18.7 | 18.2 | 17.7 | 17.2 | 16.7 | 16.3 | 15.9 | 15.4 | 15.1 | 59.1 |
| 135 | 41.3 | 39.6 | 38.0 | 36.6 | 35.2 | 33.9 | 32.6 | 31.4 | 30.3 | 29.3 | 28.3 | 27.3 | 26.4 | 25.6 | 24.7 | 24.0 | 23.2 | 22.5 | 21.8 | 21.2 | 20.6 | 20.0 | 19.4 | 18.9 | 18.3 | 17.8 | 17.4 | 16.9 | 16.5 | 16.0 | 15.6 | 61.4 |
| 140 | 42.8 | 41.1 | 39.5 | 37.9 | 36.5 | 35.1 | 33.8 | 32.6 | 31.5 | 30.4 | 29.3 | 28.3 | 27.4 | 26.5 | 25.7 | 24.9 | 24.1 | 23.3 | 22.6 | 22.0 | 21.3 | 20.7 | 20.1 | 19.6 | 19.0 | 18.5 | 18.0 | 17.5 | 17.1 | 16.6 | 16.2 | 63.6 |
| 145 | 44.3 | 42.5 | 40.9 | 39.3 | 37.8 | 36.4 | 35.0 | 33.8 | 32.6 | 31.4 | 30.4 | 29.3 | 28.4 | 27.5 | 26.6 | 25.7 | 24.9 | 24.2 | 23.5 | 22.8 | 22.1 | 21.5 | 20.8 | 20.3 | 19.7 | 19.2 | 18.7 | 18.2 | 17.7 | 17.2 | 16.8 | 65.9 |
| 150 | 45.9 | 44.0 | 42.3 | 40.6 | 39.1 | 37.6 | 36.2 | 34.9 | 33.7 | 32.5 | 31.4 | 30.4 | 29.4 | 28.4 | 27.5 | 26.6 | 25.8 | 25.0 | 24.3 | 23.5 | 22.9 | 22.2 | 21.6 | 21.0 | 20.4 | 19.8 | 19.3 | 18.8 | 18.3 | 17.8 | 17.4 | 68.2 |
| 155 | 47.4 | 45.5 | 43.7 | 42.0 | 40.4 | 38.9 | 37.5 | 36.1 | 34.8 | 33.6 | 32.5 | 31.4 | 30.3 | 29.3 | 28.4 | 27.5 | 26.7 | 25.8 | 25.1 | 24.3 | 23.6 | 22.9 | 22.3 | 21.7 | 21.1 | 20.5 | 19.9 | 19.4 | 18.9 | 18.4 | 17.9 | 70.5 |
| 160 | 48.9 | 47.0 | 45.1 | 43.3 | 41.7 | 40.1 | 38.7 | 37.3 | 35.9 | 34.7 | 33.5 | 32.4 | 31.3 | 30.3 | 29.3 | 28.4 | 27.5 | 26.7 | 25.9 | 25.1 | 24.4 | 23.7 | 23.0 | 22.4 | 21.7 | 21.2 | 20.6 | 20.0 | 19.5 | 19.0 | 18.5 | 72.7 |
| 165 | 50.5 | 48.4 | 46.5 | 44.7 | 43.0 | 41.4 | 39.9 | 38.4 | 37.1 | 35.8 | 34.6 | 33.4 | 32.3 | 31.2 | 30.2 | 29.3 | 28.4 | 27.5 | 26.7 | 25.9 | 25.1 | 24.4 | 23.7 | 23.1 | 22.4 | 21.8 | 21.2 | 20.7 | 20.1 | 19.6 | 19.1 | 75.0 |
| 170 | 52.0 | 49.9 | 47.9 | 46.0 | 44.3 | 42.6 | 41.1 | 39.6 | 38.2 | 36.9 | 35.6 | 34.4 | 33.3 | 32.2 | 31.2 | 30.2 | 29.2 | 28.3 | 27.5 | 26.7 | 25.9 | 25.2 | 24.4 | 23.8 | 23.1 | 22.5 | 21.9 | 21.3 | 20.8 | 20.2 | 19.7 | 77.3 |
| 175 | 53.5 | 51.4 | 49.3 | 47.4 | 45.6 | 43.9 | 42.3 | 40.8 | 39.3 | 37.9 | 36.7 | 35.4 | 34.2 | 33.1 | 32.1 | 31.1 | 30.1 | 29.2 | 28.3 | 27.5 | 26.7 | 25.9 | 25.2 | 24.5 | 23.8 | 23.1 | 22.5 | 21.9 | 21.3 | 20.8 | 20.3 | 79.5 |
| 180 | 55.0 | 52.8 | 50.7 | 48.8 | 46.9 | 45.1 | 43.5 | 41.9 | 40.4 | 39.0 | 37.7 | 36.4 | 35.2 | 34.1 | 33.0 | 32.0 | 31.0 | 30.0 | 29.1 | 28.3 | 27.4 | 26.6 | 25.9 | 25.2 | 24.5 | 23.8 | 23.2 | 22.5 | 22.0 | 21.4 | 20.8 | 81.8 |
| 185 | 56.6 | 54.3 | 52.1 | 50.1 | 48.2 | 46.4 | 44.7 | 43.1 | 41.6 | 40.1 | 38.7 | 37.4 | 36.2 | 35.0 | 33.9 | 32.8 | 31.8 | 30.8 | 29.9 | 29.0 | 28.2 | 27.4 | 26.6 | 25.9 | 25.1 | 24.5 | 23.8 | 23.2 | 22.6 | 22.0 | 21.4 | 84.1 |
| 190 | 58.1 | 55.8 | 53.5 | 51.5 | 49.5 | 47.7 | 45.9 | 44.3 | 42.7 | 41.2 | 39.8 | 38.5 | 37.2 | 36.0 | 34.8 | 33.7 | 32.7 | 31.7 | 30.7 | 29.8 | 28.9 | 28.1 | 27.3 | 26.6 | 25.8 | 25.1 | 24.4 | 23.8 | 23.2 | 22.6 | 22.0 | 86.4 |
| 195 | 59.6 | 57.2 | 55.0 | 52.8 | 50.8 | 48.9 | 47.1 | 45.4 | 43.8 | 42.3 | 40.8 | 39.5 | 38.2 | 36.9 | 35.7 | 34.6 | 33.5 | 32.5 | 31.5 | 30.6 | 29.7 | 28.9 | 28.0 | 27.3 | 26.5 | 25.8 | 25.1 | 24.4 | 23.8 | 23.2 | 22.6 | 88.6 |
| 200 | 61.2 | 58.7 | 56.4 | 54.2 | 52.1 | 50.2 | 48.3 | 46.6 | 44.9 | 43.4 | 41.9 | 40.5 | 39.1 | 37.9 | 36.7 | 35.5 | 34.4 | 33.4 | 32.3 | 31.4 | 30.5 | 29.6 | 28.8 | 28.0 | 27.2 | 26.4 | 25.7 | 25.0 | 24.4 | 23.8 | 23.2 | 90.9 |
| 205 | 62.7 | 60.2 | 57.8 | 55.5 | 53.4 | 51.4 | 49.5 | 47.7 | 46.1 | 44.5 | 42.9 | 41.5 | 40.1 | 38.8 | 37.6 | 36.4 | 35.3 | 34.2 | 33.2 | 32.2 | 31.2 | 30.3 | 29.5 | 28.7 | 27.9 | 27.1 | 26.4 | 25.7 | 25.0 | 24.4 | 23.7 | 93.2 |
| 210 | 64.2 | 61.6 | 59.2 | 56.9 | 54.7 | 52.7 | 50.7 | 48.9 | 47.2 | 45.5 | 44.0 | 42.5 | 41.1 | 39.8 | 38.5 | 37.3 | 36.1 | 35.0 | 34.0 | 33.0 | 32.0 | 31.1 | 30.2 | 29.4 | 28.5 | 27.8 | 27.0 | 26.3 | 25.6 | 25.0 | 24.3 | 95.5 |
| 215 | 65.7 | 63.1 | 60.6 | 58.2 | 56.0 | 53.9 | 51.9 | 50.1 | 48.3 | 46.6 | 45.0 | 43.5 | 42.1 | 40.7 | 39.4 | 38.2 | 37.0 | 35.9 | 34.8 | 33.7 | 32.8 | 31.8 | 30.9 | 30.0 | 29.2 | 28.4 | 27.7 | 26.9 | 26.2 | 25.5 | 24.9 | 97.7 |
| 220 | 67.3 | 64.6 | 62.0 | 59.6 | 57.3 | 55.2 | 53.2 | 51.2 | 49.4 | 47.7 | 46.1 | 44.5 | 43.1 | 41.7 | 40.3 | 39.1 | 37.8 | 36.7 | 35.6 | 34.5 | 33.5 | 32.6 | 31.6 | 30.7 | 29.9 | 29.1 | 28.3 | 27.6 | 26.8 | 26.1 | 25.5 | 100.0 |
| 225 | 68.8 | 66.0 | 63.4 | 60.9 | 58.6 | 56.4 | 54.4 | 52.4 | 50.5 | 48.8 | 47.1 | 45.5 | 44.0 | 42.6 | 41.2 | 39.9 | 38.7 | 37.5 | 36.4 | 35.3 | 34.3 | 33.3 | 32.4 | 31.4 | 30.6 | 29.7 | 28.9 | 28.2 | 27.4 | 26.7 | 26.1 | 102.3 |
| 230 | 70.3 | 67.5 | 64.8 | 62.3 | 59.9 | 57.7 | 55.6 | 53.6 | 51.7 | 49.9 | 48.2 | 46.6 | 45.0 | 43.5 | 42.2 | 40.8 | 39.6 | 38.4 | 37.2 | 36.1 | 35.0 | 34.0 | 33.1 | 32.1 | 31.3 | 30.4 | 29.6 | 28.8 | 28.1 | 27.3 | 26.6 | 104.5 |
| 235 | 71.9 | 69.0 | 66.2 | 63.7 | 61.2 | 58.9 | 56.8 | 54.7 | 52.8 | 51.0 | 49.2 | 47.6 | 46.0 | 44.5 | 43.1 | 41.7 | 40.4 | 39.2 | 38.0 | 36.9 | 35.8 | 34.8 | 33.8 | 32.8 | 31.9 | 31.1 | 30.2 | 29.4 | 28.7 | 27.9 | 27.2 | 106.8 |
| 240 | 73.4 | 70.4 | 67.6 | 65.0 | 62.5 | 60.2 | 58.0 | 55.9 | 53.9 | 52.0 | 50.3 | 48.6 | 47.0 | 45.4 | 44.0 | 42.6 | 41.3 | 40.0 | 38.8 | 37.7 | 36.6 | 35.5 | 34.5 | 33.5 | 32.6 | 31.7 | 30.9 | 30.1 | 29.3 | 28.5 | 27.8 | 109.1 |
| 245 | 74.9 | 71.9 | 69.0 | 66.4 | 63.8 | 61.5 | 59.2 | 57.1 | 55.0 | 53.1 | 51.3 | 49.6 | 47.9 | 46.4 | 44.9 | 43.5 | 42.1 | 40.9 | 39.6 | 38.5 | 37.3 | 36.3 | 35.2 | 34.2 | 33.3 | 32.4 | 31.5 | 30.7 | 29.9 | 29.1 | 28.4 | 111.4 |
| 250 | 76.4 | 73.4 | 70.5 | 67.7 | 65.1 | 62.7 | 60.4 | 58.2 | 56.2 | 54.2 | 52.4 | 50.6 | 48.9 | 47.3 | 45.8 | 44.4 | 43.0 | 41.7 | 40.4 | 39.2 | 38.1 | 37.0 | 35.9 | 34.9 | 34.0 | 33.1 | 32.2 | 31.3 | 30.5 | 29.7 | 29.0 | 113.6 |
| | 1.22 | 1.24 | 1.27 | 1.30 | 1.32 | 1.35 | 1.37 | 1.40 | 1.42 | 1.45 | 1.47 | 1.50 | 1.52 | 1.55 | 1.57 | 1.60 | 1.63 | 1.65 | 1.68 | 1.70 | 1.73 | 1.75 | 1.78 | 1.80 | 1.83 | 1.85 | 1.88 | 1.91 | 1.93 | 1.96 | 1.98 | |

**Height in meters**

**Key**

| Morbid obesity | Grade 2 obesity | Grade 1 obesity | Acceptable |
|---|---|---|---|

Name_____Section_____Date_____

## Assess Your Cardiovascular Disease Risk

To assess your cardiovascular disease risk, find out your waist/hip ratio. Use the following directions to obtain your waist and hip circumferences. Both measurements should be taken while you are standing.

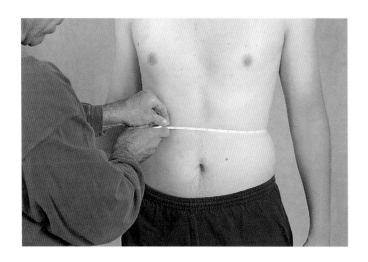

Waist: This is a horizontal measurement taken with a tape measure halfway between the navel and the lowest portion of the breastbone. The tape should be snug but not compressing the skin.

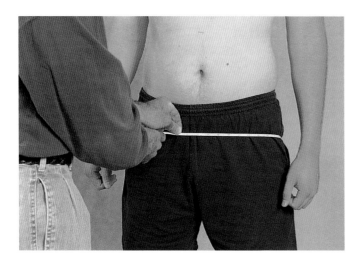

Hip: This is a horizontal measurement taken at the largest circumference of the buttocks/hip area. Again, make sure the tape is snug but not indenting the skin.

What is your waist circumference? _____

What is your hip circumference? _____

What is your waist/hip ratio? (Divide waist circumference by hip circumference.) _____

The American Heart Association recommends that males have a ratio under 1.00 and females a ratio under 0.80. How do your results compare with these recommendations?

_____

_____

## Estimate Your Percent Body Fat

Follow the directions and use the photos as references to take your skinfold measurements.

**Skinfold Measurements for College-Age Men**

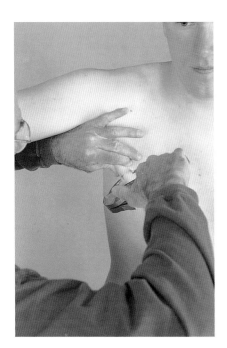

Chest: Stand with arms relaxed at sides. For the side of the chest that is being measured, place that hand on the shoulder of the person taking the measurement (this allows for easier access to the measuring point). The measurement is taken diagonally, halfway between the anterior axillary line (armpit) and the nipple.

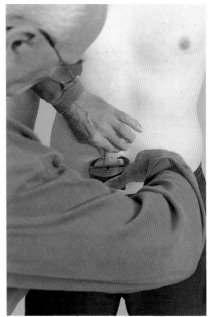

Abdomen: Stand and relax the abdominal muscles. Breathe normally. The vertical measurement is taken about 1 inch to the right side of the navel.

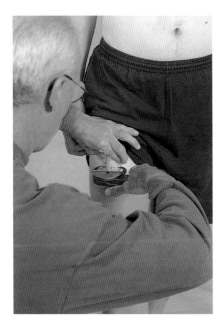

Thigh: This vertical measurement is taken at the midpoint of the right thigh, with the right leg relaxed and slightly bent (shift your weight to your left leg as you remain standing).

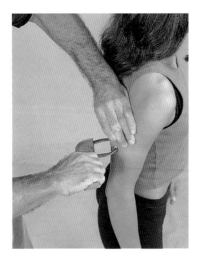

Triceps: This vertical measurement is taken at the midpoint of the back of the right arm, with the arm hanging comfortably at the side.

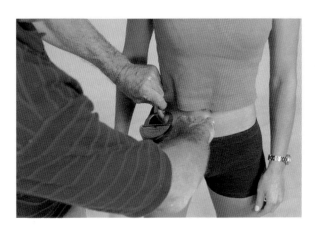

Suprailiac: This measurement is taken at a 45-degree angle while you are standing. The site is just above and in front of the hip bone.

Thigh: Same as for men.

Record the three measurements here.

| **Men** | **Women** |
|---|---|
| Chest: _____ | Triceps: _____ |
| Abdomen: _____ | Suprailiac: _____ |
| Thigh: _____ | Thigh: _____ |

Add the three measurements together and refer to the tables on page 111 (men) or 112 (women) to estimate your percent fat.

What is your percent body fat? _____

How does your percent fat compare with the values in the table?

_____

_____

_____

# Percent Fat Estimate for Men: Sum of Chest, Abdomen, and Thigh Skinfolds

**Age to Last Year**

| Sum of Skinfolds (mm) | Under 22 | 23-27 | 28-32 | 33-37 | 38-42 | 43-47 | 48-52 | 53-57 | Over 57 |
|---|---|---|---|---|---|---|---|---|---|
| 8-10 | 1.3 | 1.8 | 2.3 | 2.9 | 3.4 | 3.9 | 4.5 | 5.0 | 5.5 |
| 11-13 | 2.2 | 2.8 | 3.3 | 3.9 | 4.4 | 4.9 | 5.5 | 6.0 | 6.5 |
| 14-16 | 3.2 | 3.8 | 4.3 | 4.8 | 5.4 | 5.9 | 6.4 | 7.0 | 7.5 |
| 17-19 | 4.2 | 4.7 | 5.3 | 5.8 | 6.3 | 6.9 | 7.4 | 8.0 | 8.5 |
| 20-22 | 5.1 | 5.7 | 6.2 | 6.8 | 7.3 | 7.9 | 8.4 | 8.9 | 9.5 |
| 23-25 | 6.1 | 6.6 | 7.2 | 7.7 | 8.3 | 8.8 | 9.4 | 9.9 | 10.5 |
| 26-28 | 7.0 | 7.6 | 8.1 | 8.7 | 9.2 | 9.8 | 10.3 | 10.9 | 11.4 |
| 29-31 | 8.0 | 8.5 | 9.1 | 9.6 | 10.2 | 10.7 | 11.3 | 11.8 | 12.4 |
| 32-34 | 8.9 | 9.4 | 10.0 | 10.5 | 11.1 | 11.6 | 12.2 | 12.8 | 13.3 |
| 35-37 | 9.8 | 10.4 | 10.9 | 11.5 | 12.0 | 12.6 | 13.1 | 13.7 | 14.3 |
| 38-40 | 10.7 | 11.3 | 11.8 | 12.4 | 12.9 | 13.5 | 14.1 | 14.6 | 15.2 |
| 41-43 | 11.6 | 12.2 | 12.7 | 13.3 | 13.8 | 14.4 | 15.0 | 15.5 | 16.1 |
| 44-46 | 12.5 | 13.1 | 13.6 | 14.2 | 14.7 | 15.3 | 15.9 | 16.4 | 17.0 |
| 47-49 | 13.4 | 13.9 | 14.5 | 15.1 | 15.6 | 16.2 | 16.8 | 17.3 | 17.9 |
| 50-52 | 14.3 | 14.8 | 15.4 | 15.9 | 16.5 | 17.1 | 17.6 | 18.2 | 18.8 |
| 53-55 | 15.1 | 15.7 | 16.2 | 16.8 | 17.4 | 17.9 | 18.5 | 19.1 | 19.7 |
| 56-58 | 16.0 | 16.5 | 17.1 | 17.7 | 18.2 | 18.8 | 19.4 | 20.0 | 20.5 |
| 59-61 | 16.9 | 17.4 | 17.9 | 18.5 | 19.1 | 19.7 | 20.2 | 20.8 | 21.4 |
| 62-64 | 17.6 | 18.2 | 18.8 | 19.4 | 19.9 | 20.5 | 21.1 | 21.7 | 22.2 |
| 65-67 | 18.5 | 19.0 | 19.6 | 20.2 | 20.8 | 21.3 | 21.9 | 22.5 | 23.1 |
| 68-70 | 19.3 | 19.9 | 20.4 | 21.0 | 21.6 | 22.2 | 22.7 | 23.3 | 23.9 |
| 71-73 | 20.1 | 20.7 | 21.2 | 21.8 | 22.4 | 23.0 | 23.6 | 24.1 | 24.7 |
| 74-76 | 20.9 | 21.5 | 22.0 | 22.6 | 23.2 | 23.8 | 24.4 | 25.0 | 25.5 |
| 77-79 | 21.7 | 22.2 | 22.8 | 23.4 | 24.0 | 24.6 | 25.2 | 25.8 | 26.3 |
| 80-82 | 22.4 | 23.0 | 23.6 | 24.2 | 24.8 | 25.4 | 25.9 | 26.5 | 27.1 |
| 83-85 | 23.2 | 23.8 | 24.4 | 25.0 | 25.5 | 26.1 | 26.7 | 27.3 | 27.9 |
| 86-88 | 24.0 | 24.5 | 25.1 | 25.7 | 26.3 | 26.9 | 27.5 | 28.1 | 28.7 |
| 89-91 | 24.7 | 25.3 | 25.9 | 26.5 | 27.1 | 27.6 | 28.2 | 28.8 | 29.4 |
| 92-97 | 26.1 | 26.7 | 27.3 | 27.9 | 28.5 | 29.1 | 29.7 | 30.3 | 30.9 |
| 98-100 | 26.9 | 27.4 | 28.0 | 28.6 | 29.2 | 29.8 | 30.4 | 31.0 | 31.6 |
| 101-103 | 27.5 | 28.1 | 28.7 | 29.3 | 29.9 | 30.5 | 31.1 | 31.7 | 32.3 |
| 104-106 | 28.2 | 28.8 | 29.4 | 30.0 | 30.6 | 31.2 | 31.8 | 32.4 | 33.0 |
| 107-109 | 28.9 | 29.5 | 30.1 | 30.7 | 31.3 | 31.9 | 32.5 | 33.1 | 33.7 |
| 110-112 | 29.6 | 30.2 | 30.8 | 31.4 | 32.0 | 32.6 | 33.2 | 33.8 | 34.4 |
| 113-115 | 30.2 | 30.8 | 31.4 | 32.0 | 32.6 | 33.2 | 33.8 | 34.5 | 35.1 |
| 116-118 | 30.9 | 31.5 | 32.1 | 32.7 | 33.3 | 33.9 | 34.5 | 35.1 | 35.7 |
| 119-121 | 31.5 | 32.1 | 32.7 | 33.3 | 33.9 | 34.5 | 35.1 | 35.7 | 36.4 |
| 122-124 | 32.1 | 32.7 | 33.3 | 33.9 | 34.5 | 35.1 | 35.8 | 36.4 | 37.0 |
| 125-127 | 32.7 | 33.3 | 33.9 | 34.5 | 35.1 | 35.8 | 36.4 | 37.0 | 37.6 |

The margin of error is approximately ±3%

**Key**

| Very low | Low | Optimal | Moderately high | High (obese) | Very high |
|---|---|---|---|---|---|

Adapted from A.S. Jackson and M.L. Pollock, 1985, "Practical assessment of body composition," *The Physician and Sportsmedicine* 13(5): 85. Reproduced with permission of McGraw-Hill, Inc.

# Percent Fat Estimate for Women: Sum of Triceps, Suprailiac, and Thigh Skinfolds

## Age to Last Year

| Sum of Skinfolds (mm) | Under 22 | 23-27 | 28-32 | 33-37 | 38-42 | 43-47 | 48-52 | 53-57 | Over 57 |
|---|---|---|---|---|---|---|---|---|---|
| 23-25 | 9.7 | 9.9 | 10.2 | 10.4 | 10.7 | 10.9 | 11.2 | 11.4 | 11.7 |
| 26-28 | 11.0 | 11.2 | 11.5 | 11.7 | 12.0 | 12.3 | 12.5 | 12.7 | 13.0 |
| 29-31 | 12.3 | 12.5 | 12.8 | 13.0 | 13.3 | 13.5 | 13.8 | 14.0 | 14.3 |
| 32-34 | 13.6 | 13.8 | 14.0 | 14.3 | 14.5 | 14.8 | 15.0 | 15.3 | 15.5 |
| 35-37 | 14.8 | 15.0 | 15.3 | 15.5 | 15.8 | 16.0 | 16.3 | 16.5 | 16.8 |
| 38-40 | 16.0 | 16.3 | 16.5 | 16.7 | 17.0 | 17.2 | 17.5 | 17.7 | 18.0 |
| 41-43 | 17.2 | 17.4 | 17.7 | 17.9 | 18.2 | 18.4 | 18.7 | 18.9 | 19.2 |
| 44-46 | 18.3 | 18.6 | 18.8 | 19.1 | 19.3 | 19.6 | 19.8 | 20.1 | 20.3 |
| 47-49 | 19.5 | 19.7 | 20.0 | 20.2 | 20.5 | 20.7 | 21.0 | 21.2 | 21.5 |
| 50-52 | 20.6 | 20.8 | 21.1 | 21.3 | 21.6 | 21.8 | 22.1 | 22.3 | 22.6 |
| 53-55 | 21.7 | 21.9 | 22.1 | 22.4 | 22.6 | 22.9 | 23.1 | 23.4 | 23.6 |
| 56-58 | 22.7 | 23.0 | 23.2 | 23.4 | 23.7 | 23.9 | 24.2 | 24.4 | 24.7 |
| 59-61 | 23.7 | 24.0 | 24.2 | 24.5 | 24.7 | 25.0 | 25.2 | 25.5 | 25.7 |
| 62-64 | 24.7 | 25.0 | 25.2 | 25.5 | 25.7 | 26.0 | 26.7 | 26.4 | 26.7 |
| 65-67 | 25.7 | 25.9 | 26.2 | 26.4 | 26.7 | 26.9 | 27.2 | 27.4 | 27.7 |
| 68-70 | 26.6 | 26.9 | 27.1 | 27.4 | 27.6 | 27.9 | 28.1 | 28.4 | 28.6 |
| 71-73 | 27.5 | 27.8 | 28.0 | 28.3 | 28.5 | 28.8 | 29.0 | 29.3 | 29.5 |
| 74-76 | 28.4 | 28.7 | 28.9 | 29.2 | 29.4 | 29.7 | 29.9 | 30.2 | 30.4 |
| 77-79 | 29.3 | 29.5 | 29.8 | 30.0 | 30.3 | 30.5 | 30.8 | 31.0 | 31.3 |
| 80-82 | 30.1 | 30.4 | 30.6 | 30.9 | 31.1 | 31.4 | 31.6 | 31.9 | 32.1 |
| 83-85 | 30.9 | 31.2 | 31.4 | 31.7 | 31.9 | 32.2 | 32.4 | 32.7 | 32.9 |
| 86-88 | 31.7 | 32.0 | 32.2 | 32.5 | 32.7 | 32.9 | 33.2 | 33.4 | 33.7 |
| 89-91 | 32.5 | 32.7 | 33.0 | 33.2 | 33.5 | 33.7 | 33.9 | 34.2 | 34.4 |
| 92-94 | 33.2 | 33.4 | 33.7 | 33.9 | 34.2 | 34.4 | 34.7 | 34.9 | 35.2 |
| 95-97 | 33.9 | 34.1 | 34.4 | 34.6 | 34.9 | 35.1 | 35.4 | 35.6 | 35.9 |
| 98-100 | 34.6 | 34.8 | 35.1 | 35.3 | 35.5 | 35.8 | 36.0 | 36.3 | 36.5 |
| 101-103 | 35.3 | 35.4 | 35.7 | 35.9 | 36.2 | 36.4 | 36.7 | 36.9 | 37.2 |
| 104-106 | 35.8 | 36.1 | 36.3 | 36.6 | 36.8 | 37.1 | 37.3 | 37.5 | 37.8 |
| 107-109 | 36.4 | 36.7 | 36.9 | 37.1 | 37.4 | 37.6 | 37.9 | 38.1 | 38.4 |
| 110-112 | 37.0 | 37.2 | 37.5 | 37.7 | 38.0 | 38.2 | 38.5 | 38.7 | 38.9 |
| 113-115 | 37.5 | 37.8 | 38.0 | 38.2 | 38.5 | 38.7 | 39.0 | 39.2 | 39.5 |
| 116-118 | 38.0 | 38.3 | 38.5 | 38.8 | 39.0 | 39.3 | 39.5 | 39.7 | 40.0 |
| 119-121 | 38.5 | 38.7 | 39.0 | 39.2 | 39.5 | 39.7 | 40.0 | 40.2 | 40.5 |
| 122-124 | 39.0 | 39.2 | 39.4 | 39.7 | 39.9 | 40.2 | 40.4 | 40.7 | 40.9 |
| 125-127 | 39.4 | 39.6 | 39.9 | 40.1 | 40.4 | 40.6 | 40.9 | 41.1 | 41.4 |
| 128-130 | 39.8 | 40.0 | 40.3 | 40.5 | 40.8 | 41.0 | 41.3 | 41.5 | 41.8 |

The margin of error is approximately ±3%

## Key

| Very low | Low | Optimal | Moderately high | High (obese) | Very high |
|---|---|---|---|---|---|

Adapted from A.S. Jackson and M.L. Pollock, 1985, "Practical assessment of body composition," *The Physician and Sportsmedicine* 13(5): 85. Reproduced with permission of McGraw-Hill, Inc.

## Determine Your Desirable Weight

Determine your desirable weight following this five-step formula (assuming that your desired percent body fat is less than your current percent body fat):

1. Determine fat weight by multiplying your body weight by your percent body fat.

   Your body weight _____ ✕ your percent body fat _____ = _____ fat weight

2. Find your fat-free weight by subtracting your fat weight from your total weight.

   Your total weight _____ − your fat weight _____ = _____ current fat-free weight

3. Figure your goal for fat-free mass by subtracting your goal for your body fat from 100%.

   100% − percent fat goal _____ = _____ goal for fat-free mass

4. Find your body weight goal by dividing your current fat-free mass by your new fat-free mass goal.

   Current fat-free mass _____ / goal for fat-free mass _____ = _____body weight goal

5. Determine your weight loss goal by subtracting your body weight goal from your current weight.

   Current weight _____ − body weight goal _____ = _____ weight loss goal

   What is your desirable weight? _____

   How much fat weight must you lose to achieve your goal?

   _____

   _____

   _____

# Chapter 5

# Nutrition

*Ruth Ann Carpenter, M.S., R.D., L.D.*
The Cooper Institute for Aerobics Research

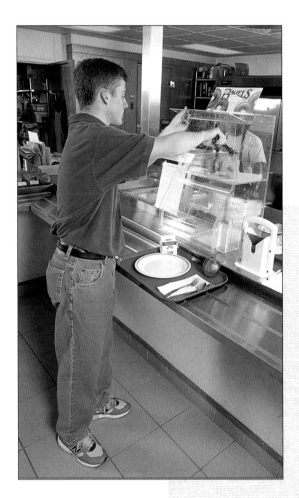

I'm finding it hard to eat what I think is a balanced diet—and in fact I'm not sure if I know what a balanced diet really is. It seems like a lot of the food choices on campus are in the categories of (a) fried and greasy, (b) bland and tasteless, (c) UFOs (unidentified food objects), or (d) all of the above. Yet my schedule is so chaotic and busy that I pretty much just grab what I can and pay for it later—in more ways than one. I'd like to first know some basic guidelines on getting good nutrition, and second figure out how I can fit good nutrition into my hectic lifestyle!

—Mike, 19-year-old sophomore

To know what constitutes a balanced diet, you first have to know what types of nutrients the body needs: carbohydrates, proteins, fats, vitamins, minerals, and water. We'll define the role of each nutrient and provide recommendations for amounts needed for health and for athletic performance. We'll show you how to use the Food Guide Pyramid and how to interpret nutrition labels. We'll give you tips on eating healthful foods in fast-food restaurants, as well as ways to plan nutritious meals and snacks. Along the way we'll explore some interesting and important issues, including iron deficiency, caffeine and alcohol, osteoporosis, carbohydrate loading, and vegetarianism.

## NUTRITION AND PHYSICAL ACTIVITY

Foods provide energy and important nutrients. We need energy to fuel body temperature regulation, chemical reactions, and muscle contractions. Energy in foods is measured in units of heat called *kilocalories*. Most people refer to kilocalories as "calories."

The nutrients that foods provide build and repair various tissues and trigger chemical reactions that are important for sustaining life. Some enzymes help break down a food into its component nutrients for easy absorption from the intestines into the blood. Others bring together various components in the body to create new substances. Our bodies are fueled by six types of nutrients, but not all are sources of energy. Following are the nutrients, with their energy value per gram where appropriate:

- Carbohydrates (4 calories per gram)
- Proteins (4 calories per gram)
- Fats (9 calories per gram)
- Vitamins
- Minerals
- Water

Notice that only carbohydrates, proteins, and fats provide calories. Alcohol also provides calories (7 per gram) but is not considered a nutrient.

## Carbohydrates

The primary function of most *carbohydrates* is to provide energy for the body. As you'll see in a moment, some carbohydrates are not a good source of energy but do provide bulk for proper digestion and elimination. There are two types of carbohydrates: *simple carbohydrates* and *complex carbohydrates*.

**KEY POINT** The primary function of most carbohydrates is to provide energy for the body.

### Simple Carbohydrates

Simple carbohydrates are often referred to as sugars because they have a simpler chemical structure than complex carbohydrates. Many sugars occur naturally in our food supply. Glucose, fructose, maltose, and sucrose are found primarily in fruits and vegetables. Lactose is a naturally occurring simple carbohydrate found in milk.

Certain plants such as sugarcane and sugar beets have very high amounts of naturally occurring sugars. Food manufacturers process these plants to make table sugar, brown sugar, molasses, and other processed sugars. These in turn are used as sweetening components for other processed foods such as soda, cookies, cakes, and pies.

### Complex Carbohydrates

When many simple carbohydrates are linked together, they form *starches* and *fiber*. These are referred to as complex carbohydrates. They are found only in plants—especially vegetables, grains, and legumes. Starch that you eat is broken down into simple sugars in your digestive tract before being absorbed into your bloodstream.

Fiber, on the other hand, is not absorbed. Fiber cannot be broken down by your digestive tract. However, various types of fiber perform important functions. *Insoluble fibers* help hold water in your lower intestines, which aids in absorption and elimination. Good sources of in-

soluble fiber are bran, fruits, vegetables, nuts, and legumes.

*Soluble fibers* have been touted as a way to reduce blood cholesterol levels. One way this may work is through binding of soluble fiber with cholesterol in the intestine, preventing the

---

**HEALTHCHECK**

**Are foods high in processed sugars bad for you?**

Not necessarily. The difference between naturally occurring and processed sugars is that foods containing naturally occurring sugars (fruits, vegetables, and milk) are often good sources of other important nutrients such as minerals, vitamins, and fiber. Foods made with processed sugars are usually void of other nutrients. For example, a 12-ounce can of regular cola has 10 teaspoons of sugar and really no other nutrients. A 12-ounce glass of orange juice has 10 teaspoons of sugar and also provides twice the vitamin C that your body needs for the day!

---

### Carbo Loading: Does It Really Work?

Yes, in addition to storing extra energy as body fat, your body also stores a ready supply of carbohydrate energy in your liver and muscles in the form of a substance called *glycogen.* Endurance athletes "carbo load" to maximize the amount of carbohydrate they have stored in their bodies before an athletic event. It's important for endurance athletes to maximize their glycogen stores because these are needed to sustain energy and ward off fatigue in events lasting 90 minutes or longer (e.g., cycling events, marathons, triathlons). Carbo loading *does* work for such events when done properly.

The best method for loading up on glycogen is to eat a high-carbohydrate diet during the weeks before your event. This will replace carbohydrate lost during daily training sessions and enable you to continue training at a high level. Then three days before your event, taper your training but maintain the high-carbohydrate diet. Because you do not need as much energy due to the reduction in training sessions, your body will "load up" on the unused carbohydrate by converting it to glycogen for storage in your muscles and liver. During the event, your body will have more glycogen (i.e., energy) to call on and therefore you will be able to sustain your effort longer before fatiguing.

cholesterol from being absorbed. Soluble fiber is found primarily in fruits, oats, and legumes. In chapter 7, you'll read about the role that cholesterol plays in the development of heart disease.

 Soluble fibers—such as are found in fruits, oats, and legumes—help reduce blood cholesterol levels.

## RECOMMENDATIONS FOR GOOD HEALTH

As shown in table 5.1, the recommendation for carbohydrate intake is 55% or more of your total daily calories. This amounts to 300 to 375 grams for most people. Most of your carbohydrates should come from complex carbohydrates rather than sugars. Try to eat between 20 and 35 grams of fiber per day. Most Americans eat about half as much fiber as they need.

## RECOMMENDATIONS FOR ATHLETIC PERFORMANCE

Athletes burn more energy than the average person; they need to replace that energy by eating more carbohydrates than the average person. Some sport nutritionists recommend that athletes get 60% to 70% of their daily calories from carbohydrates.

## Proteins

*Protein* is an important element of many body tissues including muscles, skin, internal organs, bones and teeth, and connective tissue such as ligaments and tendons. It is also important for the proper functioning of the immune system, hormones, and various chemical reactions. Protein can also provide energy, but the body prefers not to use protein for energy unless other fuels—carbohydrates and fats—are not available in adequate amounts.

Proteins are complicated structures made of building blocks called *amino acids.* The number of amino acids and order in which they are linked determine the type of protein and its specific function. For example, protein in a steak that you have for dinner has many of the same amino acid building blocks as the insulin (a hormone) that circulates in your blood. Your body breaks apart the amino acid building blocks in the steak during digestion and transports the amino acids into your bloodstream, where they become the building blocks for many new proteins, including insulin.

The body needs 20 different amino acids. It can produce 11 on its own; the other 9 must come through food. Those that come through food are called *essential amino acids.* Although all essential amino acids are important, some are

### Table 5.1 Carbohydrate Needs, Functions, and Food Sources

| | Daily dietary recommendations (>55% of daily calories) | Primary functions/ Action | Major sources |
| --- | --- | --- | --- |
| Simple sugars | Use added sugars in moderation | Provide energy | Fruits, vegetables, milk, processed sugars |
| Starches | Should be most of daily carbohydrate intake | Provide energy | Bread, pasta, rice, cereal, potatoes, peas, dried beans |
| Dietary fiber | 20-35 grams | Provide bulk for digestion and elimination | Cereals, grains, fruits, vegetables |

needed in slightly greater quantities than others. The essential amino acids include

- histidine,
- isoleucine,
- leucine,
- lysine,
- methionine,
- phenylalanine,
- threonine,
- tryptophan, and
- valine.

Protein-rich foods that contain all the essential amino acids in quantities needed by the body are called "complete" proteins. Animal proteins such as eggs, milk, fish, meat, poultry, and cheese are complete proteins.

Plant sources of protein—for example, legumes, grains, vegetables, nuts, and seeds—are called "incomplete" proteins because they have relatively low amounts of one or two essential amino acids. But not all plant proteins are low in the same amino acids. You can combine plant foods that are low in certain amino acids with other plant foods that are high in those amino acids to make a complete protein. This strategy is called *complementing proteins*; it is important for people who don't eat any animal products at all (see "Vegetarianism" on page 133). You can also complement the limited amino acids in a plant protein by combining it with an animal protein such as meat, poultry, fish, eggs, and milk products. The best plant sources of protein include dried beans, peas, grains, seeds, and nuts. See table 5.2 for various combinations of plant and animal foods that yield more complete proteins.

### Table 5.2 Complementing Proteins

| Combination | Example combination |
|---|---|
| Legumes and grains | Black beans and rice; refried beans and tortilla; peanut butter and bread |
| Legumes and nuts/seeds | Hummus (Middle Eastern recipe made with garbanzo beans and sesame butter) |
| Legumes and animal protein | Chili |
| Grains and nuts/seeds | Cereal with nuts (such as granola); bread with nuts |
| Grains and animal protein | Cereal and milk; tortilla and ground beef; bread and chicken salad; pizza with cheese; spaghetti with meatballs |
| Nuts/seeds and animal protein | Stir-fried beef with cashews; sesame chicken |

kilogram. Therefore, a 150-pound adult would need about 54 grams of protein per day (150 / 2.2 = 68.18; 68.18 × 0.8 = 54.5). *Note:* The risk of protein deficiency in this country is very low. Most Americans eat much more protein than they need.

 Most Americans eat more protein than they need. Try to limit your protein intake to 10-15% of your total daily calories.

### RECOMMENDATIONS FOR GOOD HEALTH

As shown in table 5.3, the daily recommended protein intake is 10-15% of your total daily calories. The *recommended daily allowance* for protein for most healthy adults is 0.8 grams per kilogram of body weight per day. There are 2.2 pounds in 1

### RECOMMENDATIONS FOR ATHLETIC PERFORMANCE

Many athletes mistakenly believe that they must eat extra protein to build bigger muscles. Research shows that athletes have only slightly higher protein needs than nonathletes. Depending on overall energy intake and intensity of training, athletes may require 0.9 to 1.4 grams of protein per kilogram of body weight per day. Athletes can attain adequate protein intakes by eating a well-balanced diet that includes moderate amounts of protein-rich foods (see table 5.3).

## Fats

In today's fat-conscious culture, you might think you should eliminate all *fat* from your diet. Not only would that be very difficult to do, it would also be unhealthy. Fat provides the essential fatty acids that your body needs. The body cannot manufacture linoleic acid and linolenic acid; these acids must be gained through foods. These and other fatty acids transport the fat-soluble vitamins from the digestive tract into the body. Fats are also part of all cell membranes and nerves; fat cushions your internal organs and is a rich source of energy. So a certain amount of fat is important to your health.

There are two types of fat that most people have heard of: *saturated fats* and *unsaturated fats*. *Cholesterol* technically isn't a fat, but it has many of the same characteristics as fat.

### Saturated Fats

This type of fat has gotten a lot of attention in the last several decades. Research has shown that saturated fats contribute to increased blood cholesterol, especially LDL (low density lipoprotein)-cholesterol, which is a significant risk factor for coronary heart disease. Saturated fats are typically solid at room temperature (think of butter, lard, visible fat on meat) and come primarily from animal sources. Oils from the coconut, palm, and palm kernel plants are exceptions.

### Unsaturated Fats

There are two types of unsaturated fats. *Monounsaturated fats* come from vegetable sources such as olive, canola, and peanut oils. Research suggests that when you substitute monounsaturated fats for saturated fats, you are likely to reduce your LDL-cholesterol level while keeping your HDL levels the same. HDL is your high density lipoprotein-cholesterol, known as your "good" cholesterol. However, *polyunsaturated fats* seem to reduce both LDL- and HDL-cholesterol. Corn oil and sunflower, soybean, safflower, cottonseed, and fish oils are the best sources of polyunsaturated fats.

### Cholesterol

Dietary cholesterol is a sterol that is similar in its characteristics to fat. As with fat, your body needs some cholesterol; it aids in the proper digestion of fat and is part of every cell. But you don't need to provide cholesterol through your diet, because your body manufactures all that it needs. People have been advised for decades to reduce cholesterol intake because of the association between dietary cholesterol and elevated blood cholesterol. Cholesterol is found *only* in all types of animal products, but is especially high in egg yolks, organ meats, and certain types of shellfish.

| Table 5.3 Protein Needs, Functions, and Food Sources | | |
|---|---|---|
| Daily dietary recommendations (10-15% of daily calories) | Primary functions/Action | Major sources |
| Men: about 60 grams<br>Women: about 50 grams | Protein provides amino acids for building and repairing body tissues | Meat, poultry, fish, eggs, milk products, legumes |

## RECOMMENDATIONS FOR GOOD HEALTH

As we stated earlier, some fat is necessary. But many people eat much more fat than is needed. Try to limit your fat intake to 30% of your total daily calories—and your *saturated* fat intake to less than 10% of your total daily calories (see table 5.4). For most people, that means no more than 67 grams of total fat per day, or 22 grams of saturated fat (based on 2,000 total daily calories). The next column shows recommended fat intakes for other calorie levels. The fat amount listed for each calorie level represents the *most* you should eat each day. In addition, you should eat no more than 300 milligrams of dietary cholesterol per day.

| Calorie level | Total fat (grams) | Saturated fat (grams) |
|---|---|---|
| 1,200 | 40 | 13 |
| 1,400 | 47 | 15 |
| 1,600 | 53 | 18 |
| 1,800 | 60 | 20 |
| 2,000 | 67 | 22 |
| 2,200 | 73 | 24 |
| 2,400 | 80 | 27 |
| 2,600 | 87 | 29 |
| 2,800 | 93 | 31 |
| 3,000 | 100 | 33 |

## RECOMMENDATIONS FOR ATHLETIC PERFORMANCE

Athletes should especially be concerned with keeping their fat intake at healthy levels. In fact, athletes should probably reduce their fat intake to less than 20% of their daily calories. That's because many athletes need to make room in their diets for an increased percentage of carbohydrates.

Most Americans eat more fat than they need. Try to limit your fat intake to 30% of your total calories per day and saturated fat intake to less than 10% of your total daily calories.

| | Table 5.4 Fat Needs, Functions, and Food Sources | | |
|---|---|---|---|
| | Daily dietary recommendations (< 30% of daily calories) | Primary functions/ Action | Major sources |
| Saturated fat | < 10% of daily calories | Provides energy; increases blood LDL-cholesterol level | Meat, poultry, butter and other spreads, cheese, tropical oils |
| Monounsaturated fat | < 10% of daily calories | Provides energy; decreases blood LDL-cholesterol | Canola, olive, peanut oils |
| Polyunsaturated fat | < 10% of daily calories | Provides energy; decreases blood LDL- and HDL-cholesterol | Vegetable oils except those previously mentioned |
| Dietary cholesterol | < 300 mg | Nerve function and fat digestion; increases blood LDL-cholesterol | Animal products only, especially egg yolks, organ meats, and some shellfish |

## Vitamins

The primary function of *vitamins* is to regulate various metabolic reactions. As table 5.5 shows, many vitamins perform various functions in the body; no one vitamin "does it all." In comparison to our requirement for carbohydrates, protein, and fats, we need vitamins in very minute amounts. While no single food provides all the vitamins you need, fruits and vegetables are excellent sources of most vitamins. There are two types of vitamins: *fat soluble* and *water soluble.*

Vitamins A, D, E, and K are fat soluble because they cannot be dissolved in water. In other words, they need to be "dissolved" in fat to be transported into and around the body. Table 5.5 describes the basic functions and sources of these vitamins. An important concept to note is that if you eat more of a fat-soluble vitamin than you need, the excess is stored in the body. You can even ingest toxic levels of fat-soluble vitamins; this usually doesn't occur unless you're taking high-dose vitamin supplements.

Water-soluble vitamins include the B-complex vitamins (thiamin, riboflavin, niacin, B-6, B-12, folate, biotin, pantothenic acid) and vitamin C. As the phrase implies, these vitamins dissolve

### To Supplement or Not to Supplement . . .

. . . that is the question. Most healthy people who are eating a diet in accordance with the Food Guide Pyramid (see page 129) don't need to take vitamin or mineral supplements. However, if you doubt the adequacy of your dietary habits, you may wish to take a multivitamin/mineral supplement once a day. Choose one that has only 100% of the recommended daily allowance—you don't need more—for the various nutrients. You can select a generic brand to save money. You may also benefit from taking a vitamin or mineral supplement if you

- can't or don't like to drink milk or eat dairy products;
- are a postmenopausal woman (to supplement your calcium intake by 1,000 to 1,200 milligrams);
- are on a very low calorie diet;
- are pregnant or breast-feeding (especially iron, folate, and calcium if recommended by your doctor); or
- are a vegetarian who includes no animal products in your diet (especially calcium, iron, and B-12).

When selecting a supplement, be careful not to fall prey to advertising gimmicks. While manufacturers cannot make unproven claims about their supplements, the purity, safety, and effectiveness of supplements are not regulated. Buyer beware!

## Table 5.5  Vitamin Needs, Functions, and Food Sources

| | Daily dietary recommendations | Primary functions/ Action | Major sources |
|---|---|---|---|
| **Fat-soluble** | | | |
| A | Men*: 1,000 mcg RE** Women*: 800 mcg RE | Skin health; vision; immune function; bone growth | Milk products, dark green leafy vegetables, orange fruits and vegetables |
| D | Men: 5-15 mcg Women: 5-15 mcg | Bone health | Sunlight, milk products |
| E | Men: 10 mg Women: 8 mg | Protects cell membranes from oxidative damage | Leafy green vegetables, oils from plants |
| K | Men: 70-80 mcg Women: 60-65 mcg | Promotes blood clotting | Produced in intestines; leafy green vegetables |
| **Water-soluble** | | | |
| Thiamin (B-1) | Men: 1.2 mg Women: 1.1 mg | Carbohydrate metabolism | Lean meats, whole-grain or enriched cereals, nuts, legumes |
| Riboflavin (B-2) | Men: 1.3 mg Women: 1.1 mg | Energy metabolism | Milk and milk products, enriched breads and cereals, leafy green vegetables |
| Niacin | Men: 16 mg Women: 14 mg | Carbohydrate and energy metabolism | Milk, meat, poultry, fish, and other protein-rich foods |
| B-6 | Men: 1.3-1.7 mg Women: 1.3-1.5 mg | Amino acid metabolism | Leafy green vegetables, meats, poultry, fish, legumes, fruits |
| B-12 | Men: 2.4 mcg Women: 2.4 mcg | New cell formation; nerve function | Animal products only—milk and meats |
| Folate | Men: 400 mcg Women: 400 mcg | Vital to new cell formation | Leafy green vegetables, legumes, seeds, fortified grain products |
| Biotin | Men: 30 mcg Women: 30 mcg | Fat and amino acid metabolism | Legumes, egg yolks |
| Pantothenic acid | Men: 5 mg Women: 5 mg | Energy and tissue metabolism | Lean meats, whole grains, broccoli, legumes, eggs |
| C (ascorbic acid) | Men: 60 mg Women: 60 mg | Antioxidant; amino acid metabolism; immune function; wound healing and bone metabolism | Citrus fruits, dark green vegetables, strawberries, peppers, potatoes |

* For men and women ages 19-51+; women not pregnant or breast-feeding.
** mcg = micrograms;  RE = retinol equivalents

in water. Table 5.5 describes the basic functions and sources for most of these vitamins. While the body excretes much of the extra vitamins it doesn't need, research now indicates that prolonged use of high doses of B-6 might lead to serious neurological problems. In addition, large quantities of niacin can cause side effects, and large quantities of vitamin C may reduce its effectiveness.

### RECOMMENDATIONS FOR GOOD HEALTH

Table 5.5 shows that daily intake recommendations for many vitamins are slightly higher for men than for women. This is so because men generally have a larger body mass than women. Also, some vitamins are needed in larger quantities than others (compare vitamins C and B-12). Eating a balanced diet is the best way to ensure adequate intake of vitamins.

### RECOMMENDATIONS FOR ATHLETIC PERFORMANCE

Because of increased energy requirements, athletes have a higher-than-normal need for many of the B vitamins. Athletes usually meet these needs by getting more calories from whole grains, fruits, and vegetables.

## Minerals

*Minerals* build and maintain bones and teeth, form enzymes and hormones, aid in muscle contractions, and regulate the body's water. Minerals are like vitamins in that they do not provide energy and are needed in much smaller quantities than carbohydrates, protein, and fat. They differ from vitamins in that they are simple, inorganic chemical elements whereas vitamins are complex, organic compounds.

You need anywhere from 20 to 60 minerals regularly in your diet for good health. Minerals are categorized as "major" or "trace" minerals depending on the amounts present in the body.

You need the major minerals in greater quantities than the trace minerals. Table 5.6 describes the basic functions and sources of six minerals that are of concern for most people today. Three minerals—sodium, calcium, and iron—deserve further attention.

### Sodium

This mineral is essential for adequate fluid balance in the body. It is also important for muscle contraction and nerve conduction. American diets are rarely deficient in sodium. In fact, most Americans eat more sodium than the recommended maximum of 2,400 milligrams per day. Excessive sodium may contribute to high blood pressure in some people who are sensitive to sodium. At least 75% of sodium intake comes from salt added during processing and manufacturing. You can moderate your sodium intake by not eating many salty or highly processed foods.

### Calcium

Calcium is the most abundant mineral in the body. Ninety-nine percent of the body's calcium is in the bones, but calcium is also essential for nerve conduction, muscle contraction, and blood clotting. Milk and milk products are the best sources of calcium in the food supply. Note that nonfat and low-fat milk products have as much calcium as regular, full-fat versions—and often more.

### Iron

Iron is a trace mineral that is essential for the transportation and storage of oxygen in the blood and muscles. Without oxygen, cells can't produce energy. Iron is also necessary for the metabolism of hormones and amino acids. Women have higher recommended intake levels (see table 5.6) because of iron lost through menstrual blood. Iron-poor diets can contribute to iron deficiency especially in women and young children. The best sources of iron are red meats, poultry, fish, legumes, green leafy vegetables, and dried fruit. Grain products that are fortified with iron are good sources as well.

## Table 5.6  Mineral Needs, Functions, and Food Sources

| | Daily dietary recommendations | Primary functions/Action | Major sources |
|---|---|---|---|
| Sodium | Men*: < 2,400 mg<br>Women*: < 2,400 mg | Maintains body fluid balance | Salt, processed foods |
| Calcium | Men: 1,000-1,500 mg<br>Women: 1,000-1,500 mg | Bone and teeth formation; muscle and nerve function | Milk products, green vegetables, tofu |
| Phosphorus | Men: 800-1,200 mg<br>Women: 800-1,200 mg | Bone and teeth formation; cell membranes | Meat, poultry, fish, milk |
| Magnesium | Men: 350 mg<br>Women: 280 mg | Bone and teeth formation; muscle function | Whole grains, legumes, dark green vegetables |
| Iron | Men: 10 mg<br>Women: 10-15 mg | Needed to carry oxygen in red blood cells to body tissues | Meat, poultry, fish, dried fruit, legumes, green leafy vegetables, iron-enriched grain products |
| Zinc | Men: 15 mg<br>Women: 12 mg | Immune function; protein metabolism | Meat, poultry, fish |

*For men and women ages 19-51+; women not pregnant or breast-feeding.

## Osteoporosis

You probably know or have heard of an older person who has become permanently disabled or even died prematurely due to complications of a hip fracture. Some fractures are caused by a fall, but in some cases scientists suggest that the hip breaks first, *causing* the fall. Osteoporosis is the disease that causes bones to become so brittle that they break. (For more on osteoporosis, see chapter 8.) Although it is a disease that shows up mostly in older adults, especially older women, osteoporosis actually starts at a much younger age. Throughout your lifetime, your bones are constantly changing. They become stronger and denser when you stress them through exercise. They add and lose calcium all the time. Up until about age 30, you add more calcium than you lose; after 30, you begin to lose more calcium than you add.

What can you do to minimize your risk for developing osteoporosis? Eat at least three servings of calcium-rich dairy products each day. Choose low-fat or nonfat varieties if you're concerned about fat and calories. Calcium-fortified orange juice and some cereals are good choices for people who cannot tolerate milk products. Some people, especially older women, may need to take calcium supplements.

And stay active. Any weight-bearing activity (e.g., walking, running) will help improve bone density and keep your bones healthy throughout your life.

Symptoms of iron deficiency include fatigue, reduced resistance to infection, reduced physical fitness, and reduced learning ability. It may be wise for vegetarians or people who are on weight loss diets to take a multivitamin that contains up to 15 milligrams of iron. But don't take large doses of iron in supplement form, because it can be toxic—even deadly.

### RECOMMENDATIONS FOR GOOD HEALTH

As with vitamins, the best way to ensure adequate mineral intake and avoid mineral toxicity is to eat a well-balanced diet. This is especially important with regard to minerals, because scientists know that many other minerals than those we've discussed here are important for good health but haven't been able to determine specific intake recommendations. Eating a variety of foods that aren't overly processed can help ensure that you don't become mineral deficient (with the added bonus of reducing your sodium intake).

### RECOMMENDATIONS FOR ATHLETIC PERFORMANCE

Some athletes (e.g., gymnasts, dancers, wrestlers) restrict food intake to meet weight or performance standards. Such athletes risk developing nutrient deficiencies. For example, many athletes restrict milk and meat product consumption in trying to attain a certain weight. Excessive restriction for a prolonged time could result in iron deficiency or stress fractures due to weakened bones. Obviously, an athlete's performance would be greatly diminished in either case.

Athletes who perspire heavily lose a lot of sodium through sweat. This is usually not a problem unless an athlete is consciously reducing sodium intake. Don't use salt tablets to compensate for lost sodium. The best advice is to eat a balanced diet but not be overly concerned about sodium intake. Enough sodium is normally provided in the diet.

Eating a balanced diet should ensure that you eat the recommended daily amounts of vitamins and minerals.

## Water

Water is the most abundant component of the human body, and as such is extremely important to health. Water is a component of blood and other fluids; it transports nutrients to cells and carries away waste products. It helps regulate body temperature and acts as a shock absorber in joints and around other tissues and organs (see table 5.7).

The average person loses about 5 1/2 to 11 cups of water per day through sweat, waste, and respiration. Inadequate replacement of this water loss can result in dehydration. Inadequate water balance can come from illnesses that cause vomiting or diarrhea, excessive sweat loss, and inadequate intake. Severe dehydration can lead to serious health complications and even death.

Besides water itself, other good sources of water are fruits, vegetables, and milk.

### RECOMMENDATIONS FOR GOOD HEALTH

Consuming water and other fluids is the best way to ensure adequate intake. Don't rely on coffee or other caffeinated beverages for fluid intake; caffeine causes your body to *lose* water. Also, don't rely on thirst as your only indicator for proper hydration; your body's thirst mechanism often lags behind its needs. Make it a habit to drink plenty of fluids (at least 7 to 11 cups) throughout the day.

### RECOMMENDATIONS FOR ATHLETIC PERFORMANCE

For athletes, the main function of water during activity is to remove heat created by exercise. If water balance is inadequate, performance will suffer; if the inadequate water balance is prolonged, serious heat-related injury can occur. Vigorous exercise tends to

## Table 5.7  Water Needs, Functions, and Sources

|  | Daily dietary recommendations | Primary functions/Action | Major sources |
| --- | --- | --- | --- |
| Water | Depends on total energy expenditure; about 4 to 6 cups per 1,000 calories of energy expenditure | Carries nutrients and wastes; acts as a joint lubricant; maintains body temperature | Water and other beverages, fruits, vegetables, milk |

blunt the body's thirst mechanism, so it is extremely important for athletes to drink on a predetermined schedule. A practical way to prevent dehydration when exercising in hot weather is to weigh yourself before you start exercising and again immediately after you finish. For every pound of weight you lose, drink 2 cups (16 ounces) of water. For example, if you lose 3 pounds, you should drink 6 cups of water within a few hours of finishing your workout.

## Caffeine

Caffeine is not a nutrient, but it is a substance found in commonly consumed foods such as coffee, tea, and chocolate. It is a natural stimulant that causes the heart rate to increase slightly, may elevate blood pressure, and can enhance alertness in some people. Excessive caffeine intake may lead to irritability, nervousness, headaches, diarrhea, and stomach upset. Caffeine is also a diuretic (i.e., it causes fluid loss) and as such can be very detrimental to hydration status, performance, and overall health. Consume caffeine in moderation if at all. Athletes should avoid beverages that contain caffeine prior to and during training and athletic events.

## Alcohol

Alcohol, like caffeine, is not a nutrient. If used in moderation (no more than one or two drinks per day), alcohol doesn't appear to be detrimental to health. In fact, moderate alcohol intake may slightly reduce heart disease risk. However, the possible benefit of moderate alcohol intake is *not* a reason to start drinking if you currently don't drink alcohol.

Like caffeine, alcohol is a diuretic. Consuming alcoholic beverages can be detrimental to athletic training and performance because it can cause excessive fluid losses. Don't consume alcohol both before an event and after an event until your body has been fully rehydrated with water.

## NUTRITION GUIDELINES

Until the last 50 years, nutrition scientists focused mainly on preventing diseases associated with nutrient deficiencies. More recently, the overconsumption of certain dietary components has become a major concern for Americans. On average, our diets have improved since the late 1970s, but as figure 5.1 shows, we haven't reached all of our public nutritional goals.

Since 1980, several federal agencies have provided recommendations for choosing a healthful diet. *Nutrition and Your Health: Dietary Guidelines for Americans* (1995) takes the latest scientific information and transforms it into easily understood recommendations. The most recent recommendations are that we

- eat a variety of foods;
- balance the food we eat with physical activity to attain or maintain a healthy weight;
- eat plenty of grain products, vegetables, and fruits;
- eat a diet that's low in fat, saturated fat, and cholesterol;

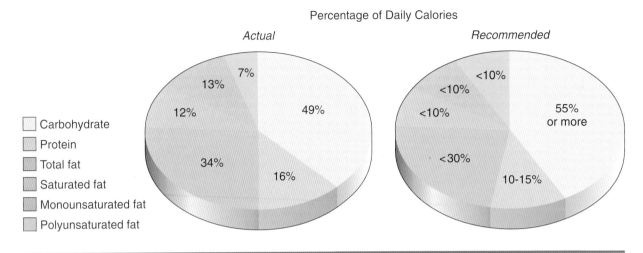

**FIGURE 5.1** Actual versus recommended nutrient intake for persons two months of age and older.

Data for actual percentages is from NHANES III (phase 1), 1988-91.

- eat a diet that's moderate in sugars, salt, and sodium; and
- drink alcohol in moderation if we do drink alcohol.

However, these are general recommendations. The Food Guide Pyramid takes these recommendations a step further.

## Food Guide Pyramid

The Food Guide Pyramid (see figure 5.2) details what we should eat daily. As you look at the pyramid, notice the placement of the various food groups, the number of servings recommended for each food group, and the circles and triangles scattered throughout the groupings. Next we'll explain these three facets of the Food Guide Pyramid.

### Food Groups and Recommended Servings

Your food choices should begin with the foods at the base of the pyramid and at the level just above the base. The foundation for a healthy diet consists of the bread, cereal, rice, and pasta group and the vegetable and fruit groups. These three groups are excellent sources of complex carbohydrates (starches and fiber), vitamins, and minerals. Most of what you eat every day should come from these three groups.

The foundation for a healthy diet lies in the bread, cereal, rice, and pasta group and the vegetable and fruit groups.

The milk, yogurt, and cheese group provides protein, calcium, phosphorus, and other nutrients, but you don't need as much of these foods as you do of the first three groups. The same is true for the meat, poultry, fish, dry beans, eggs, and nuts group, which is a good source of protein, iron, and zinc.

At the tip of the pyramid are fats, oils, and sweets. These aren't considered a group because they don't provide much besides calories. Butter, margarine, soft drinks, sweet desserts, candy, salad dressings, oils, and similar foods are included in this category. As these foods are at the top of the pyramid, they should make up the smallest part of your diet.

The Food Guide Pyramid gives a range for numbers of servings within each group because people have varying energy needs. The more energy you burn, the more servings you need in

# Food Guide Pyramid

A Guide to Daily Food Choices

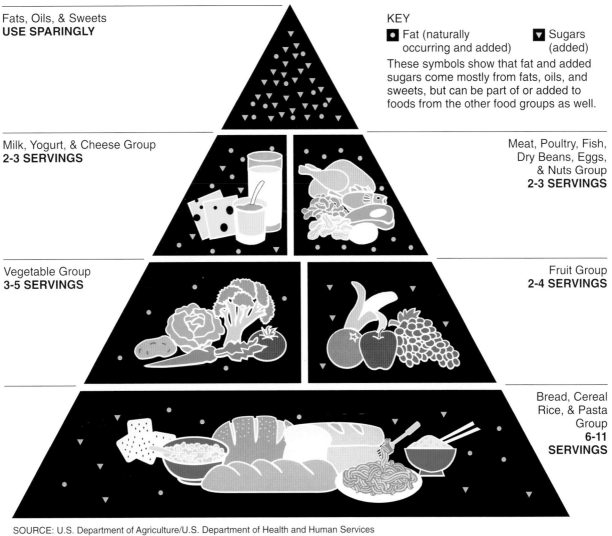

Fats, Oils, & Sweets
**USE SPARINGLY**

KEY
◻ Fat (naturally occurring and added)    ▽ Sugars (added)

These symbols show that fat and added sugars come mostly from fats, oils, and sweets, but can be part of or added to foods from the other food groups as well.

Milk, Yogurt, & Cheese Group
**2-3 SERVINGS**

Meat, Poultry, Fish, Dry Beans, Eggs, & Nuts Group
**2-3 SERVINGS**

Vegetable Group
**3-5 SERVINGS**

Fruit Group
**2-4 SERVINGS**

Bread, Cereal Rice, & Pasta Group
**6-11 SERVINGS**

SOURCE: U.S. Department of Agriculture/U.S. Department of Health and Human Services

**FIGURE 5.2**   The Food Guide Pyramid.

most groups. Table 5.8 shows the appropriate serving numbers for people in various categories.

Many people are surprised by the number of servings recommended—thinking that a serving is the amount they put on their plate. Not so! For example, a 3-cup pile of spaghetti may fit onto a plate, but it counts as *six* servings rather than one. Check out the following list for amounts that are equal to one serving for each food group.

## Food Group Serving Sizes

### Bread, Cereal, Rice, and Pasta Group

- 1 slice of regular bread (2 slices diet bread)
- 1/2 English muffin
- 1/3 to 1/2 bagel

| | Women and some older adults | Children, teen girls, active women, most men | Teen boys and active men |
|---|---|---|---|
| **Table 5.8 Recommended Number of Servings Per Day** | | | |
| Approximate calorie level | 1,600 | 2,200 | 2,800 |
| ***Servings per day*** | | | |
| Bread group | 6 | 9 | 11 |
| Vegetable group | 3 | 4 | 5 |
| Fruit group | 2 | 3 | 4 |
| Milk group | 2-3* | 2-3* | 2-3* |
| Meat group | 2, for a total of 5 ounces | 2, for a total of 6 ounces | 3, for a total of 7 ounces |

*Women who are pregnant or breast-feeding, teenagers, and young adults to age 24 need 3 servings.

- 1/2 cup cooked rice or pasta
- 1/2 cup cooked cereal
- 1 ounce ready-to-eat cereal

**Vegetable Group**

- 1/2 cup chopped raw or cooked vegetables
- 1 cup leafy raw vegetables
- 3/4 cup vegetable juice

**Fruit Group**

- 1 medium-size piece of fruit or melon wedge
- 1/2 cup canned fruit
- 1/4 cup dried fruit
- 3/4 cup fruit juice

**Milk, Yogurt, and Cheese Group**

- 1 cup milk or yogurt
- 1 1/2 to 2 ounces of cheese

**Meat, Poultry, Fish, Dry Beans, Eggs, and Nuts Group**

- 2 1/2 to 3 ounces of cooked lean meat, poultry, or fish (about the size of a deck of playing cards)
- 1 1/2 cups cooked legumes
- 3 eggs
- 6 tablespoons of peanut butter

**Fats, Oils, and Sweets**

- Use sparingly; limit calories from these especially if you need to lose weight.

Here's another example of serving sizes. Say that within the bread group you want to eat nine servings a day. You could reach nine servings by eating

- 2 ounces of cereal and a slice of toast for breakfast (three servings),
- a bagel for a snack (two servings),
- 2 slices of bread from a sandwich for lunch (two servings), and
- 1 cup of rice with stir-fry for dinner (two servings).

See how quickly it adds up?

### Food Guide Symbols ( • ▽ )

As you've noted, the Food Guide Pyramid has two symbols scattered throughout the food groups: circles and triangles. Circles alert you to food groups that may contain fat, either naturally occurring or added; triangles denote food groups that may contain added sugars. As you can see, most of the fat and added sugars are found in the fats, oils, and sweets category. Fat is also found in the milk and meat groups. You can limit fat intake from these two groups by choosing low-fat and nonfat milk products and lean meats, poultry without skin, and fish.

The bread and vegetable groups may have some fat, depending on how the food is prepared.

## ⚪ OF INTEREST

### The "Five-a-Day" Campaign

The "Five-a-Day" campaign was a public health promotion launched in the mid-1990s to encourage people to eat adequate amounts of vegetables and fruits. Through the campaign, people were encouraged to eat at least three servings of vegetables and two servings of fruits per day.

Why the need for such a promotion? Because currently most Americans eat only three and a half servings of vegetables and fruits per day. That may not seem too bad, but over a year that adds up to 548 missed servings of vegetables and fruits! That's a *lot* of missed nutrients. How do *you* compare with the average American in consumption of fruits and vegetables? (The lab at the end of this chapter will give you a chance to determine your current intake of foods from all the groups.)

### HEALTHCHECK

**Can I count canned or frozen fruits and vegetables as part of my Five-a-Day quota?**

Absolutely. Just be sure to choose fruits canned in fruit juice; frozen fruits without added sugar; reduced-sodium canned vegetables; and frozen vegetables without added fat, cheese sauces, or salt.

Croissants, certain crackers, and heavily buttered popcorn are all high-fat foods found in the bread group. Likewise, vegetables cooked in cream or cheese sauces are high in fat. But there are numerous low-fat and nonfat choices in each of these groups. Make most of your choices in these groups low-fat.

As for added sugars, you can find them in almost any food group—in cereals from the bread group; fruits processed with sugar; and yogurt and chocolate milk with sugar added. Although sugar itself isn't associated with any health problems (besides dental cavities), it is a source of extra calories with little nutritional value.

Again, the Food Guide Pyramid is a simple way to help you make wise food choices. Use the pyramid to plan meals. If you're lacking in a food group, include foods from that group in your next meal or snack.

## Nutrition Labels

They say you can't judge a book by its cover—but you can learn a lot about food before you open the can or package. And you can trust the label contents description because all food manufacturers now must follow the same labeling rules.

Take a look at the label in figure 5.3. Nearly all foods carry this or a similar label. The "Nutrition Facts" give the nutrient contents of a single serving of the food.

Food manufacturers know that many health-conscious Americans are swayed by nutrition claims on packages—"fat-free," "cholesterol-free," "low in sodium," and so on. Can you believe these claims? Yes. Such claims can be made only when the food meets specific criteria set by the Food and Drug Administration, as described in the following list.

- **Free (none)**
  - **Fat-free (nonfat):** Fewer than 0.5 grams of fat per serving.
  - **Calorie-free:** Fewer than 5 calories per serving.
  - **Sugar-free:** Fewer than 0.5 grams of sugar per serving.
  - **Cholesterol-free:** Fewer than 2 milligrams of cholesterol and 2 grams (or less) of saturated fat per serving.

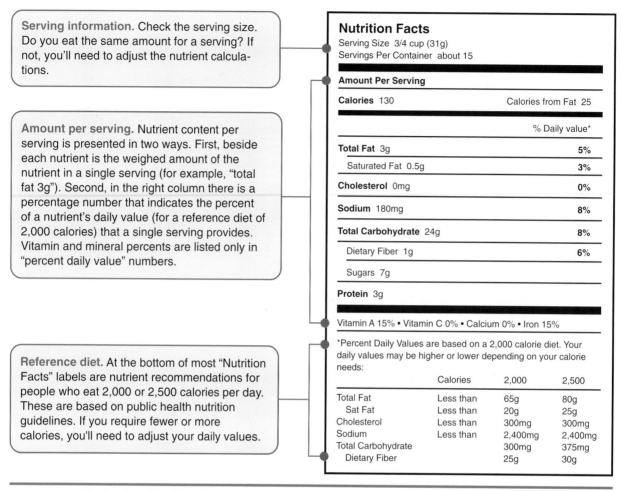

Serving information. Check the serving size. Do you eat the same amount for a serving? If not, you'll need to adjust the nutrient calculations.

Amount per serving. Nutrient content per serving is presented in two ways. First, beside each nutrient is the weighed amount of the nutrient in a single serving (for example, "total fat 3g"). Second, in the right column there is a percentage number that indicates the percent of a nutrient's daily value (for a reference diet of 2,000 calories) that a single serving provides. Vitamin and mineral percents are listed only in "percent daily value" numbers.

Reference diet. At the bottom of most "Nutrition Facts" labels are nutrient recommendations for people who eat 2,000 or 2,500 calories per day. These are based on public health nutrition guidelines. If you require fewer or more calories, you'll need to adjust your daily values.

**Nutrition Facts**

Serving Size  3/4 cup (31g)
Servings Per Container  about 15

**Amount Per Serving**

| Calories  130 | Calories from Fat  25 |
|---|---|

| | % Daily value* |
|---|---|
| **Total Fat**  3g | 5% |
| Saturated Fat  0.5g | 3% |
| **Cholesterol**  0mg | 0% |
| **Sodium**  180mg | 8% |
| **Total Carbohydrate**  24g | 8% |
| Dietary Fiber  1g | 6% |
| Sugars  7g | |
| **Protein**  3g | |

Vitamin A 15% • Vitamin C 0% • Calcium 0% • Iron 15%

*Percent Daily Values are based on a 2,000 calorie diet. Your daily values may be higher or lower depending on your calorie needs:

| | | Calories | 2,000 | 2,500 |
|---|---|---|---|---|
| Total Fat | Less than | | 65g | 80g |
| Sat Fat | Less than | | 20g | 25g |
| Cholesterol | Less than | | 300mg | 300mg |
| Sodium | Less than | | 2,400mg | 2,400mg |
| Total Carbohydrate | | | 300mg | 375mg |
| Dietary Fiber | | | 25g | 30g |

**FIGURE 5.3**  A typical "Nutrition Facts" label.

- **Sodium-free:** Fewer than 5 milligrams of sodium per serving.
- Low
  - **Low-fat:** 3 grams of fat (or less) per serving.
  - **Low-calorie:** Fewer than 40 calories per serving.
  - **Low cholesterol:** Fewer than 20 milligrams of cholesterol and 2 grams (or less) of saturated fat per serving.
  - **Low sodium:** Fewer than 40 milligrams per serving.
- **Reduced or less:** When compared to the higher-fat (-calorie, -sodium, etc.) version, at least 25% less fat (calories, sodium, etc.) per serving.
- **Light (or lite):** If a food normally derives 50% or more of its calories from fat, it can be labeled light or lite if it is reduced in fat by 50%. If a food derives less than 50% of its calories from fat, the food must be reduced in fat by at least 50% or reduced in calories by at least 1/3.
- **Lean (meat, fish, poultry):** Fewer than 10 grams of fat, 4 grams of saturated fat, and 95 milligrams of cholesterol per serving.
- **Extra lean:** Fewer than 5 grams of fat, 2 grams of saturated fat, and 95 milligrams of cholesterol per serving.
- **High or good source:** High is 20% or more of the daily reference value (DRV); good is 10% to 19%. For example, to be high in fiber, a cereal must have 5 grams because the DRV is 25 grams.
- **Fresh:** Food labeled fresh must be in its raw state, having not been frozen or subjected to

## A Tale of Two Potatoes

Want to know how a low-fat food such as a potato can turn into a source of high calories, fat, and cholesterol? It's all in the preparation.

Here's what you get from one medium potato, baked with 2 tablespoons of chives and 3 tablespoons of salsa:

Calories: 247
Fat: 0.2 grams
Saturated fat: 0.0 grams
Cholesterol: 0 grams

Now take a similar potato, and apply 1 tablespoon of butter, 2 tablespoons of sour cream, and 2 tablespoons of bacon bits. Here's what you get:

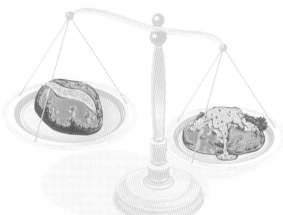

Calories: 434
Fat: 20.6 grams
Saturated fat: 10.8 grams
Cholesterol: 38 grams

No wonder they're called "stuffed" potatoes!

other forms of processing. Fresh does not apply to processed food such as fresh milk or bread.

So how do you make nutrition labels work for you? Here are five tips.

1. Make a habit of reading nutrition labels. Compare similar products to help you make the best choices.

2. Use labels to help you track your nutrient intake. Just how many calories or grams of fat do you eat in a day? One way to find out is to log what you eat, using the nutrition labels to keep track of various nutrient totals. You'll see how this works in the lab for this chapter.

3. Choose foods that have low percentage daily values for fat, saturated fat, cholesterol, and sodium. Shoot for a daily value sum of less than 100% in these areas.

4. Accumulate 100% of the daily value for vitamins, minerals, fiber, and carbohydrates.

5. Be wary of health claims on supplements. The federal government doesn't regulate manufacturers of nutrient supplements such as protein powders, vitamin and mineral pills, and herbal remedies as well as it does food manufacturers.

## Vegetarianism

Vegetarians derive most of their nutrition from plant foods. There are many types of vegetarian diets; most can be quite healthy if the diet is planned carefully enough. Because vegetarians consume less fat and cholesterol than non-vegetarians, they are less likely to develop coronary heart disease. Here's a brief look at different types of vegetarians, with potential dietary concerns noted:

- **Semi-vegetarian:** Includes some, but not all, animal products (e.g., avoids red meats but eats fish).
- **Lacto-ovo vegetarian:** Excludes all meat and flesh foods but eats milk products (lacto) and eggs (ovo). Must make sure iron intake is adequate.
- **Lacto vegetarian:** Excludes all meat, flesh foods, and eggs; eats milk products. Must watch iron and zinc intake to ensure adequate amounts.
- **Vegan:** Excludes all animal foods; eats only grains, legumes, fruits, vegetables, and their derivatives. Not recommended for pregnant women, infants, and children because of the difficulty in consuming enough calories and enough vitamin B-12, calcium, zinc, and iron.

 Most vegetarian diets can be quite healthy if adequate care is taken. Because vegetarians consume less fat and cholesterol than nonvegetarians, they are less likely to develop coronary heart disease.

## NUTRITION TIPS

We've provided information on basic nutritional needs, food groups, and recommended servings within those food groups; now we want to give some tips that help put that information into context for you. That is, how do you use that information to help you choose healthy meals and snacks and make nutritious selections in fast-food restaurants?

### Eating Healthy Meals and Snacks

Eating well while living the typical harried life of a college student probably won't happen unless you *plan* for it to happen! Here we'll provide tips to help you develop healthy meal patterns with these goals in mind:

- Reduce fat intake and increase intake of whole grains, fruits, and vegetables.
- Aim for balance and variety in food choices.
- Make food preparation easy even for the "kitchen-challenged."
- Keep the pleasure in eating.

### Maximizing Nutrients When Cooking

Cooking foods for a long time at high temperatures can destroy some nutrients. What are some other ways that you can preserve as many nutrients as possible when preparing food?

▮ Thoroughly clean but leave the edible skins on fruits and vegetables such as apples, carrots, pears, peaches, and potatoes.

▮ Use very little water when cooking vegetables. Better yet, place the vegetables in a microwave bowl and add 1 to 2 tablespoons of water. Cover with plastic wrap and zap for 2 to 4 minutes (depending on amount and type of vegetable).

▮ Drink the liquid that is left after cooking vegetables, or save it to use as a base for a hearty soup.

▮ Cook vegetables only until they are tender but still crisp.

▮ Cut vegetables that have longer cooking times (e.g., beets, turnips, and carrots) into large pieces. This will help retain more of the nutrients in the interior of the food.

### Breakfast Tips

Breakfast is a great time to get a good start on foods from the bread, fruit, and milk groups.

- **Eat breakfast every day.** It gives your body a needed energy boost.
- **Prepare what you can the night before.** "I don't have time" is the excuse given by most who skip breakfast. Cut up fruit, pour juice (but keep it in the fridge!), and get out cereal boxes before you go to bed.
- **Choose a high-fiber cereal.** This means at least 5 grams of fiber per serving. This is a good way to get a jump on your fiber intake for the day.
- **Be nontraditional.** You don't have to eat cereal every morning. Leftover low-fat pizza or a sandwich is a quick and easy way to "break your fast."
- **Put your blender to work.** Toss in low-fat vanilla yogurt, strawberries, and bananas or other fruit and let it fly! In less than 15 seconds you have a frothy, healthful meal you can eat on the run.
- **Try to get at least one serving of fruit at breakfast.** A 6-ounce glass of orange juice (3/4 cup) is all it takes. Use the calcium-fortified varieties for an added nutritional boost.
- **Add 1/4 cup of dried fruit to your hot or cold cereal.** Use raisins, apricots, peaches, or figs to add flavor and get in one fruit serving.
- **Try jam or jelly instead of butter or margarine on your toast.** You won't even miss the fat!

- **Drink at least one 8-ounce cup of 1% or skim milk.** As table 5.9 shows, 2% milk is hardly low-fat! By changing from a daily 8-ounce glass of 2% milk to 1%, you'll save 764 grams of fat and 6,916 calories in just one year!
- **Partake in a parfait.** Alternate layers of cut-up fruit with low-fat vanilla yogurt and eat with toast, a bagel, or a muffin for a healthy breakfast.

### Lunch Tips

Lunch is your chance to boost your servings of all food groups.

- **Take your lunch with you if you can.** That way you control the amount of fat and calories. Use insulated containers to keep hot things hot and cold things cold.
- **Pack your lunch the night before.** Use leftovers from dinner. Or grab a healthful frozen dinner and canned or fresh fruit.
- **Pack in the vegetables.** Whether you take your lunch or eat out, use lunch as a chance to "veg out." Pack cut-up vegetables and low-fat salad dressing for dipping. Order steamed veggie plates and dark green salads when eating out.
- **Use a microwave.** Zap a low-fat frozen entree in the microwave. Add a few crackers and a container of low-fat yogurt and you have a balanced—and quick—meal.
- **Make wise selections at salad and baked potato bars.** You can do a lot of fat and calorie damage with the dressings, mayonnaise-based salads, cheeses, sour cream, and bacon

| Table 5.9  Dairy Decisions | | | | |
|---|---|---|---|---|
| One cup (8 oz) | Calories | Total fat (g) | Saturated fat | Cholesterol (mg) |
| Whole milk | 150 | 8.2 | 5.1 | 33 |
| 2% milk | 121 | 4.7 | 2.9 | 18 |
| 1% milk | 102 | 2.6 | 1.6 | 10 |
| Skim milk | 86 | 0.4 | 0.3 | 4 |

that are often available. Stick with the fresh veggies and fruits. Use potato toppers such as salsa, cottage cheese, lemon juice, and chives.

- **Have another 8-ounce cup of 1% or skim milk or have a low-fat yogurt.**
- **Choose sandwiches made with lean meats.** Limit the amount of meat to 2 or 3 ounces.

### Dinner Tips

With dinner, you can balance out your food intake for the day.

- **Take a mental diet inventory.** How many bread servings, milk servings, fruit servings, and so on have you already eaten for the day? What are you missing? Plan your dinner around the food groups that you have yet to complete.

- **Use pre-cut frozen vegetables as the basis for a quick, nutritious stir-fry.** Add a little lean meat or poultry. If you buy a premade stir-fry kit, watch out—some have seasoning packets that are very high in fat and sodium. Read the labels to find the best choices.
- **Share the dinner preparation chores.** Invite friends over for healthy potluck dinners. Or rotate dinner preparation with roommates or friends who live nearby.
- **Make several dinners on the weekends and refrigerate or freeze them for use later in the week.** Check out low-fat cookbooks to gather recipe ideas.
- **Use "quick and easy" produce to boost your fruit and vegetable intake.** Prepackaged salads, peeled baby carrots, presliced vegetables, and frozen vegetables and fruit are all great time-savers.

### The Scoop on Pesticides

Many people worry about residues from chemical pesticides that may remain on the products they eat. Pesticides are used to keep insects, weeds, molds, and fungi from damaging or destroying crops, both while they're growing and during storage after harvest. The pesticides are necessary for maximizing crop yields, thereby keeping food prices low. But how much of that chemical can trickle down to you?

The residues left on food crops vary depending on many factors, including the plant, time of year, and soil conditions; however, it is likely that most plant crops will have some minuscule amount of residue. Federal and state governments monitor and regulate pesticide use and safety very closely, and it is our opinion that the health benefits of eating a variety of fruits and vegetables far outweigh any risks that pesticide residues may impose.

To minimize any residues that may remain on food you purchase,

- pick produce that is fresh with skin intact (no cuts, holes, or scrapes) and free of mold,
- wash the food thoroughly, and
- remove outer leaves of leafy vegetables.

By the way, the wax you may feel on apples and cucumbers is safe to eat. Simply wash the outside thoroughly using a vegetable brush.

• **Make dessert count.** This is a great time to get in an extra serving of fruit. Choose what is in season or eat frozen fruit without added sugar.

• **Minimize clean-up by creating one-pot meals.** Lightly saute lots of vegetables, add beaten eggs and extra egg whites, and stir until egg is thoroughly cooked. Have toast and skim milk, and have fruit for dessert. Or boil pasta, toss a bunch of frozen vegetables in for last few minutes, drain, and put the pasta and vegetables in a pot; add your favorite low-fat spaghetti sauce.

• **Max out on your veggies.** If you haven't eaten vegetables all day, now is your chance to catch up by eating a double or triple serving.

• **Drink another glass of 1% or skim milk.** Remember, it takes three 8-ounce cups of skim milk or yogurt to get you close to the minimum daily calcium recommendations.

### Snack Tips

Snack time is often "high-fat" time for many people who head to the nearest vending machine or convenience store when they get the midmorning or midafternoon munchies. Here are some tips for healthful snacking.

• **Carry a bag of dried fruit with you.** Dried apples, apricots, or prunes are sweet and full of lots of great nutrients.

• **Drink a can of fruit or tomato juice.** You'll get many more nutrients and usually fewer calories than from a can of soda.

• **Enjoy low-fat versions of popcorn.** Choose one that has less than 2 grams of fat per 3-cup serving. Cut the calories by sharing a bag with a friend.

• **Boost your calcium intake with a glass of 1% or skim milk or a serving of low-fat yogurt.**

• **Snack on frozen fruit.** Try freezing bananas (peeled), grapes, strawberries, and other berries. They make for great snacks in the summertime or any time you're looking for a sweet treat.

• **Look for low-fat cookies and crackers.** They're simple to carry and satisfying to the taste buds.

---

**HEALTHCHECK**

**I often need a quick "pick-me-up" snack in the afternoon on my way to my workout. Is a candy bar a good choice?**

Not unless you don't mind a letdown shortly after your "pick-up." As large quantities of sugar enter the blood, the increase in glucose levels stimulates the release of the hormone insulin. This helps the blood glucose levels return to normal. This drop in blood sugar levels may leave you feeling fatigued. A better snack would be two slices of whole wheat bread and an ounce of mozzarella cheese. This will provide B vitamins, fiber, and carbohydrates (in the bread), as well as calcium and protein (in the cheese)—and the cheese will help slow the release of insulin so that you don't experience drastic fluctuations in your blood sugar levels.

---

## Eating Well While Eating Out

Is eating out doing your diet in? Many fast-food items are high in calories, fat, and sodium (see the table starting on page 154 for a sampling of items at popular fast-food restaurants). If you find yourself eating out often, your calorie, fat, and sodium intakes will likely soar, no matter how diligently you watch them when you eat at home. But you can take measures to make sure you keep your intakes in these areas at reasonable levels even when you eat out. Here's how:

• **Have it your way.** Ask for salad dressings, sauces, and gravies on the side. That way you control the amounts you eat.

• **Make it plain and simple.** Skip the specialty burgers. Choose the regular hamburger, roast beef, or grilled chicken sandwich.

- **Read the fine print.** Find out how menu items are prepared. Choose foods that are broiled, grilled, baked, poached, or steamed. Try to avoid items described with terms such as "creamed," "au gratin," "in a cheese sauce," "fried," "sauteed," or "crispy." They're indicators of high-fat foods.
- **Milk it for all it's worth.** Request 1% or skim milk. You may be surprised at how many restaurants (even fast-food restaurants) serve low-fat milk.

- **Don't pass up pizza.** Just order it with lots of veggies. If you must have meat on your pizza, try Canadian bacon instead of pepperoni—it's lower in fat.
- **For breakfast, choose pancakes or cold cereal.** Omelettes, biscuit sandwiches, and croissants are loaded with fat.

You can eat healthful meals when you eat out by watching your calorie, fat, and sodium intakes.

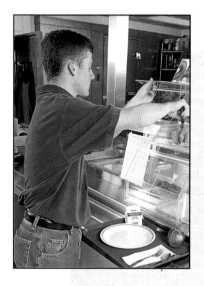

# Health Concepts

As you'll remember from the beginning of the chapter, Mike wondered just *what* a balanced diet consisted of—and if eating a balanced diet was possible while living the life of a busy college student. A balanced diet consists of about 55% to 60% of nutrition through carbohydrates, 10% to 15% through protein, and 25% to 30% through fat. You can attain a balanced diet—even on campus!—by eating a variety of foods, by including plenty of grain products, vegetables, and fruits, and by eating a diet that's low in fat, saturated fat, and cholesterol.

## SUMMARY

▌ Our bodies are fueled by six types of nutrients: carbohydrates, proteins, fats, vitamins, minerals, and water. Only carbohydrates, proteins, and fats provide calories. Carbohydrates provide energy for the body. It is recommended for most people that about 55% of their diet come from carbohydrates; some sport nutritionists recommend that athletes get 60% to 70% of their calories from carbohydrates.

▌ Protein is important for many body tissues, including muscle, skin, internal organs, bones and teeth, and connective tissue. Proteins are made of building blocks called amino acids. The body needs 20 different amino acids; it produces 11 on its own but must gain the other 9 from foods. Most Americans eat more protein than they need.

▌ Americans also eat more fat than they need. A certain amount of fat is important to the body, but fat intake should be limited to 30% of total daily caloric intake—and most of that intake should come from *unsaturated fats* rather than *saturated fats.*

▌ By eating a balanced diet, you can attain the recommended daily amounts of vitamins and minerals. The Food Guide Pyramid provides recommendations for servings from these food groups: breads, vegetables, fruits, milk, and meat.

▌ If you find yourself eating out often, your calorie, fat, and sodium intakes will likely soar, no matter how diligently you watch them when you eat at home. But you can take measures to make sure you keep your intakes in these areas at reasonable levels even when you eat out.

*In this chapter you learned the basics of sound nutrition and the ways in which nutrition affects physical activity. In the next chapter we'll look at the keys to weight control. We'll also give you some guidelines to help you determine a weight that's good for you and some strategies to help you get and stay there.*

## KEY TERMS

| | |
|---|---|
| carbohydrates | minerals |
| cholesterol | protein |
| complementing proteins | recommended daily allowance |
| complex carbohydrates | saturated fats |
| essential amino acids | simple carbohydrates |
| fat-soluble vitamins | soluble fiber |
| fats | unsaturated fats |
| insoluble fiber | vitamins |
| kilocalories | water-soluble vitamins |

**5**

# Determining Nutrient Intake

## THE PURPOSES OF THIS LAB EXPERIENCE ARE TO

▌ determine your intake for several important nutrients,

▌ determine the number of servings you currently eat from each of the food groups, and

▌ identify areas of your diet that you can improve.

## Determine Your Nutrient Intake

One of the best ways to assess your nutrient intake is to keep a daily food diary. Use the Food Diary Form to help you track your intake. You might want to photocopy the page so you can record your diet for several days.

Use food labels, the tables at the end of this lab, and other food reference books to identify the nutrient content for each food. List calorie, carbohydrate, protein, and fat amounts on the form. There is an extra column for a nutrient that may be of particular interest to you (e.g., iron or vitamin C). Total the numbers at the end of each day.

### Tips for Keeping a Food Diary

• It's best to pick a day that's typical in terms of what you eat. Don't change your diet just because you're recording it.

• Write down everything you eat and drink for the entire day. Record your intake immediately so you don't forget things.

• Describe everything in detail—remember the mayonnaise on sandwiches and the dressings on salads!

• Be accurate on portions. If possible, weigh and measure your foods.

Which foods contributed the most carbohydrate grams?

_____

Which foods contributed the most protein grams?

_____

Which foods contributed the most fat grams?

_____

## Judging Dietary Quality

Now calculate the proportions of your diet that come from carbohydrate, protein, and fat.

   **Carbohydrate:** Multiply your total carbohydrate grams by 4. Divide by your total calories.

   **Protein:** Multiply your total protein grams by 4. Divide by your total calories.

   **Fat:** Multiply your total fat grams by 9. Divide by your total calories.

   How do your carbohydrate, protein, and fat intakes compare to the daily recommended values in tables 5.1, 5.3, and 5.4?

---

### Legend for Nutrient Values of Common Foods

| | | |
|---|---|---|
| E | = | energy |
| P | = | protein |
| C | = | carbohydrate |
| DF | = | dietary fiber |
| CH | = | cholesterol |
| CA | = | calcium |
| I | = | iron |
| S | = | sodium |
| kcal | = | kilocalories |
| g | = | grams |
| mg | = | milligrams |
| t | = | trace amounts |

| Food Diary Form | | | | | | |
|---|---|---|---|---|---|---|
| **Food description** | **Amount consumed** | **Calories** | **Carbohydrate (grams)** | **Protein (grams)** | **Fat (grams)** | **Other** |
| *Example:* 1% milk | 1 cup | 102 | 12.0 | 8.0 | 3.0 | |
| | | | | | | |
| | | | | | | |
| | | | | | | |
| | | | | | | |
| | | | | | | |
| | | | | | | |
| | | | | | | |
| | | | | | | |
| | | | | | | |
| | | | | | | |
| | | | | | | |
| | | | | | | |
| | | | | | | |
| | | | | | | |
| | | | | | | |
| | | | | | | |
| | | | | | | |
| | | | | | | |
| **TOTAL** | | | | | | |

**Assess Your Food Group Servings**

Review the food group serving sizes on page 129. Go back through your food diary and count the number of servings for each food group. Use the space below to keep track of your count.

Bread group          _____

Vegetable group    _____

Fruit group            _____

Milk group            _____

Meat group           _____

How often did you eat foods in the fats, oils, and sweets category?

_____

Compare your food group results with the numbers in table 5.8. Would you say that your food group intake is in line with the Food Guide Pyramid recommendations?

## Identify Dietary Improvement Areas

Review your

- food diary;
- percentages of calories from carbohydrate, protein, and fat; and
- food group balance.

How would you rate your diet?

— Excellent
— Good
— Fair
— Poor
— Very poor

In the space below, list strategies you can use at each meal that will help you improve your diet.

**Breakfast**

**Lunch**

**Dinner**

**Snacks**

## Nutrient Values of Common Foods

| | Measure | E (kcal) | P (g) | C (g) | DF (g) | Fat Total | Fat Sat | Mono | CH (mg) | CA (mg) | I (mg) | S (mg) |
|---|---|---|---|---|---|---|---|---|---|---|---|---|
| **Beverages** | | | | | | | | | | | | |
| Beer | | | | | | | | | | | | |
|   Regular (12 fl oz) | 1 1/2 c | 146 | 1 | 13 | 3 | 0 | 0 | 0 | 0 | 18 | .11 | 18 |
|   Light (12 fl oz) | 1 1/2 c | 99 | 1 | 5 | 1 | 0 | 0 | 0 | 0 | 18 | .14 | 11 |
| Gin, rum, vodka, whiskey (80 proof) | 1 1/2 fl oz | 97 | 0 | 0 | 0 | 0 | 0 | 0 | 0 | 0 | .02 | <1 |
| Wine | | | | | | | | | | | | |
|   Red | 3 1/2 fl oz | 74 | <1 | 2 | 0 | 0 | 0 | 0 | 0 | 8 | .44 | 5 |
|   White | 3 1/2 fl oz | 70 | <1 | 1 | 0 | 0 | 0 | 0 | 0 | 9 | .33 | 5 |
| Carbonated | | | | | | | | | | | | |
|   Cola beverage (12 fl oz) | 1/2 c | 152 | 0 | 38 | 0 | <1 | .02 | .03 | 0 | 11 | .11 | 15 |
|   Diet cola w/aspartame (12 fl oz) | 1/2 c | 4 | <1 | <1 | 0 | 0 | 0 | 0 | 0 | 14 | .11 | 21 |
| Coffee, brewed | 1 c | 5 | <1 | 1 | 0 | <1 | 0 | 0 | 0 | 5 | .12 | 5 |
| Gatorade | 1 c | 60 | 0 | 15 | 0 | 0 | 0 | 0 | 0 | 0 | .12 | 96 |
| Tea | | | | | | | | | | | | |
|   Brewed, regular | 1 c | 2 | 0 | 1 | 0 | <1 | 0 | 0 | 0 | 0 | .05 | 7 |
|   From instant, sweetened | 1 c | 89 | <1 | 22 | 0 | <1 | t | 0 | 0 | 5 | .05 | 8 |
| **Dairy** | | | | | | | | | | | | |
| Cheese, natural | | | | | | | | | | | | |
|   Cheddar | 1 oz | 114 | 7 | <1 | 0 | 9 | 6 | 2.7 | 30 | 204 | .19 | 176 |
|   Cottage: small curd, low fat 2% | 1 c | 203 | 31 | 8 | 0 | 4 | 2.8 | 1.2 | 19 | 155 | .36 | 918 |
|   Cream | 1 oz | 99 | 2 | 1 | 0 | 10 | 6.2 | 2.8 | 31 | 23 | .34 | 84 |
|   Cream, low fat | 1 oz | 65 | 3 | 2 | 0 | 5 | 3.1 | 1.4 | 16 | 32 | .48 | 84 |
|   Feta | 1 oz | 75 | 4 | 1 | 0 | 6 | 4.2 | 1.3 | 25 | 140 | .18 | 316 |
| Mozzarella, part-skim milk, low moisture | 1 oz | 79 | 8 | 1 | 0 | 5 | 3.1 | 1.4 | 15 | 207 | .07 | 149 |
| Swiss | 1 oz | 106 | 8 | 1 | 0 | 8 | 5 | 2.1 | 26 | 272 | .05 | 74 |
| Pasteurized, processed American | 1 oz | 106 | 6 | <1 | 0 | 9 | 5.6 | 2.5 | 27 | 174 | .11 | 405 |
| Half & half (cream & milk) | 1 tbs | 19 | <1 | 1 | 0 | 2 | 1.1 | .5 | 6 | 16 | .01 | 6 |
| Cream, sour, cultured | 1 tbs | 30 | <1 | 1 | 0 | 3 | 1.8 | .8 | 6 | 16 | .01 | 7 |
| Milk, fluid | | | | | | | | | | | | |
|   Whole | 1 c | 150 | 8 | 11 | 0 | 8 | 5.1 | 2.3 | 33 | 290 | .12 | 120 |
|   2% low-fat | 1 c | 121 | 8 | 12 | 0 | 5 | 2.9 | 1.3 | 18 | 298 | .12 | 122 |
|   1% low-fat | 1 c | 102 | 8 | 12 | — | 3 | 1.6 | .8 | 10 | 300 | .12 | 123 |
|   Nonfat, vitamin A added | 1 c | 86 | 8 | 12 | 0 | <1 | .3 | .1 | 4 | 301 | .1 | 126 |
| Ice cream, vanilla (about 10% fat) | | | | | | | | | | | | |
|   Hardened, 1/2 gallon | 1 c | 267 | 5 | 31 | <1 | 15 | 9 | 4.2 | 59 | 170 | .12 | 106 |
|   Soft serve | 1 c | 372 | 7 | 38 | <1 | 22 | 12.9 | 6 | 157 | 227 | .36 | 106 |
| Chocolate pudding (5 oz can, .55 c) | 1 ea | 189 | 4 | 32 | 1 | 6 | 1 | 2.4 | 4 | 128 | .72 | 183 |
| Vanilla pudding, instant | 1/2 c | 148 | 4 | 26 | <1 | 4 | 2.3 | 1.1 | 14 | 131 | .09 | 372 |
| Yogurt, frozen, low-fat | 1 c | 276 | 6 | 42 | 0 | 10 | 6 | 2.8 | 4 | 248 | .52 | 152 |
| **Eggs** | | | | | | | | | | | | |
| Whole, w/o shell (raw, large) | 1 ea | 74 | 6 | 1 | 0 | 5 | 1.5 | 1.9 | 213 | 25 | .72 | 63 |
| White (raw, large) | 1 ea | 17 | 4 | <1 | 0 | 0 | 0 | 0 | 0 | 2 | .01 | 54 |
| Egg Beaters, Fleischmann's | 1/4 c | 30 | 6 | 1 | 0 | 0 | 0 | 0 | 0 | 40 | 1.08 | 100 |

*(continued)*

5

(continued)

| | Measure | E (kcal) | P (g) | C (g) | DF (g) | Fat (g) Total | Sat | Mono | CH (mg) | CA (mg) | I (mg) | S (mg) |
|---|---|---|---|---|---|---|---|---|---|---|---|---|
| **Fats and Oils** | | | | | | | | | | | | |
| Butter: stick | 1 tbs | 100 | <1 | <1 | 0 | 11 | 7.1 | 3.4 | 31 | 3 | .02 | 117 |
| Margarine: regular, soft (about 80% fat) | 1 tbs | 100 | <1 | <1 | 0 | 11 | 1.9 | 5.1 | 0 | 4 | 0 | 103 |
| Oils | | | | | | | | | | | | |
| Canola | 1 tbs | 124 | 0 | 0 | 0 | 14 | 1 | 8.2 | 0 | 0 | 0 | 0 |
| Corn | 1 tbs | 124 | 0 | 0 | 0 | 14 | 1.8 | 3.4 | 0 | 0 | 0 | 0 |
| Olive | 1 tbs | 124 | 0 | 0 | 0 | 14 | 1.9 | 10.3 | 0 | <1 | .05 | <1 |
| Salad dressings/sandwich spreads | | | | | | | | | | | | |
| French, regular | 1 tbs | 69 | <1 | 3 | <1 | 9 | 1.5 | 1.2 | 9 | 2 | .06 | 219 |
| French, low calorie | 1 tbs | 21 | <1 | 3 | <1 | 1 | .1 | .2 | 1 | 2 | .06 | 126 |
| Italian, regular | 1 tbs | 70 | <1 | 1 | <1 | 9 | 1 | 1.6 | 0 | 2 | .03 | 118 |
| Italian, low calorie | 1 tbs | 16 | <1 | 1 | <1 | 1 | .2 | .3 | 1 | <1 | .03 | 118 |
| Mayonnaise | | | | | | | | | | | | |
| Regular (soybean) | 1 tbs | 100 | <1 | <1 | 0 | 11 | 1.6 | 3.1 | 8 | 3 | .07 | 80 |
| Regular, low calorie | 1 tbs | 37 | <1 | 3 | 0 | 3 | .5 | .7 | 4 | <1 | 0 | 80 |
| Ranch, regular | 1/2 c | 436 | 4 | 6 | 0 | 45 | 6.7 | 19.4 | 47 | 119 | .31 | 522 |
| Ranch, low calorie | 1 tbs | 32 | 0 | 1 | 0 | 3 | .5 | — | 5 | 11 | 0 | 150 |
| Vinegar & oil | 1 tbs | 72 | 0 | <1 | 0 | 8 | 1.5 | 2.4 | 0 | 0 | 0 | <1 |
| **Fruits and Fruit Juices** | | | | | | | | | | | | |
| Apples: fresh, raw, w/peel, 2 3/4" diam (about 3 per lb w/cores) | 1 ea | 81 | <1 | 21 | 3 | <1 | .1 | t | 0 | 10 | .25 | 0 |
| Apple juice, bottled or canned | 1 c | 116 | <1 | 29 | <1 | <1 | <1 | t | 0 | 17 | .92 | 7 |
| Bananas, raw, w/o peel: whole, 8 3/4" long (175g w/peel) | 1 ea | 104 | 1 | 27 | 2 | 1 | .2 | t | 0 | 7 | .35 | 1 |
| Grapefruit: pink/red, half fruit | 1 ea | 37 | 1 | 9 | 2 | <1 | t | t | 0 | 13 | .15 | 0 |
| Grapes: Thompson seedless, raw | 10 ea | 35 | <1 | 9 | <1 | <1 | .1 | t | 0 | 6 | .13 | 1 |
| Kiwi fruit, raw, peeled (88g w/peel) | 1 ea | 46 | 1 | 11 | 1 | <1 | t | .1 | 0 | 20 | .31 | 4 |
| Cantaloupe, 5" diam (2 1/3 lb whole w/refuse), orange flesh | 1/2 ea | 93 | 2 | 22 | 2 | 1 | .1 | .1 | 0 | 29 | .56 | 24 |
| Oranges, raw: whole w/o peel & seeds, 2 5/8" diam (180 g w/peel & seeds) | 1 ea | 62 | 1 | 15 | 3 | <1 | t | t | 0 | 52 | .13 | 0 |
| Orange juice: fresh, all varieties | 1 c | 112 | 2 | 26 | <1 | <1 | t | .1 | 0 | 27 | .5 | 2 |
| Orange juice frozen concentrate: diluted w/3 parts water by volume | 1 c | 112 | 2 | 27 | <1 | <1 | t | t | 0 | 22 | .25 | 3 |
| Peaches: raw, whole, 2 1/2" diam, peeled, pitted (about 4 per lb whole) | 1 ea | 37 | 1 | 10 | 2 | <1 | t | t | 0 | 4 | .1 | 0 |
| Pears: fresh, w/skin, cored: Bosc, 2 1/5" diam (about 3 per lb) | 1 ea | 83 | 1 | 21 | 3 | 1 | t | .1 | 0 | 16 | .35 | 0 |
| Pineapple: fresh chunks, diced | 1 c | 76 | 1 | 19 | 2 | 1 | t | .1 | 0 | 11 | .57 | 2 |
| Raisins, seedless | 1 c | 435 | 5 | 115 | 5 | 1 | .2 | t | 0 | 71 | 3.02 | 17 |
| Strawberries: fresh, whole, capped | 1 c | 45 | 1 | 10 | 2 | 1 | t | .1 | 0 | 21 | .57 | 1 |
| Watermelon: raw, w/o rind & seeds, diced | 1 c | 51 | 1 | 11 | 1 | 1 | .2 | .1 | 0 | 13 | .27 | 3 |
| **Baked Goods: Breads, Cakes, Cookies, Crackers, Pies** | | | | | | | | | | | | |
| Bagels, plain, enriched, 3 1/2" diam | 1 ea | 187 | 7 | 36 | 2 | 1 | .1 | .1 | 0 | 50 | 2.43 | 363 |
| Biscuits from refrigerated dough | 1 ea | 75 | 1 | 9 | <1 | 4 | .2 | 1 | 1 | 24 | .44 | 158 |

| | | | | | | | | | | | | |
|---|---|---|---|---|---|---|---|---|---|---|---|---|
| **Breads** | | | | | | | | | | | | |
| French/Vienna, enriched | 1 slice | 68 | 2 | 13 | 1 | 1 | .2 | .3 | 0 | 19 | .63 | 152 |
| Mixed grain, enriched | 1 slice | 62 | 3 | 12 | 1 | 1 | .2 | .4 | 0 | 23 | .87 | 122 |
| Pita pocket, enriched, 6 1/2" round | 1 ea | 165 | 5 | 33 | 1 | 1 | .1 | .1 | 0 | 52 | 1.58 | 322 |
| Rye, light (1/3 rye & 2/3 enriched wheat flour) | 1 slice | 65 | 2 | 12 | 2 | 1 | .2 | .3 | 0 | 18 | .71 | 165 |
| White, enriched | 1 slice | 67 | 2 | 12 | 1 | 1 | .2 | .4 | <1 | 27 | .71 | 135 |
| Whole-wheat | 1 slice | 69 | 3 | 13 | 2 | 1 | .3 | .5 | 0 | 20 | .94 | 147 |
| **Cakes, prepared from mixes** | | | | | | | | | | | | |
| Angel food | 1 pce (1/12) | 137 | 3 | 31 | 1 | <1 | .1 | t | 0 | 74 | .28 | 397 |
| Devil's food, choc. frosting | 1 pce (1/16) | 253 | 3 | 38 | 2 | 11 | 3.2 | 6.2 | 32 | 30 | 1.52 | 230 |
| Pound cake (from recipe w/enriched flour) | 1/2" slice | 109 | 2 | 14 | <1 | 6 | .3 | 1.5 | 0 | 5 | .1 | 88 |
| Cheesecake | 1 pce (1/12) | 295 | 5 | 23 | 2 | 21 | 10.6 | 7.1 | 51 | 47 | .58 | 190 |
| Cheese puffs/Cheetos | 1 oz | 155 | 2 | 15 | <1 | 10 | 1.9 | 5.8 | 1 | 16 | .67 | 294 |
| **Cookies made w/enriched flour** | | | | | | | | | | | | |
| Chocolate chip (home recipe, 2 1/4" diam) | 4 ea | 195 | 2 | 23 | 1 | 11 | 3.2 | 4.2 | 13 | 16 | .99 | 144 |
| Fig bars | 4 ea | 195 | 2 | 40 | 3 | 4 | .7 | 2.2 | 0 | 36 | 1.63 | 196 |
| Peanut butter (home recipe, 2 5/8" diam) | 4 ea | 228 | 4 | 28 | 1 | 11 | 2.1 | 5.2 | 15 | 19 | 1.08 | 249 |
| Shortbread, commercial, small | 4 ea | 161 | 2 | 21 | 1 | 8 | .2 | 4.3 | 6 | 11 | .88 | 146 |
| Corn chips | 1 oz | 151 | 2 | 16 | 1 | 9 | 1.3 | 2.7 | 0 | 36 | .37 | 179 |
| **Crackers** | | | | | | | | | | | | |
| Graham | 2 ea | 59 | 1 | 11 | <1 | 1 | .4 | .7 | 0 | 3 | .52 | 85 |
| Saltine | 4 ea | 52 | 1 | 9 | <1 | 1 | .3 | .8 | 0 | 14 | .65 | 156 |
| Croissants, 4 1/2 x 4 x 1 3/4" | 1 ea | 231 | 5 | 26 | 1 | 12 | 6.7 | 3.2 | 43 | 21 | 1.16 | 424 |
| Doughnuts: cake type, plain, 3 1/4" diam | 1 ea | 211 | 3 | 25 | 1 | 11 | 1.9 | 4.8 | 18 | 22 | .98 | 273 |
| English muffin: plain, enriched | 1 ea | 134 | 4 | 26 | 2 | 1 | .1 | .2 | 0 | 99 | 1.43 | 264 |
| **Muffins, 2 1/2" diam, 1 1/2" high (from commercial mix)** | | | | | | | | | | | | |
| Blueberry | 1 ea | 135 | 2 | 22 | 1 | 4 | .7 | 1.6 | 21 | 11 | .51 | 197 |
| Bran, wheat | 1 ea | 124 | 3 | 21 | 4 | 4 | 1.1 | 2.1 | 31 | 14 | 1.14 | 210 |
| Cornmeal | 1 ea | 144 | 3 | 22 | 2 | 5 | 1.3 | 2.4 | 28 | 34 | .88 | 358 |
| Pancakes, 4" diam: plain, from mix: egg, milk, oil added | 1 ea | 52 | 1 | 10 | <1 | 1 | .1 | .2 | 3 | 34 | .42 | 170 |
| **Pies, 9" diam; crust made w/vegetable shortening, enriched flour** | | | | | | | | | | | | |
| Apple | 1 pce (1/6) | 374 | 3 | 54 | 3 | 17 | 3.3 | 9.4 | 0 | 17 | .71 | 420 |
| Chocolate cream | 1 pce (1/6) | 561 | 10 | 62 | 1 | 32 | 10 | 13 | 105 | 161 | 2.04 | 487 |
| Custard | 1 pce (1/6) | 319 | 8 | 32 | 2 | 18 | 4.2 | 8.8 | 50 | 122 | .88 | 365 |
| Lemon meringue | 1 pce (1/6) | 375 | 2 | 66 | 2 | 12 | 2.2 | 5.1 | 63 | 78 | .85 | 204 |
| Pecan | 1 pce (1/6) | 552 | 6 | 79 | 5 | 25 | 5.2 | 14.9 | 44 | 23 | 1.45 | 585 |
| Pumpkin | 1 pce (1/6) | 433 | 8 | 56 | 6 | 20 | 4.2 | 10.3 | 41 | 124 | 1.63 | 581 |
| Pretzels: thin twists, 3 1/4 x 2 1/4 x 1/4" | 10 ea | 229 | 5 | 47 | 2 | 2 | .4 | .8 | 0 | 22 | 2.59 | 1029 |
| Toaster pastries, fortified (Poptarts) | 1 ea | 212 | 3 | 38 | 1 | 6 | .8 | 2.2 | 0 | 14 | 1.89 | 226 |
| **Tortilla chips** | | | | | | | | | | | | |
| Plain | 1 oz | 140 | 2 | 18 | 2 | 6 | .2 | 4.4 | 0 | 0 | 0 | 135 |
| Nacho flavor | 1 oz | 139 | 2 | 18 | 1 | 7 | 1.4 | 4.3 | 1 | 42 | .4 | 198 |
| **Tortillas** | | | | | | | | | | | | |
| Corn, enriched, 6" diam | 1 ea | 67 | 2 | 14 | 2 | 1 | .1 | .2 | 0 | 52 | .42 | 48 |
| Flour, 8" diam | 1 ea | 115 | 3 | 20 | 1 | 2 | .4 | 1 | 0 | 44 | 1.17 | 169 |
| Taco shells | 1 ea | 66 | 1 | 9 | 1 | 3 | .4 | 1.5 | 0 | 22 | .35 | 51 |

*(continued)*

(continued)

150

## Grain Products: Cereal, Flour, Grain, Pasta and Noodles, Popcorn

| | Measure | E (kcal) | P (g) | C (g) | DF (g) | Fat Total | Fat Sat | Mono | CH (mg) | CA (mg) | I (mg) | S (mg) |
|---|---|---|---|---|---|---|---|---|---|---|---|---|
| Oatmeal or rolled oats | | | | | | | | | | | | |
| Plain, from packet | 3/4 c | 104 | 4 | 18 | 3 | 2 | .3 | .6 | 0 | 162 | 6.3 | 283 |
| Flavored, from packet | 3/4 c | 167 | 4 | 33 | 2 | 2 | .3 | .6 | 0 | 172 | 7 | 235 |
| Breakfast cereals, ready-to-eat | | | | | | | | | | | | |
| All-Bran | 1/3 c | 70 | 4 | 21 | 10 | 1 | .1 | .1 | 0 | 23 | 4.52 | 315 |
| Cap'n Crunch | 1 c | 156 | 2 | 30 | 1 | 3 | 2.2 | .4 | 0 | 6 | 9.81 | 278 |
| Cheerios | 1 c | 90 | 3 | 16 | 2 | 1 | .3 | .5 | 0 | 39 | 3.66 | 249 |
| Corn Chex | 1 c | 110 | 2 | 25 | <1 | 1 | .1 | .2 | 0 | 3 | 1.8 | 268 |
| Corn Flakes, Kellogg's | 1 1/4 c | 109 | 2 | 24 | 1 | <1 | t | t | 0 | 1 | 1.8 | 286 |
| Cracklin' Oat Bran | 1 c | 229 | 6 | 41 | 10 | 9 | 2.1 | 2.3 | 0 | 40 | 3.78 | 487 |
| Frosted Flakes | 1 c | 133 | 2 | 32 | 1 | <1 | t | t | 0 | 1 | 2.21 | 283 |
| Grape Nuts | 1/2 c | 203 | 7 | 47 | 6 | <1 | t | t | 0 | 5 | 2.47 | 396 |
| Kix | 1 c | 74 | 2 | 16 | <1 | <1 | .1 | .1 | 0 | 24 | 5.44 | 194 |
| Lucky Charms | 1 c | 125 | 3 | 26 | 1 | 1 | .2 | .4 | 0 | 36 | 5.09 | 227 |
| Product 19 | 1 c | 125 | 3 | 27 | 1 | <1 | t | t | 0 | 4 | 21 | 378 |
| Raisin Bran, Kellogg's | 1 c | 152 | 5 | 37 | 5 | <1 | .2 | .1 | 0 | 17 | 22.2 | 271 |
| Rice Krispies, Kellogg's | 1 c | 114 | 2 | 25 | <1 | <1 | t | t | 0 | 5 | 1.83 | 213 |
| Special K | 1 c | 83 | 4 | 16 | 1 | <1 | t | t | <1 | 6 | 3.39 | 196 |
| Total, wheat, w/added calcium | 1 c | 116 | 3 | 26 | 4 | 1 | .1 | .1 | 0 | 282 | 21 | 326 |
| Macaroni, cooked, enriched | 1 c | 197 | 7 | 40 | 2 | 1 | .1 | .1 | 0 | 10 | 1.96 | 1 |
| Egg noodles, cooked, enriched | 1 c | 213 | 8 | 40 | 2 | 2 | .5 | .7 | 53 | 19 | 2.54 | 11 |
| Popcorn | | | | | | | | | | | | |
| Air popped, plain | 1 c | 31 | 1 | 6 | 1 | <1 | <.1 | .1 | 0 | 1 | .21 | <1 |
| Microwaved, low fat, low sodium | 1 c | 24 | 1 | 4 | 1 | 1 | .1 | .2 | 0 | 1 | .13 | 28 |
| Popped in vegetable oil, salted | 1 c | 55 | 1 | 6 | 1 | 3 | .5 | .9 | 0 | 1 | .31 | 97 |
| Rice, white: regular/long grain, cooked | 1 c | 267 | 6 | 58 | 1 | <1 | .2 | .2 | 0 | 20 | 2.48 | 2 |
| Spaghetti, w/o salt, enriched | 1 c | 197 | 7 | 40 | 2 | 1 | .1 | .1 | 0 | 10 | 1.96 | 1 |

## Meats: Fish and Shellfish

| | Measure | E (kcal) | P (g) | C (g) | DF (g) | Fat Total | Fat Sat | Mono | CH (mg) | CA (mg) | I (mg) | S (mg) |
|---|---|---|---|---|---|---|---|---|---|---|---|---|
| Catfish, breaded/flour fried | 4 oz | 325 | 21 | 14 | 1 | 20 | 5 | 9 | 92 | 40 | 1.44 | 597 |
| Cod, batter fried | 4 oz | 196 | 20 | 8 | <1 | 9 | 2.2 | 3.6 | 64 | 43 | .9 | 124 |
| Cod, poached, no added fat | 4 oz | 116 | 25 | 0 | 0 | 1 | .2 | .1 | 61 | 23 | .54 | 69 |
| Fish sticks, breaded pollock | 2 ea | 155 | 9 | 14 | <1 | 7 | 1.8 | 2.9 | 64 | 11 | .42 | 331 |
| Halibut, baked or broiled | 4 oz | 158 | 30 | 0 | 0 | 3 | .5 | 1.1 | 47 | 68 | 1.21 | 78 |
| Salmon, baked or broiled | 4 oz | 244 | 31 | 0 | 0 | 13 | 2.2 | 6 | 99 | 8 | .62 | 75 |
| Shrimp | | | | | | | | | | | | |
| Cooked, boiled, 2 large (11g) | 16 ea | 85 | 18 | 0 | 0 | 1 | .2 | .2 | 167 | 33 | 2.65 | 192 |
| Fried, 2 large (15g) | 12 ea | 218 | 19 | 10 | <1 | 11 | 1.9 | 3.6 | 159 | 60 | 1.13 | 309 |
| Swordfish, baked or broiled | 4 oz | 176 | 29 | 0 | 0 | 6 | 1.6 | 2.2 | 57 | 7 | 1.18 | 130 |
| Tuna, light, canned, drained, water packed | 3 oz | 98 | 22 | 0 | 0 | 1 | .2 | .1 | 25 | 9 | 1.3 | 287 |

## Meats: Beef, Lamb, Pork, and Others

| | Measure | E (kcal) | P (g) | C (g) | DF (g) | Fat Total | Fat Sat | Mono | CH (mg) | CA (mg) | I (mg) | S (mg) |
|---|---|---|---|---|---|---|---|---|---|---|---|---|
| Beef, cooked | | | | | | | | | | | | |
| Ground beef, broiled, patty (3 x 5/8") lean, 21% fat | 4 oz | 316 | 32 | 0 | 0 | 20 | 7.9 | 8.7 | 114 | 14 | 2.78 | 101 |
| Steak, broiled, choice sirloin, lean only | 4 oz | 228 | 34 | 0 | 0 | 9 | 3.5 | 3.9 | 101 | 12 | 3.81 | 75 |

| Food | Amount | | | | | | | | | | | |
|---|---|---|---|---|---|---|---|---|---|---|---|---|
| **Steak, broiled, relatively fat, choice T-bone** | | | | | | | | | | | | |
| Lean and fat | 4 oz | 337 | 28 | 0 | 0 | 24 | 9.7 | 10.1 | 94 | 9 | 3.01 | 69 |
| Lean only | 4 oz | 242 | 32 | 0 | 0 | 12 | 4.7 | 4.7 | 91 | 8 | 3.4 | 74 |
| **Pork, cured, cooked** | | | | | | | | | | | | |
| Bacon, medium slices | 3 pce | 109 | 6 | <1 | 0 | 9 | 3.3 | 4.5 | 16 | 2 | .31 | 303 |
| Canadian-style bacon | 2 pce | 87 | 11 | 1 | 0 | 4 | 1.3 | 1.9 | 27 | 5 | .38 | 726 |
| Ham, roasted, lean only | 4 oz | 177 | 24 | 0 | 0 | 6 | 2 | 3 | 62 | 8 | 1 | 1500 |
| **Pork, fresh, cooked** | | | | | | | | | | | | |
| Chops, loin (cut 3 per lb w/bone) | | | | | | | | | | | | |
| Broiled, lean and fat | 1 ea | 211 | 24 | 0 | 0 | 12 | 4.6 | 5.4 | 70 | 17 | .76 | 54 |
| Broiled, lean only | 1 ea | 151 | 21 | 0 | 0 | 7 | 2.6 | 3.4 | 57 | 12 | .66 | 46 |
| **Meats: Poultry and Poultry Products** | | | | | | | | | | | | |
| **Chicken, cooked** | | | | | | | | | | | | |
| Fried, batter dipped | | | | | | | | | | | | |
| Breast (5.6 oz w/bones) | 1 ea | 364 | 35 | 13 | <1 | 18 | 4.9 | 7.6 | 119 | 28 | 1.75 | 385 |
| Drumstick (3.4 oz w/bones) | 1 ea | 192 | 16 | 6 | <1 | 11 | 3 | 4.6 | 62 | 12 | .97 | 193 |
| Thigh | 1 ea | 238 | 19 | 8 | <1 | 14 | 3.8 | 5.8 | 80 | 15 | 1.25 | 247 |
| Roasted | | | | | | | | | | | | |
| Breast, w/o skin | 1 ea | 141 | 27 | 0 | 0 | 3 | .9 | 1.1 | 73 | 13 | .89 | 64 |
| Drumstick | 1 ea | 95 | 12 | 0 | 0 | 5 | 1.4 | 2 | 41 | 5 | .57 | 40 |
| Thigh, w/o skin | 1 ea | 108 | 13 | 0 | 0 | 6 | 1.6 | 2.2 | 49 | 6 | .68 | 46 |
| **Turkey** | | | | | | | | | | | | |
| Roasted, meat only | | | | | | | | | | | | |
| Dark meat | 4 oz | 250 | 31 | 0 | 0 | 13 | 4 | 4 | 101 | 37 | 2.64 | 86 |
| Light meat | 4 oz | 223 | 32 | 0 | 0 | 9 | 2.7 | 3.8 | 86 | 24 | 1.53 | 71 |
| **Meats: Sausages and Lunchmeats** | | | | | | | | | | | | |
| **Bologna** | | | | | | | | | | | | |
| Beef | 1 pce | 72 | 3 | <1 | 0 | 7 | 2.8 | 3.2 | 13 | 3 | .38 | 226 |
| Healthy Favorites | 2 ea | 45 | 7 | 2 | 0 | 1 | 0 | — | 15 | — | .36 | 510 |
| Turkey | 1 pce | 56 | 4 | <1 | 0 | 4 | 1.4 | 1.4 | 28 | 24 | .43 | 246 |
| **Frankfurters** | | | | | | | | | | | | |
| Beef, large link, 8/package | 1 ea | 180 | 7 | 1 | 0 | 16 | 6.9 | 7.7 | 35 | 11 | .81 | 585 |
| Turkey, 10/package | 1 ea | 101 | 6 | 1 | 0 | 8 | 2.7 | 2.5 | 39 | 48 | .83 | 641 |
| Ham lunchmeat, regular | 2 pce | 103 | 10 | 2 | 0 | 6 | 1.9 | 2.8 | 32 | 4 | .56 | 746 |
| Turkey breast, fat free | 1 pce | 25 | 4 | 1 | 0 | 0 | 0 | 0 | 10 | 0 | 0 | 310 |
| Turkey pastrami | 2 pce | 80 | 10 | 1 | 0 | 4 | 1 | 1.2 | 31 | 5 | .95 | 595 |
| **Mixed Dishes and Fast Foods** | | | | | | | | | | | | |
| Beef stew w/vegetables, homemade | 1 c | 218 | 16 | 15 | 2 | 10 | 4.9 | 4.5 | 64 | 29 | 2.94 | 292 |
| Buffalo wings/spicy chicken wings | 2 ea | 98 | 8 | <1 | <1 | 7 | 1.8 | 2.8 | 26 | 5 | .4 | 61 |
| Chicken chow mein, canned | 1 c | 95 | 6 | 18 | 2 | 1 | 0 | .1 | 8 | 45 | 1.25 | 725 |
| Chicken fajitas | 1 ea | 344 | 17 | 43 | 4 | 11 | 2 | .5 | 35 | 71 | 3 | 372 |
| Chicken salad w/celery | 2 c | 268 | 11 | 1 | <1 | 25 | 4 | 7.2 | 47 | 16 | .62 | 201 |
| Chili w/beans, canned | 1 c | 286 | 15 | 30 | 11 | 14 | 6 | 5.9 | 43 | 120 | 8.75 | 1331 |
| Coleslaw | 1 c | 178 | 2 | 15 | 2 | 13 | 2 | 2.9 | 6 | 41 | .88 | 324 |
| Egg roll, w/meat | 1 ea | 114 | 5 | 9 | 1 | 6 | 1.6 | 2.9 | 38 | 12 | .77 | 305 |
| Lasagna (w/meat, homemade) | 1 pce | 382 | 22 | 39 | 3 | 15 | 7.7 | 5 | 56 | 258 | 3.43 | 745 |
| Macaroni & cheese, homemade | 1 c | 430 | 17 | 40 | 1 | 22 | 8.9 | 8.8 | 42 | 362 | 1.8 | 1086 |
| Meat loaf, beef | 1 pce | 185 | 14 | 5 | <1 | 11 | 4 | 4.8 | 72 | 35 | 1.61 | 329 |

*(continued)*

**5**

(continued)

| | Measure | E (kcal) | P (g) | C (g) | DF (g) | Fat (g) Total | Fat (g) Sat | Mono | CH (mg) | CA (mg) | I (mg) | S (mg) |
|---|---|---|---|---|---|---|---|---|---|---|---|---|
| Potato salad w/mayonnaise & eggs | 1/2 c | 179 | 3 | 14 | 2 | 10 | 1.8 | 3.1 | 85 | 24 | .81 | 661 |
| Fried rice (meatless) | 1 c | 264 | 5 | 34 | 1 | 11 | 1.7 | 2.9 | 42 | 30 | 1.84 | 286 |
| Spaghetti (enriched) in tomato sauce, with cheese | | | | | | | | | | | | |
|   Canned | 1 c | 190 | 5 | 38 | 2 | 1 | 0 | .4 | 8 | 40 | 2.75 | 955 |
|   Homemade | 1 c | 260 | 9 | 37 | 2 | 9 | 2 | 5.4 | 8 | 80 | 2.25 | 955 |
| Sandwiches (on part whole wheat) | | | | | | | | | | | | |
|   Avocado, cheese, tomato, lettuce | 1 ea | 454 | 14 | 33 | 5 | 31 | 9 | 12.6 | 32 | 277 | 3.01 | 525 |
|   Bacon, lettuce, tomato | 1 ea | 398 | 13 | 32 | 3 | 25 | 6 | 9.5 | 27 | 73 | 2.6 | 753 |
|   Cheese, grilled | 1 ea | 389 | 18 | 27 | 2 | 24 | 12.3 | 7.7 | 53 | 405 | 2.08 | 1143 |
|   Chicken salad | 1 ea | 366 | 10 | 27 | 2 | 25 | 4 | 7 | 31 | 67 | 2.13 | 461 |
|   Egg salad | 1 ea | 375 | 9 | 27 | 2 | 26 | 4.5 | 8 | 146 | 77 | 2.36 | 521 |
|   Ham | 1 ea | 257 | 17 | 22 | 2 | 11 | 2.3 | 4.1 | 35 | 56 | 2.09 | 1274 |
|   Ham & cheese | 1 ea | 384 | 22 | 27 | 3 | 21 | 7.8 | 6.9 | 57 | 236 | 2.49 | 1578 |
|   Peanut butter & jelly | 1 ea | 341 | 11 | 46 | 4 | 14 | 2.8 | 6.6 | 0 | 73 | 2.52 | 305 |
|   Reuben; grilled: corned beef, swiss cheese, sauerkraut on rye | 1 ea | 639 | 29 | 40 | 5 | 40 | 13.7 | 12.8 | 114 | 411 | 3.68 | 1685 |
|   Roast beef | 1 ea | 311 | 23 | 25 | 2 | 13 | 2.8 | 4.3 | 34 | 56 | 3.33 | 1254 |
|   Tuna salad | 1 ea | 326 | 13 | 30 | 3 | 17 | 3 | 5 | 14 | 67 | 2.35 | 557 |
|   Turkey | 1 ea | 267 | 19 | 21 | 2 | 11 | 2 | 3.5 | 34 | 53 | 1.8 | 1249 |
| Vegetarian burger, no salt added (Worthington) | 1/2 c | 150 | 22 | 7 | — | 4 | — | — | — | — | 1.80 | 170 |
| **Nuts, Seeds, and Products** | | | | | | | | | | | | |
| Almonds: whole, dried, unsalted | 1 oz | 165 | 6 | 6 | 3 | 15 | 1.4 | 9.6 | 0 | 75 | 1.04 | 3 |
| Cashew nuts: oil roasted, salted | 1 oz | 161 | 5 | 8 | 1 | 14 | 2.7 | 8 | 0 | 11 | 1.16 | 175 |
| Macadamias: oil roasted, salted | 1 oz | 201 | 2 | 4 | 3 | 21 | 3.2 | 16.9 | 0 | 13 | .5 | 73 |
| Peanuts: oil roasted, salted | 1 oz | 163 | 7 | 5 | 2 | 14 | 1.9 | 6.9 | 0 | 25 | .52 | 123 |
| Peanut butter | 2 tbs | 188 | 8 | 7 | 2 | 16 | 3.1 | 7.6 | 0 | 11 | .54 | 153 |
| Sunflower seed kernels: oil roasted | 1/4 c | 209 | 7 | 5 | 2 | 19 | 2 | 3.7 | 0 | 19 | 2.28 | 1 |
| English walnuts, chopped | 1 oz | 180 | 4 | 5 | 1 | 17 | 1.6 | 4 | 0 | 27 | .69 | 3 |
| **Sweets** | | | | | | | | | | | | |
| Almond Joy candy bar | 1 oz | 130 | 1 | 16 | 2 | 8 | 4.7 | 1.5 | 1 | 22 | .34 | 38 |
| Milk chocolate | | | | | | | | | | | | |
|   Plain | 1 oz | 143 | 2 | 17 | 1 | 9 | 5.2 | 2.8 | 6 | 54 | .39 | 23 |
|   With almonds | 1 oz | 147 | 3 | 15 | 2 | 10 | 4.8 | 3.8 | 5 | 63 | .46 | 21 |
| Gumdrops | 1 oz | 108 | 0 | 28 | 0 | <1 | 0 | t | 0 | 1 | .11 | 12 |
| Jellybeans | 1 oz | 104 | 0 | 26 | 0 | <1 | 0 | t | 0 | 1 | .31 | 7 |
| Milky Way candy bar | 1 ea | 251 | 3 | 43 | 1 | 9 | 4.7 | 3.3 | 12 | 78 | .46 | 144 |
| Reese's peanut butter cups | 2 ea | 218 | 5 | 21 | 2 | 14 | 10.4 | .9 | 7 | 35 | .49 | 131 |
| Snickers candy bar (2.2 oz) | 1 ea | 278 | 6 | 37 | 2 | 14 | 7.3 | 4.1 | 7 | 70 | .48 | 164 |
| Chocolate syrup | | | | | | | | | | | | |
|   Hot fudge type | 2 tbs | 131 | 2 | 22 | <1 | 5 | 2.2 | 1.4 | 5 | 38 | .46 | 49 |
|   Thin type | 2 tbs | 83 | 1 | 22 | 1 | <1 | .2 | .1 | 0 | 5 | .81 | 36 |
| **Vegetables and Legumes** | | | | | | | | | | | | |
| Asparagus, green, cooked, from fresh, cuts and tips | 1/2 c | 22 | 2 | 4 | 2 | <1 | .1 | t | 0 | 18 | .66 | 10 |

| Food | Serving | | | | | | | | | | | |
|---|---|---|---|---|---|---|---|---|---|---|---|---|
| Black beans, cooked | 1/2 c | 114 | 8 | 20 | 7 | <1 | .1 | t | 0 | 23 | 1.81 | 1 |
| Green string beans, cooked from frozen | 1/2 c | 17 | 1 | 4 | 2 | <1 | t | t | 0 | 30 | .55 | 9 |
| Broccoli, cooked from frozen, chopped | 1 c | 51 | 6 | 10 | 5 | <1 | t | t | 0 | 94 | 1.12 | 44 |
| Carrots, raw, whole, 7 1/2 x 1 1/8" | 1 ea | 31 | 1 | 7 | 2 | <1 | t | t | 0 | 19 | .36 | 25 |
| Carrots, cooked, from frozen, sliced, drained | 1/2 c | 26 | 1 | 6 | 3 | <1 | t | t | 0 | 20 | .34 | 43 |
| Cauliflower, flowerets, cooked from frozen, drained | 1/2 c | 17 | 1 | 3 | 2 | <1 | t | t | 0 | 15 | .37 | 16 |
| Celery, pascal type, raw, diced | 1 c | 19 | 1 | 4 | 2 | 1 | t | t | 0 | 48 | .48 | 104 |
| Corn, cooked, drained | | | | | | | | | | | | |
| From fresh, on cob, 5" long | 1 ea | 83 | 3 | 19 | 2 | 1 | .3 | .3 | 0 | 2 | .47 | 13 |
| Kernels, cooked from frozen | 1/2 c | 66 | 2 | 17 | 2 | <1 | t | t | 0 | 2 | .25 | 4 |
| Corn, canned | | | | | | | | | | | | |
| Cream style | 1/2 c | 92 | 2 | 23 | 2 | 1 | .2 | .2 | 0 | 4 | .49 | 364 |
| Whole kernel, vacuum pack | 1/2 c | 83 | 3 | 20 | 6 | 1 | .2 | .2 | 0 | 5 | .44 | 286 |
| Cucumber slices w/peel | 7 pce | 4 | <1 | 1 | <1 | <1 | t | t | 0 | 4 | .07 | 1 |
| Lettuce: iceberg/crisphead, wedge, 1/4 head | 1 ea | 18 | 1 | 3 | 1 | <1 | t | t | 0 | 25 | .67 | 12 |
| Mushrooms, raw, sliced | 1/2 c | 9 | 1 | 2 | <1 | <1 | t | t | 0 | 2 | .43 | 1 |
| Onions | | | | | | | | | | | | |
| Raw, chopped | 1 c | 61 | 2 | 14 | 3 | <1 | t | t | 0 | 32 | .35 | 5 |
| Cooked, drained, chopped | 1/2 c | 46 | 1 | 11 | 1 | <1 | t | t | 0 | 23 | .25 | 3 |
| Peas | | | | | | | | | | | | |
| Black-eyed, cooked from frozen, drained | 1/2 c | 112 | 7 | 20 | 7 | 1 | .2 | .1 | 0 | 20 | 1.8 | 4 |
| Green, canned, drained | 1/2 c | 59 | 4 | 11 | 3 | <1 | .1 | t | 0 | 17 | .81 | 186 |
| Peppers, sweet, green: whole pod (90 g w/refuse), raw | 1 ea | 20 | 1 | 5 | 1 | <1 | t | t | 0 | 7 | .34 | 1 |
| Potatoes | | | | | | | | | | | | |
| Baked in oven, 4 3/4" x 2 1/3" diam | | | | | | | | | | | | |
| With skin | 1 ea | 220 | 5 | 51 | 5 | <1 | .1 | 1 | 0 | 20 | 2.75 | 16 |
| Flesh only | 1 ea | 145 | 3 | 34 | 2 | <1 | t | t | 0 | 8 | .55 | 8 |
| French fried in vegetable oil, strips 2-3 1/2" long | 10 ea | 155 | 2 | 19 | 2 | 8 | 2.5 | 4 | 0 | 8 | .68 | 82 |
| Mashed | | | | | | | | | | | | |
| Home recipe w/milk & marg | 1/2 c | 111 | 2 | 18 | 2 | 4 | 1.1 | 1.9 | 2 | 27 | .27 | 310 |
| Prepared from flakes: water, milk, margarine, salt added | 1/2 c | 124 | 2 | 17 | 1 | 6 | 1.6 | 2.5 | 4 | 54 | .24 | 365 |
| Potato chips | 14 ea | 150 | 2 | 15 | 1 | 10 | 3.1 | 2.8 | 0 | 7 | .46 | 166 |
| Refried beans, canned | 1/2 c | 135 | 8 | 23 | 7 | 1 | .5 | .6 | 0 | 58 | 2.24 | 534 |
| Spinach: raw, chopped | 1 c | 12 | 2 | 2 | 2 | <1 | .5 | .6 | 0 | 55 | 1.52 | 44 |
| Zucchini, cooked | 1/2 c | 14 | 1 | 4 | 1 | <1 | t | t | 0 | 12 | .31 | 3 |
| Acorn squash, baked, mashed | 1/2 c | 68 | 1 | 18 | 5 | <1 | t | t | 0 | 54 | 1.14 | 5 |
| Sweet potatoes: baked in skin, peeled, 5 x 2" diam | 1 ea | 140 | 3 | 28 | 4 | <1 | t | t | 0 | 32 | 2 | 11 |
| Tomatoes: raw, chopped | 1 c | 38 | 2 | 8 | 2 | 1 | t | .1 | 0 | 9 | .81 | 16 |
| Tomato juice, canned | 1 c | 41 | 2 | 10 | 1 | <1 | .1 | t | 0 | 22 | 1.42 | 881 |
| Tomato paste, canned | 1 c | 220 | 10 | 49 | 11 | 2 | t | .4 | 0 | 92 | 7.83 | 2070 |
| Tomato sauce, canned | 1 c | 73 | 3 | 18 | 3 | <1 | .1 | .1 | 0 | 34 | 1.89 | 1482 |

## Nutrient Values at Popular Fast-Food Restaurants

| Food item | Calories | Total fat (g) | Saturated fat (g) | Cholesterol (mg) | Protein (g) | Sodium (mg) | Carbohydrate (g) |
|---|---|---|---|---|---|---|---|
| *Arby's* | | | | | | | |
| Beef n' Cheddar | 487 | 28 | 9 | 50 | 25 | 1216 | 40 |
| Giant Roast Beef | 555 | 28 | 11 | 71 | 35 | 1561 | 43 |
| Regular Roast Beef | 388 | 19 | 7 | 43 | 23 | 1009 | 33 |
| Junior Roast Beef | 324 | 14 | 5 | 30 | 17 | 779 | 35 |
| Breaded Chicken Filet | 536 | 28 | 5 | 45 | 28 | 1016 | 46 |
| Ham n' Cheese | 359 | 14 | 5 | 53 | 24 | 1283 | 34 |
| Curly Fries | 300 | 15 | 3 | 0 | 4 | 853 | 38 |
| Potato Cakes | 204 | 12 | 2 | 0 | 2 | 397 | 20 |
| Baked Potato (plain) | 355 | .3 | 0 | 0 | 7 | 26 | 82 |
| Deluxe Baked Potato | 736 | 36 | 16 | 59 | 19 | 499 | 86 |
| Plain Biscuit | 280 | 15 | 3 | 0 | 6 | 730 | 34 |
| Blueberry Muffin | 230 | 9 | 2 | 25 | 2 | 290 | 35 |
| Garden Salad | 61 | .5 | | 0 | 3 | 40 | 12 |
| Roast Chicken Salad | 149 | 2 | | 29 | 20 | 418 | 12 |
| Side Salad | 23 | .3 | | 0 | 1 | 15 | 4 |
| Reduced-Calorie Italian Dressing | 20 | 1 | 0 | 0 | 0 | 1000 | 3 |
| Reduced-Calorie Buttermilk Ranch Dressing | 50 | 0 | 0 | 0 | 0 | 710 | 12 |
| *Burger King* | | | | | | | |
| Whopper Sandwich (with cheese) | 730 | 46 | 16 | 115 | 33 | 1350 | 46 |
| Hamburger | 330 | 15 | 6 | 55 | 20 | 530 | 28 |
| Cheeseburger | 380 | 19 | 9 | 65 | 23 | 770 | 28 |
| BK Broiler Chicken Sandwich | 530 | 26 | 5 | 105 | 29 | 1060 | 5 |
| Croissan'wich with Sausage, Egg, and Cheese | 600 | 46 | 16 | 260 | 22 | 1140 | 25 |
| French Toast Sticks | 500 | 27 | 7 | 0 | 4 | 490 | 60 |
| Hash Browns (small) | 240 | 15 | 6 | 0 | 2 | 440 | 25 |
| French Fries (medium, salted) | 400 | 21 | 8 | 0 | 3 | 820 | 50 |
| Broiled Chicken Salad | 190 | 8 | 4 | 75 | 20 | 500 | 9 |
| Garden Salad | 100 | 5 | 3 | 15 | 6 | 115 | 8 |
| Side Salad | 60 | 3 | 2 | 5 | 3 | 55 | 4 |
| Reduced-Calorie Light Italian Dressing | 15 | .5 | 0 | 0 | 0 | 50 | 3 |
| *Kentucky Fried Chicken* | | | | | | | |
| Original Recipe | | | | | | | |
| Wing | 140 | 10 | 2.5 | 55 | 9 | 414 | 5 |
| Breast | 400 | 24 | 6 | 135 | 29 | 1116 | 16 |
| Drumstick | 140 | 9 | 2 | 75 | 13 | 422 | 4 |
| Thigh | 250 | 18 | 4.5 | 95 | 16 | 747 | 6 |
| Tender Roast With Skin | | | | | | | |
| Wing | 121 | 7.7 | 2.1 | 74 | 12.2 | 331 | 1 |
| Breast | 251 | 10.8 | 3 | 151 | 37 | 830 | 2 |
| Thigh | 207 | 12 | 3.8 | 120 | 18.4 | 504 | < 2 |
| Drumstick | 97 | 4.3 | 1.2 | 85 | 14.5 | 271 | < 1 |
| Tender Roast Without Skin | | | | | | | |
| Breast | 169 | 4.3 | 1.2 | 112 | 31.4 | 797 | 1 |
| Thigh | 106 | 5.5 | 1.7 | 84 | 12.9 | 312 | < 1 |
| Drumstick | 67 | 2.4 | .7 | 63 | 11 | 259 | < 1 |
| Chunky Chicken Pot Pie | 770 | 42 | 13 | 70 | 29 | 2160 | 69 |
| BBQ Flavored Chicken Sandwich | 256 | 8 | 1 | 57 | 17 | 782 | 28 |
| Mashed Potatoes and Gravy | 120 | 6 | 1 | < 1 | 1 | 440 | 17 |
| Cole Slaw | 180 | 9 | 1.5 | 5 | 2 | 280 | 21 |
| Potato Salad | 230 | 14 | 2 | 15 | 4 | 540 | 23 |
| Corn on the Cob | 150 | 1.5 | 0 | 0 | 5 | 20 | 35 |
| Green Beans | 45 | 1.5 | .5 | 5 | 1 | 730 | 7 |
| BBQ Baked Beans | 190 | 3 | 1 | 5 | 6 | 760 | 33 |
| Mean Greens | 70 | 3 | 1 | 10 | 4 | 650 | 11 |

Nutrient values were obtained from each restaurant's website.
Colorized items denote healthy choices.

154

| Food item | Calories | Total fat (g) | Saturated fat (g) | Cholesterol (mg) | Protein (g) | Sodium (mg) | Carbohydrate (g) |
|---|---|---|---|---|---|---|---|
| *Long John Silver's* | | | | | | | |
| Batter-Dipped Fish (1 piece) | 170 | 11 | 2.5 | 30 | 11 | 470 | 12 |
| Batter-Dipped Chicken (1 piece) | 120 | 6 | 1.5 | 15 | 8 | 400 | 11 |
| Batter-Dipped Shrimp (1 piece) | 35 | 2.5 | .5 | 10 | 1 | 95 | 2 |
| Flavorbaked Fish | 90 | 2.5 | 1 | 35 | 14 | 320 | 1 |
| Flavorbaked Chicken | 110 | 3 | 1 | 55 | 19 | 600 | < 1 |
| Flavorbaked Fish Sandwich | 320 | 14 | 7 | 55 | 23 | 930 | 28 |
| Flavorbaked Chicken Sandwich | 290 | 10 | 2 | 60 | 24 | 970 | 27 |
| Wraps | 730 | 36 | 7 | 25 | 18 | 1780 | 83 |
| Fries | 250 | 15 | 2.5 | 0 | 3 | 500 | 28 |
| Hushpuppy (1 piece) | 60 | 2.5 | 0 | 0 | 1 | 25 | 9 |
| Corn Cobbette (without butter) | 80 | .5 | 0 | 0 | 3 | 0 | 19 |
| Rice Pilaf | 140 | 3 | 1 | 0 | 3 | 210 | 26 |
| Baked Potato | 210 | 0 | 0 | 0 | 4 | 10 | 49 |
| Garden Salad | 45 | 0 | 0 | 0 | 3 | 25 | 9 |
| Grilled Chicken Salad | 140 | 2.5 | .5 | 45 | 20 | 260 | 10 |
| Ocean Chef Salad | 130 | 2 | 0 | 60 | 14 | 540 | 15 |
| Side Salad | 25 | 0 | 0 | 0 | 1 | 15 | 4 |
| Fat-Free Ranch dressing | 50 | 0 | 0 | 0 | 2 | 380 | 13 |
| Fat-Free French dressing | 50 | 0 | 0 | 0 | 0 | 360 | 14 |
| *McDonald's* | | | | | | | |
| Big Mac | 560 | 31 | 10 | 85 | 26 | 1070 | 45 |
| Quarter Pounder With Cheese | 530 | 30 | 13 | 95 | 28 | 1290 | 38 |
| Hamburger | 260 | 9 | 3.5 | 30 | 13 | 580 | 34 |
| Cheeseburger | 320 | 13 | 6 | 40 | 15 | 820 | 35 |
| Fish Filet Deluxe | 560 | 28 | 6 | 60 | 23 | 1060 | 54 |
| Grilled Chicken Deluxe | 440 | 20 | 3 | 60 | 27 | 1040 | 38 |
| Egg McMuffin | 290 | 12 | 4.5 | 235 | 17 | 710 | 27 |
| Bacon, Egg, and Cheese Biscuit | 470 | 28 | 8 | 235 | 18 | 1250 | 36 |
| Hash Browns | 130 | 8 | 1.5 | 0 | 1 | 330 | 14 |
| Hotcakes (plain) | 310 | 7 | 1.5 | 15 | 9 | 610 | 53 |
| Cheese Danish | 410 | 22 | 8 | 70 | 7 | 340 | 47 |
| French Fries (large) | 450 | 22 | 4 | 0 | 6 | 290 | 57 |
| Garden Salad | 35 | 0 | 0 | 0 | 2 | 20 | 7 |
| Grilled Chicken Salad Deluxe | 120 | 1.5 | 0 | 45 | 21 | 240 | 7 |
| Fat-Free Herb Vinaigrette | 50 | 0 | 0 | 0 | 0 | 330 | 11 |
| Low-Fat Apple Bran Muffin | 300 | 3 | .5 | 0 | 6 | 380 | 61 |
| Vanilla Reduced-Fat Ice Cream Cone | 150 | 4.5 | 3 | 20 | 4 | 75 | 23 |
| 1% Low-Fat Milk | 100 | 2.5 | 1.5 | 10 | 8 | 115 | 13 |
| Orange Juice | 80 | 0 | 0 | 0 | 1 | 20 | 20 |
| *Pizza Hut* | | | | | | | |
| Supreme (per slice) | | | | | | | |
| Thin n' Crispy | 250 | 11 | 5 | 20 | 13 | 710 | 24 |
| Pan | 300 | 13 | 5 | 25 | 13 | 670 | 32 |
| Chicken Supreme | | | | | | | |
| Thin n' Crispy | 220 | 7 | 2.5 | 25 | 14 | 550 | 26 |
| Hand Tossed | 240 | 6 | 3 | 25 | 14 | 660 | 31 |
| Meat Lover's | | | | | | | |
| Thin n' Crispy | 310 | 16 | 7 | 35 | 16 | 900 | 25 |
| Pan | 360 | 19 | 6 | 40 | 17 | 870 | 30 |
| Veggie Lover's | | | | | | | |
| Thin n' Crispy | 170 | 6 | 2 | 10 | 7 | 460 | 23 |
| Hand Tossed | 240 | 7 | 3 | 20 | 11 | 650 | 34 |

*(continued)*

*(continued)*

| Food item | Calories | Total fat (g) | Saturated fat (g) | Cholesterol (mg) | Protein (g) | Sodium (mg) | Carbohydrate (g) |
|---|---|---|---|---|---|---|---|
| **Cheese** | | | | | | | |
| Thin n' Crispy | 210 | 9 | 4.5 | 20 | 12 | 530 | 21 |
| Hand Tossed | 280 | 10 | 5 | 25 | 16 | 770 | 32 |
| **Ham** | | | | | | | |
| Thin n' Crispy | 190 | 6 | 3 | 15 | 10 | 560 | 23 |
| Hand Tossed | 230 | 6 | 3 | 25 | 13 | 710 | 30 |
| **Italian Sausage** | | | | | | | |
| Thin n' Crispy | 300 | 16 | 6 | 35 | 15 | 740 | 24 |
| Pan | 350 | 18 | 6 | 40 | 16 | 740 | 31 |
| Garlic Bread (1 slice) | 150 | 8 | 1.5 | 0 | 3 | 240 | 16 |
| Breadstick | 130 | 4 | 1 | 0 | 3 | 170 | 20 |
| | | | | | | | |
| ***Subway*** | | | | | | | |
| **Cold Subs (6 inch)*** | | | | | | | |
| Veggie Delight | 222 | 3 | 0 | 0 | 9 | 582 | 38 |
| Turkey Breast | 273 | 4 | 1 | 19 | 17 | 1391 | 40 |
| Ham | 287 | 5 | 1 | 28 | 18 | 1308 | 39 |
| Subway Club | 297 | 5 | 1 | 26 | 21 | 1341 | 40 |
| Roast Beef | 288 | 5 | 1 | 20 | 19 | 928 | 39 |
| Cold Cut Trio | 362 | 13 | 4 | 64 | 19 | 1401 | 39 |
| Spicy Italian | 467 | 24 | 9 | 57 | 20 | 1592 | 38 |
| **Hot Subs (6 inch)*** | | | | | | | |
| Roasted Chicken Breast | 332 | 6 | 1 | 48 | 26 | 967 | 41 |
| Meatball | 404 | 16 | 6 | 33 | 18 | 1035 | 44 |
| Steak and Cheese (+) | 383 | 10 | 6 | 70 | 29 | 1106 | 41 |
| Cheese (2 triangles) | 41 | 3 | 2 | 10 | 2 | 201 | 0 |
| Mayonnaise | 37 | 4 | 1 | 3 | 0 | 27 | 0 |
| Light Mayonnaise | 18 | 2 | 0 | 2 | 0 | 33 | 0 |
| Mustard | 8 | 0 | 0 | 0 | 1 | 0 | 1 |

* Cheese and condiments not included unless indicated with a (+).

| Food item | Calories | Total fat (g) | Saturated fat (g) | Cholesterol (mg) | Protein (g) | Sodium (mg) | Carbohydrate (g) |
|---|---|---|---|---|---|---|---|
| ***Taco Bell*** | | | | | | | |
| **Supreme Gordita** | | | | | | | |
| Beef | 300 | 13 | 6 | 35 | 14 | 390 | 31 |
| Chicken | 290 | 12 | 5 | 55 | 15 | 420 | 30 |
| Steak | 280 | 11 | 5 | 35 | 18 | 310 | 28 |
| **Fiesta Gordita** | | | | | | | |
| Beef | 290 | 13 | 4 | 25 | 14 | 880 | 31 |
| Chicken | 280 | 12 | 3 | 45 | 14 | 910 | 29 |
| Steak | 270 | 10 | 2.5 | 25 | 17 | 800 | 28 |
| **Santa Fe Gordita** | | | | | | | |
| Beef | 380 | 20 | 4 | 35 | 14 | 440 | 33 |
| Chicken | 360 | 19 | 2.5 | 55 | 15 | 470 | 32 |
| Steak | 350 | 18 | 2.5 | 35 | 18 | 360 | 31 |
| Burrito Supreme | 440 | 19 | 8 | 35 | 17 | 1230 | 51 |
| Bean Burrito | 380 | 12 | 4 | 10 | 13 | 1100 | 55 |
| Chili Cheese Burrito | 330 | 13 | 6 | 35 | 14 | 870 | 37 |
| Grilled Chicken Burrito | 410 | 15 | 4.5 | 55 | 17 | 1380 | 50 |
| 7-Layer Burrito | 530 | 23 | 7 | 25 | 16 | 1280 | 66 |
| Taco Supreme | 220 | 14 | 7 | 35 | 10 | 350 | 14 |
| Taco | 180 | 10 | 4 | 25 | 9 | 330 | 12 |
| Soft Taco | 220 | 10 | 4.5 | 25 | 11 | 580 | 21 |
| Grilled Steak Soft Taco | 230 | 10 | 2.5 | 25 | 15 | 1020 | 20 |
| Grilled Chicken Soft Taco | 240 | 12 | 3.5 | 45 | 12 | 1110 | 21 |
| Mexican Pizza | 570 | 35 | 10 | 45 | 21 | 1040 | 42 |
| Tostada | 300 | 15 | 5 | 15 | 10 | 650 | 31 |
| Cheese Quesadilla | 350 | 18 | 9 | 50 | 16 | 860 | 32 |
| Country Breakfast Burrito | 270 | 14 | 5 | 195 | 8 | 690 | 26 |
| Grande Breakfast Burrito | 420 | 22 | 7 | 205 | 13 | 1050 | 43 |
| Nachos | 320 | 18 | 4 | 30 | 5 | 570 | 34 |
| Pintos n' Cheese | 190 | 9 | 4 | 15 | 9 | 650 | 18 |
| Cinnamon Twists | 140 | 6 | 0 | 0 | 1 | 190 | 19 |

# Chapter 6

# Weight Control

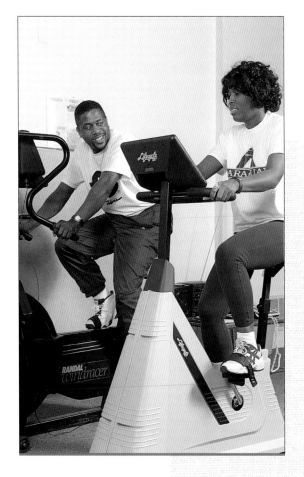

I don't get it. I've gained 15 pounds since I moved into the dorm three months ago even though I'm just as active as I was in high school—maybe even more active. I have to walk all over campus to get to classes, I play intramural basketball, and I work out with my girlfriend on weekends. She noticed I'd gained weight and she talked me into a low-calorie, high-protein diet a couple of weeks ago, one she saw in a magazine. I stayed on it for a week and actually lost about 4 pounds, but I didn't like the diet and once I went off it I immediately gained the weight back. I know I probably need to make better food choices, but I've never really had to watch my weight before. I'm not sure what to do differently. I just know I want to lose the extra pounds to feel and look better.

—Jarrod, 18-year-old freshman

*What do you think?*

Would Jarrod's diet have worked—and been healthy for him—if he'd kept with it? There are numerous weight loss diet plans available, with different nutritional (and not so nutritional) focuses. Does *any* weight loss diet work? What is Jarrod not taking into account as he tries to lose weight?

In this chapter we'll look at the factors affecting weight control and consider why Americans are getting fatter generation by generation. We'll explore the key to weight control: caloric balance, which consists of metabolic rate, genetics, and lifestyle (including physical activity). And we'll examine sound weight management guidelines, including information on modifying eating habits and on strategies for losing, and gaining, weight.

## FACTORS AFFECTING WEIGHT CONTROL

As we showed in chapter 4, Americans young and old are becoming fatter than previous generations, and over 30% of adults are overweight. Among youth, 20% of boys and 22% of girls are overweight, a 6% increase in less than a decade. The more appropriate term might be *overfat* rather than overweight. This condition is largely a function of lifestyle behavioral changes. Advanced technology has resulted in our being less physically active on our jobs and in our lives than we used to be, and changes in dietary patterns have added to the problem.

As we have become more reliant on technology to assist us in our work and provide entertainment for us in our homes, we have become less active. According to the U.S. Centers for Disease Control and Prevention, 26% of men and 30% of women reported no leisure-time physical activity. Among overweight people, these percentages were even higher: a government study showed that 33% of overweight men and 41% of overweight women were inactive during their leisure time. James (1995) estimates that technological enhancements such as automatic doors and windows, escalators, elevators, and remote controls have resulted in 800 calories less in daily energy expenditure for the average person.

Lack of sufficient physical activity and increased caloric intake result in increased body weight. Studies show that body weight is an independent risk factor in mortality, and the American Heart Association recently declared obesity to be a major risk factor for coronary heart disease. At first it was thought that excess weight was simply related to hypertension (high blood pressure) and to other diseases or conditions such as diabetes and high cholesterol. It is now known that obesity is directly related to increased mortality. Those who maintain healthy levels of fat weight are at less risk of dying prematurely from heart disease. An important lifelong goal for *everyone* should be to attain and maintain a healthy weight and body fat percent as described in chapter 4.

The main factor that affects weight control is *caloric balance*, which consists of metabolic rates, genetics, and lifestyle choices. We discussed caloric balance—or *energy balance*—in chapter 4. A positive energy balance means you consume more calories than you expend; a negative energy balance means you expend more calories than you consume. Of course, if you have a positive energy balance, you'll gain weight; if you are attempting to lose weight, you'll need to achieve a negative energy balance. Your energy balance is affected not only by the calories you consume, but also by your genetics and by how physically active you are.

**KEY POINT** Three main factors that affect weight control are caloric balance, metabolic rates, and lifestyle behaviors including physical activity.

Next we'll look at the other two factors: metabolic rates and exercise.

## Metabolic Rates

Your caloric balance is determined in part by your metabolic rates—your *basal metabolic rate (BMR)* and your *resting metabolic rate (RMR)*. Your BMR indicates the energy (and calories) you expend by simply being alive; BMR depends on your gender, age, body size, metabolic functions, and body characteristics. But even people with the same characteristics can vary widely in their BMR. Men generally have higher metabolic rates than women because they are bigger and have more muscle mass. The larger your body, generally the higher your BMR. However, various body functions (e.g., thyroid and pituitary) can accelerate or reduce your BMR. Some people become overweight as a result of thyroid conditions that slow their metabolic rates and cause them to gain weight. However, most people who are overweight or obese don't suffer from thyroid problems, but rather have developed a long-term positive caloric balance.

Your body composition also affects your basal metabolism. If you have an abundance of lean tissue, your BMR will be higher than if you had an abundance of fat tissue. Lean tissue is "metabolically active," causing you to expend more calories. Ideally, your BMR should account for about 65% of your daily caloric expenditure, with physical activity accounting for about 25% and digestion 10% (see figure 6.1). You can easily see what will happen if physical activity is missing from your lifestyle—BMR and digestion are the only calorie-burning activities left, and it becomes easy to maintain a positive caloric balance.

Because most people don't just "exist" on a daily basis, researchers often use the RMR to

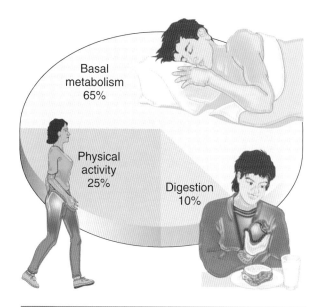

**FIGURE 6.1** Daily energy expenditure for the average person.

reflect daily caloric needs. Your RMR is the caloric expenditure for a typical inactive day—that is, it's caloric expenditure resulting from rest plus your BMR. A typical RMR is about 1,500 calories per day. Thus, if you're basically inactive all day, performing minimal physical work or activity, you will likely expend less than 2,000 calories. If you consume 2,500 calories, you will create a positive caloric balance for that day—and if this becomes a pattern, you'll gain weight over the months and years. As you can see in figure 6.2, your RMR drops as you age—which

### HEALTHCHECK

**Why do metabolic rates change as we age?**

Our metabolic rates decrease as we age for several reasons. As we age, our bodies generally replace lean tissue (i.e., metabolically active tissue) with fat (i.e., less metabolically active tissue). Additionally, we generally become more sedentary as we age and the ultimate effect is that our RMR declines. Our metabolic rates decline because of the physiological and lifestyle changes we experience through the years.

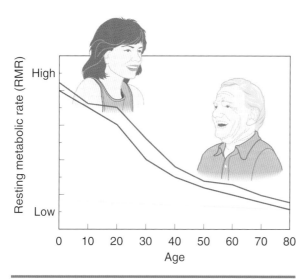

FIGURE 6.2 Relationship between resting metabolic rate (RMR) and age for males and females.

means that in order to not gain weight you'll have to consume less calories and be more physically active to burn the calories you do consume.

Another factor that affects metabolic rates is *thermogenesis*. This refers to the change in body temperature brought about by eating and by the body's attempt to maintain a healthy body temperature. Research continues to identify the role thermogenesis plays in obesity and weight control. Its role is probably minor compared to those of caloric intakes and expenditures and exercise.

## Physical Activity

As we said, physical activity should account for about 25% of your daily metabolic expenditure, so lifestyle physical activity and exercise are key factors in controlling weight. The best way to develop a negative caloric balance is to reduce calories and increase exercise. Numerous studies have shown that people who initiate a weight loss program through diet and exercise can maintain that weight loss if they continue their regimen of diet and exercise. However, those who lose weight through diet and exercise and then stop the exercise while continuing on their diet gain back most of the weight they lost.

People who repeatedly lose weight and then gain it back because of changes to their diet and

 The best way to develop a negative caloric balance is to reduce caloric intake and increase exercise and lifestyle physical activity.

exercise experience "weight cycling." This may happen in part because their diets and exercise regimens are too extreme and they can't maintain those patterns for long. Or people may simply lose motivation and slip back into less healthy lifestyle behaviors. Whatever the reason, this "yo-yoing" of weight may negatively affect their health. It may reduce their metabolic rate (thus reducing caloric needs), and it has been related to increased risk of heart disease and death.

Table 6.1 provides examples of caloric expenditures associated with a variety of activities (including some pretty sedentary ones for comparison). On the basis of your weight, you can determine how many calories you expend in 1 minute for each activity. Obviously, the more intensely you perform the activities, the more calories you'll expend. These values are rough estimates of the average caloric expenditures associated with the activities. In the lab at the end of this chapter, you'll see how a small amount of regular physical activity can impact your weight over the long term.

Compare the caloric expenditures in table 6.1 with the 100-calorie list in table 6.2. This list shows approximate amounts of foods that equal 100 calories (see the table on page 147 for more calorie values). You can see that in many cases it doesn't take much! That's another reason why exercise is so important in weight control. In the lab at the end of the chapter you'll learn more about how portion size can affect your weight.

## WEIGHT MANAGEMENT GUIDELINES

To avoid the yo-yo effect of losing and then regaining (or gaining and then losing) weight, you need to follow wise guidelines. There is no "quick fix" to losing or gaining weight. To effect a lasting change, you need to make lifestyle

## Table 6.1 Approximate Energy Expenditure for Selected Activities

| Activity | Calories per minute per kilogram* |
|---|---|
| Badminton | 0.097 |
| Baseball (except pitching) | 0.060 |
| Basketball | 0.138 |
| Billiards | 0.043 |
| Bowling | 0.094 |
| Canoeing (leisurely pace) | 0.045 |
| Card playing | 0.025 |
| Carpet sweeping | 0.046 |
| Circuit training | 0.185 |
| Cooking | 0.046 |
| Cycling | |
|   5.5 mph | 0.064 |
|   9.4 mph | 0.100 |
| Dancing | |
|   Aerobic (moderate) | 0.102 |
|   Modern | 0.072 |
| Eating | 0.023 |
| Field hockey | 0.138 |
| Fishing | 0.064 |
| Food shopping | 0.060 |
| Football | 0.132 |
| Frisbee | 0.100 |
| Gardening | 0.090 |
| Grass mowing | 0.112 |
| Golf | 0.085 |
| Ice hockey | 0.157 |
| Judo | 0.196 |
| Jumping rope | |
|   70 per minute | 0.162 |
|   125 per minute | 0.177 |
|   145 per minute | 0.198 |
| Karate | 0.202 |
| Lacrosse | 0.149 |
| Lying at ease | 0.022 |
| Mopping | 0.060 |
| Jogging 5.3 mph (11:30 minutes/mile) | 0.135 |
| Jogging 6.7 mph (9 minutes/mile) | 0.193 |
| Jogging 7.5 mph (8 minutes/mile) | 0.209 |
| Sitting quietly | 0.021 |
| Standing quietly | 0.026 |
| Tennis | 0.109 |
| Walking, normal pace | 0.080 |
| Writing (sitting) | 0.029 |

*Divide your weight in pounds by 2.2 to calculate your weight in kilograms.

Data from F.I. Katch and W.D. McArdle, 1983. *Nutrition, weight control, and exercise*, (Philadelphia: Lea & Febiger).

## Table 6.2 List of Approximately 100-Calorie Foods

| | |
|---|---|
| Almonds (salted) | 15 nuts |
| Apple | 1 medium size |
| Bacon | 2 strips |
| Banana | 1 medium size |
| Beans (fresh green) | 3 cups |
| Beer (light) | 12 oz |
| Bread (wheat) | 2 slices |
| Butter | 1 tbsp |
| Carrots (fresh) | 5 (6-in) |
| Chicken (fried) | 1.6 oz |
| Cornflakes | 1 cup |
| Cottage cheese (regular) | 1/2 cup |
| Fruit pie | 1/3 slice |
| Ham (boiled) | 1.6 oz |
| Ice cream | 1/3 cup |
| Ice cream (low fat) | 1/2 cup |
| Milk (whole) | 2/3 cup |
| Milk (low fat) | 1 cup |
| Peanuts (roasted) | 1/10 cup |
| Peas (fresh) | 8/10 cup |
| Pecans | 2 tbsp |
| Popcorn | 1 1/2 cups |
| Potato chips | 8-9 |
| Tomato | 3 medium size |

behavior changes in diet and exercise. If you want to lose weight, you need to have a negative caloric balance, expending more calories than you take in. If you want to gain weight, you need to take in more calories than you expend. But you need to undertake such a plan wisely, making sure you're providing your body proper nutrition. Otherwise you'll likely experience the yo-yo effect yourself.

Following are guidelines for managing your weight. We'll look at tips not only on how to lose weight, but also on how to *gain* weight (there are some people who want to gain weight, and who could derive health benefits from doing so).

## Effective Weight Loss Strategies

Losing weight isn't easy. Millions of people have lost weight only to gain it (and more) back, despite the $33 billion Americans spend annually on weight loss products and services. Therefore, you must consider effective strategies that will help you reduce body weight (actually, body fat) and keep it off. The first key to consider is that you must change your lifestyle behaviors if you expect to lose weight. Consider the lifestyle behaviors you can implement that will result in a negative caloric balance. Actually, there are only three:

1. Consuming fewer calories
2. Expending more calories
3. A combination of 1 and 2

Sounds simple! But what steps can *you* take to modify your lifestyle behaviors that will help you stick to your weight loss program? Let's classify these recommendations in three ways: psychological and behavioral, caloric intake, and caloric expenditure.

### Psychological and Behavioral Considerations

Make a commitment to yourself, set reasonable goals, and learn to reward yourself for progress. Remember—it may have taken you 10 years to put the weight on, so don't expect to lose it over the weekend. A reasonable and healthy goal is to lose 1 to 2 pounds (0.45 to 0.90 kilograms) per week.

Realize that you will have setbacks. However, consider the long-term goal that you have in mind. Minor setbacks should not cause you to stop seeking your long-term goal.

You'll be more likely to succeed if you set a moderate pace. Don't try to starve yourself to reach your target weight. Not only can this be dangerous to your health, it simply isn't a good long-term effective strategy for weight loss. Such methods lead to the yo-yo effect on your weight that we discussed earlier. As another part of pacing, don't check on your progress too often: don't weigh yourself daily. After setting your goal, follow your plan, and weigh yourself weekly at the same time of day and in the same type of clothing.

Make reinforcement a part of your plan. Reward yourself in a variety of ways when you reach specific goals. Perhaps a new outfit, shopping (walking, of course!), or an evening out on the town would be a good reward. Along the way, share your goals with close friends and family. They can encourage you and reinforce healthy behaviors.

### Caloric Intake

It will also help to have a plan for when, what, and how you eat. Set specific times for eating. Don't snack while watching TV or just talking with friends during the day. Make a conscious effort to avoid standing next to the food table at receptions. In general, plan meals ahead to help you identify healthier foods that contain less fat. When you prepare your own meals, cook foods in ways that reduce fat intake (e.g., broil, steam, or stir-fry meats and vegetables rather than frying them).

At mealtime, eat smaller amounts of healthy foods, and don't have second helpings on the table. Choose fruits and vegetables when possible. Eat slowly—put down your fork or spoon between bites and take a 2-minute break during the meal. When eating out, you don't have to empty your plate or eat all of the food prepared by the restaurant. Take some home for another meal to get your money's worth.

Finally, be prepared to counter tempting situations like the last piece of pie or just one more cookie. These cravings will occur, so prepare to face them and focus on your weight loss goal. If you must snack, choose low-fat foods or better yet, consider exercising or drinking a glass of water to fill your stomach.

### Caloric Expenditure

Look for ways to increase your caloric expenditure in your daily lifestyle behaviors. For example, leave your car farther out in the parking lot and take the stairs every day. Find reasons to take brief walks throughout the day. For example, personally deliver a note to a friend or colleague who is working two floors below you (and take the stairs!) rather than sending an e-mail or using the phone.

## "Quick Fixes" in Weight Loss: Fad Diets, Cellulite, and Spot Reduction

A new (or recycled) fad diet seems to pop up every few weeks—at least according to the supermarket tabloids. Fad diets vary greatly in their approach, but they all have two things in common. One, they deprive the body of essential nutrients; two, they don't work.

They may "work" for the short haul—that is, a starvation diet or a very low calorie diet may result in a rapid loss of water weight and lean protein tissue—but when any type of "normal" diet is resumed, the weight returns. The danger with very low calorie or fad diets is that they use body fat for energy as desired but also, if followed for too long, they cause the body to use protein and lean tissue from the liver, heart, muscles, and blood for energy. This can lead to serious—and even fatal—health problems.

Two other topics that are often targeted for quick fixes are *cellulite* and *spot reduction*. Cellulite is advertised as a special type of fat on the thighs and backs of arms, where the fat can be seen to "ripple." Advertisers sell special equipment, medications, and diets to "attack" the cellulite—to no avail. The best attack is a healthy diet and physical activity to cause a negative caloric balance. This will result in decreased overall body fat.

Which brings us to the next topic: spot reduction. People can't reduce fat where they want to—they can't target the fat on their thighs or the backs of their arms! They can only lose fat overall. People who want to "spot reduce" perform exercises for, say, the hips and stomach; but research shows that this doesn't work. In one study, people performed over 5,000 sit-ups in 27 days. They had fat biopsied from three different sites on their bodies before and after the sit-up regimen; the change in fat cells was the same in all three sites. Exercise can help reduce fat, but exercise is blind—it doesn't know where it's taking the fat from!

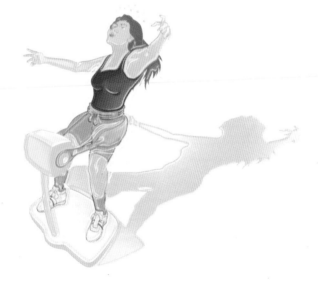

Determine a specific time of day when it is good for you to work exercise into your daily routine. Consider how much time you waste sitting around. For example, try taking a brief walk every day after lunch. Focus on your goal and work toward taking steps to meet your goal. To maintain a long-term negative caloric balance, try to exercise five to seven days per week for 20 to 60 minutes.

Remember that people engage in physical activity for a variety of reasons but the end result in all cases is that they become healthier. Some enjoy the social aspects; if that fits you, find someone to walk with you. Others enjoy the aesthetic aspects of activity; if that sounds more like you, take a walk through a park, or any setting you find appealing.

## HEALTHCHECK

**I tend to limit my calories pretty well throughout the day, but then at night I often just "lose it" and eat whatever I want—nachos, ice cream, chips, or whatever's there. Do I just need more willpower in order to lose weight?**

No, you need a better plan. Limiting calories too much during the day usually results in mild bingeing at the end of the day. It's much better to eat in moderation throughout the day—up to six smaller meals (rather than the "three square meals" approach, or the mild starvation/bingeing approach that you describe). Several smaller meals is easier on your digestion system and is less likely to result in the unhealthy bingeing, which is typically high in both calorie and fat intake.

## POINT OF INTEREST

### Fen-Phen: A Big No-No

Fen-Phen (a combination of fenfluramine and phentermine) became available on the American market in the early 1980s as a way to combat obesity. Fenfluramine (which goes by the brand name Pondimin) is a sympathomimetic amine, meaning it produces central nervous system depression and a feeling of satiation (thus acting as an appetite suppressant). Its side effects include depression, diarrhea, nausea, impotence, and drowsiness. Phentermine is also a sympathomimetic amine; it acts like an amphetamine, increasing metabolism. It can cause nervousness, dizziness, and insomnia. Fenfluramine was combined with phentermine to decrease the unwanted side effects of the latter.

The use of Fen-Phen escalated greatly in the early and mid-1990s after Michael Weintraub, a former pharmacologist at the University of Rochester, published a series of articles in 1992 extolling the benefits of Fen-Phen based on a series of studies that found no adverse effects among people who had taken Fen-Phen for more than three years.

Unfortunately, these studies didn't tell the real story: in 1997, Fen-Phen was pulled off the market by the Food and Drug Administration because it was found not only to cause weight loss, but also to carry the high risks of primary pulmonary hypertension (an often fatal condition), valvular heart disease (occurring when one of the four heart valves is damaged and cannot open properly or does not close all the way, resulting in blood leaking backward, leading to severe heart or lung complications), and permanent brain damage (by altering the brain's neurotransmission process). The link between Fen-Phen, Pondimin, and valvular heart disease is what prompted the Food and Drug Administration to pull Fen-Phen and Pondimin off the market. But not before the drugs caused extensive damage among the estimated 20 million people who used them in hopes of losing weight.

The moral to the story is quite simple: there is no shortcut to losing weight, there is no quick fix. A sound diet and regular, physician-approved physical activity is the real answer.

**KEY POINT** To lose weight, you must expend more calories than you consume. You can do this by consuming fewer calories, expending more calories, or a combination of the two.

## Gaining Weight the Healthy Way

While our discussion has focused primarily on weight control or weight reduction, there are some who will want to gain weight and to do so without becoming overweight. Here again, the issue is one of caloric balance. If you want to gain weight, do it carefully so that you gain lean weight and don't simply add fat weight.

Obviously, one way to increase caloric balance is to eat more. However, this can result in gaining fat unless you take the steps to ensure that the increased weight is added as lean tissue. The best way to gain weight is to increase your caloric intake through healthy foods, and continue to exercise. You should also consider increasing the amount of strength training you do—increased caloric intake with increased weight training will result in lean weight gain.

Some people think that a special potion is needed to help you gain weight (for example, high-protein diets, special foods, medications, or vitamins). This simply is not true. Eating a well-balanced diet and increasing your level of training result in weight gain, as long as your caloric intake exceeds the caloric expenditure.

A safe goal for weight gain is about 1 pound (0.45 kilograms) per week. Since muscle tissue

---

### Disordered Eating

*Bulimia* and *anorexia nervosa* are eating disorders that are fueled by our cultural obsession to be thin. Bulimia involves bingeing and purging; anorexia nervosa is a form of starvation that can result in lean body tissue loss and a multitude of health problems—and in severe cases it can be fatal. Both disorders are predominantly found in females; about 95% of those who suffer from anorexia nervosa are female. The American Psychiatric Association estimates that about 500,000 individuals have disordered eating habits, which means about 1% to 4% of all adolescents and young adults. The annual death rate from eating disorders in the United States is almost 4,000.

Although bulimia is the more common of the two disorders, the onset of bulimic behaviors usually occurs later in life than that of anorexic behaviors. About 14% of high school girls have forced themselves to vomit in an attempt to lose or maintain weight. (About 4% of boys have done likewise.) Bulimic behaviors usually begin to surface around the ages of 16 to 20. Behaviors include using laxatives, stringently modifying diets, and exercising excessively to counteract caloric intake.

Symptoms of anorexia nervosa include "starvation" eating; obsessive exercise; calorie and fat gram counting; an extreme fascination with food and health; self-induced vomiting; use of laxatives, diuretics, or diet pills; and constant concern with body image.

Disordered eating has genetic, environmental, and psychological components that require immediate expert medical evaluation and treatment.

contains less fat and more water than other tissue, it takes about 2,500 calories to gain a pound of lean tissue. Thus, a positive caloric balance of approximately 400-500 calories per day, coupled with an appropriate strength-training program, should result in healthy lean weight gain.

As with losing weight, it is important to set reasonable goals, make lifestyle behavior changes that will influence your weight, follow your exercise program regularly, and monitor your weight gain weekly.

 **KEY POINT** To gain about 1 pound (0.45 kilograms) per week, eat about 400-500 more calories per day than you expend, and continue to exercise regularly and include weight training to ensure that the gain is in lean weight.

## HEALTHCHECK

**I'm trying to gain weight but apparently have trouble eating more calories than I expend. I don't really want to eat a lot of junk food, but it has more calories than other foods. Is it okay to increase calories through junk food?**

It's much better to increase caloric intake through foods that offer good nutrition—fruits, vegetables, cereals and grains, dairy products, and nuts and meats. Focus on these foods, and try to incorporate healthy snacking throughout the day to increase your calories.

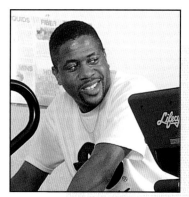

## Health Concepts

At the beginning of the chapter, we met Jarrod, who had briefly tried a diet and had initial success, only to gain the weight back as soon as he went off the diet. Jarrod is physically active, but he's been paying attention to only one aspect of weight control, without taking nutrition into account.

Jarrod's weight will likely continue to yo-yo if he tries fad diets. Permanent weight loss comes through lifestyle behavioral diet and exercise changes, not through a quick-fix program. Weight loss hinges on whether your caloric balance is negative or positive. A positive balance means you take in more calories than you expend, and you gain weight; a negative balance means you expend more calories than you consume, and you lose weight. It's that simple.

## SUMMARY

▌ The way to lose weight is to establish a negative caloric balance, which occurs when you expend more calories than you take in. Combining good nutrition and exercise along with a negative caloric balance will help you lose weight in a safe and healthy fashion. Permanent weight loss is attained by changing lifestyle eating and exercising behaviors, not by adhering to a quick-fix diet for a short time.

▌ The way to *gain* weight is to establish a positive caloric balance—taking in more calories than you expend. As with weight loss, you should adhere to good nutrition principles and exercise while gaining weight. High-protein diets, special foods, medications, or vitamins are not necessary to help you gain weight.

▌ Metabolism affects weight gain and loss. The higher your metabolic rate, the quicker you "burn" calories. Your basal metabolic rate depends on your age, gender, body size, metabolic functions, and body characteristics.

▌ Physical activity is a key component to weight loss.

▌ *Bulimia* and *anorexia nervosa* are eating disorders that are fueled by our cultural obsession to be thin. Bulimia involves bingeing and purging; anorexia nervosa is a form of starvation that can result in lean body tissue loss and a multitude of health problems—and in severe cases it can be fatal.

*You've now learned how to manage your weight. Just as exercise is an important facet of weight management, it plays an important role in the next topic we'll look at: physical activity and cardiovascular disease.*

## KEY TERMS

| | |
|---|---|
| anorexia nervosa | overfat |
| basal metabolic rate (BMR) | resting metabolic rate (RMR) |
| bulimia | spot reduction |
| caloric balance | thermogenesis |
| cellulite | |

# 6

# Determining the Effect of Physical Activity on Weight

**THE PURPOSE OF THIS LAB EXPERIENCE IS TO**

▌help you determine how a little change in physical activity or diet can have a long-term effect on your weight.

**1.** Determine your weight in kilograms by dividing your weight in pounds by 2.2. Now let's consider the year-long effects of watching television (i.e., sitting quietly) or taking a half-hour walk each day. Use the values from table 6.1 to determine how many calories are expended during various activities. The numbers below are illustrative of a 220-pound person.

220 pounds / 2.2 = 100 kilograms (kg)

Sitting caloric expenditure for one year is
100 kg × 30 minutes × 0.021 calories × 365 days = 22,995 calories per year

Walking caloric expenditure for one year is
100 kg × 30 minutes × 0.080 calories × 365 days = 87,600 calories per year

Note that the caloric difference is 64,605 calories; 64,605 / 3,500 (the number of calories needed to lose 1 pound of fat) = 18.46 pounds weight difference per year.

Now make these calculations for your weight, choosing different activities and intensities. Note the impact that as little as 30 minutes of activity per day can have on your weight change in one year.

**2.** Now let's look at the other component of weight control, caloric intake. Use table 6.2 to determine the effects of increasing the size of the portion of food that you eat in a meal. Assume your meal consists of the following:

|  | **Calories** |
|---|---|
| 1/2 cup cottage cheese | 100 |
| 1 cup of fresh green beans | 33 |
| 1 slice of wheat bread | 50 |
| 1 tablespoon of butter | 100 |
| 1.6 oz boiled ham | 100 |
| Fruit pie (1/3 of a slice) | 100 |
| 1/2 cup low-fat ice cream | 100 |
| 1-12 oz beer (light) | 100 |
| **Total calories consumed:** | **683** |

Note that this meal is rather small. Now consider that you probably could have easily doubled each of the portion sizes. If you had, the total caloric intake would have increased to 1,366 calories. If you ate twice the portion size each day, the weekly caloric intake for this meal would be 9,562 calories (or approximately 2.73 pounds of added weight per week). This example, of course, suggests that you aren't engaging in any additional physical activity to reduce this positive caloric balance. Extrapolate this for a month and then a year, and you'll see that small increases in portion sizes have a great long-term effect on body weight.

Choose some foods you normally eat from table 6.2. Consider the portion sizes you typically eat of these foods and then adjust them up and down to see the long-term effects of portion size on your weight.

# Part III

# Physical Activity and Health

As you learned in part I, modern medicine has dramatically affected the diseases that lead to morbidity and mortality. However, no amount of medicine can "cure all our ills." In part III you'll learn about the chronic and deadly diseases that still affect our population. You'll discover the positive effects that good nutrition and physical activity can have on these diseases. You'll also examine the role of physical activity in childbearing.

In chapter 7, you'll examine the nation's number one killer, cardiovascular disease, exploring ways to prevent the disease and the impact physical activity has on it. Chapter 8 explores the effects of physical activity on musculoskeletal health. You'll examine osteoporosis, low back pain, arthritis, and soft tissue injuries. In chapter 9, you'll learn about the number two killer, cancer, as well as diabetes, which affects almost 16 million Americans. You'll explore risk factors and ways to lessen your risks of getting cancer and diabetes, as well as learning about the effect physical activity has on these diseases. Chapter 10 reveals how long and hard women can exercise while maintaining a healthy pregnancy and presents safe physical activities for pregnant women, as well as exploring the benefits of exercise during pregnancy. Chapter 11 delineates the effects of physical activity on mental health and looks into the origins of depression: is it a "state of mind," or does it have a neurological or physiological basis? In this chapter you'll also learn about the effects of stress on your body. In all, part III will help you take charge of your lifestyle through good nutrition and physical activity, thus lowering your risk of disease while improving your quality of life.

# Chapter 7

# Cardiovascular Disease

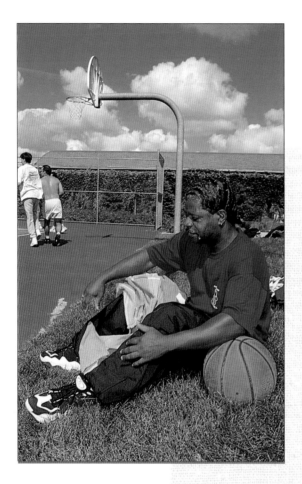

I was playing basketball the other day when my chest started to feel real tight. It was hard to take in a full breath of air because it was so painful. The sharpness only lasted a few minutes, but I still felt some tightness for about half an hour before it finally felt okay again. That was the first time I'd ever had anything like that happen.

We don't have any family history of heart problems, and I've always been in pretty decent shape. I played basketball in high school, though that was a long time ago. I do still play a lot of pick-up games. But I've heard of guys who were in real good shape and then they collapsed on the court with some kind of heart problem or other. I wonder if exercise can actually bring on a heart attack. I'm not sure if the chest pains I felt were some type of warning or not. Could I possibly be at risk for some type of heart disease?

—Mark, 42-year-old junior

## *W*hat do you think*?*

Does Mark have reason to be concerned? His family doesn't have a history of heart disease, and he's always been active. But what about those athletes who were in apparently fine physical shape, only to collapse on the court with some type of heart disease? Should Mark get checked out or should he just continue playing pick-up games and monitor how he feels? If he *does* have heart disease, does his being physically active hurt him or help him?

In this chapter we'll look at cardiovascular disease (including coronary heart disease and stroke), which is the leading cause of death in the United States. We'll explore the causes and risk factors of the disease and distinguish between the factors we *can't* change (such as age and heredity) and the ones we *can* change. We'll look at ways to prevent cardiovascular disease by working on the factors that we can change. And within those risk factors, we'll examine how physical activity affects the disease.

## CARDIOVASCULAR DISEASE

Cardiovascular disease accounts for nearly half of the deaths in this country. For every person who dies of cancer (see chapter 9), almost 2 people die of cardiovascular disease. According to the American Heart Association (1998), more than 58 million Americans have some form of cardiovascular disease. It's estimated that cardiovascular disease cost the nation more than $274 billion in treatment and lost productivity in 1998.

That's the downside. The upside is that the incidence of cardiovascular disease has actually decreased by 36% in the last two decades, and the death rate from cardiovascular disease has dropped by more than 25% in the last 10 years. This decline is due in part to an increased awareness about the risk factors of cardiovascular disease, which has prompted some people to change lifestyle behaviors to lessen their risk of developing the disease. These lifestyle behaviors in-

clude not smoking, getting regular exercise, eating well, maintaining a healthy body weight, and managing stress. In addition, better diagnostic procedures have led to earlier detection, and advances in medical technology have saved lives through improved heart transplants and artificial heart devices.

**KEY POINT**

Your risk of developing cardiovascular disease is reduced when you don't smoke, get regular exercise, eat well, maintain a healthy body weight, and manage stress.

## THE CARDIOVASCULAR SYSTEM

The heart is a truly amazing organ. It carries out its function continuously, even at "rest" contracting 60 or more times a minute for most adults; a functioning heart pumps the equivalent of 2,000 gallons of blood a day through 100,000 contractions. That is the sole function of the heart: to pump blood throughout the body. A person weighing 150 pounds has about 5 liters of blood, which circulates through the body about once every minute.

The heart has four chambers: right and left *atriums* and right and left *ventricles* (see figure 7.1). Blood that is low in oxygen and high in carbon dioxide enters the right atrium. As the heart contracts, the blood is pumped from the right atrium into the right ventricle. (The period of contraction is called *systole;* the period of relaxation is called *diastole.*) The blood is then pumped into the *pulmonary artery* and goes through the lungs, where the carbon dioxide is removed and oxygen is supplied. It then enters the *pulmonary vein* and reenters the heart through the left atrium. From the left atrium the blood is pumped into the left ventricle, which is the strongest chamber of this muscular pump. From here it is pumped through the *aorta,* the body's largest artery; from the aorta it will go through the arteries and then through the blood vessels. Blood flow is controlled by a synchronized set of contractions regulated by the heart's pacemaker, the *sinoatrial node,* and by four heart valves that force the blood to flow in the proper direction.

While the heart is the primary organ of the circulatory system, the lungs are also part of this system. As already mentioned, the lungs move oxygen into the blood and carbon dioxide out of the blood. The circulatory system includes arteries, which carry blood away from the heart, and veins, which transport blood back to the heart (see figure 7.1). Arteries are widest in diameter when they are nearest the heart; they narrow to *arterioles* (small arteries), which in turn narrow

to *capillaries* (extremely small blood vessels). It is through the capillaries that oxygen moves from the blood to the body's cells and carbon dioxide moves from the body's cells to the blood. These capillaries widen to form *venules* (small veins) and widen further to form veins, through which the blood returns to the heart to repeat the cycle.

## TYPES OF CARDIOVASCULAR DISEASES AND CONDITIONS

Many people may translate "cardiovascular disease" as heart disease leading to a heart attack. This is one type of cardiovascular disease, but there are in fact a number of distinct diseases that have been identified and that are targeted for prevention or treatment. These diseases include

- heart attack,
- atherosclerosis,
- angina pectoris,
- arrhythmias,
- congenital heart defects,

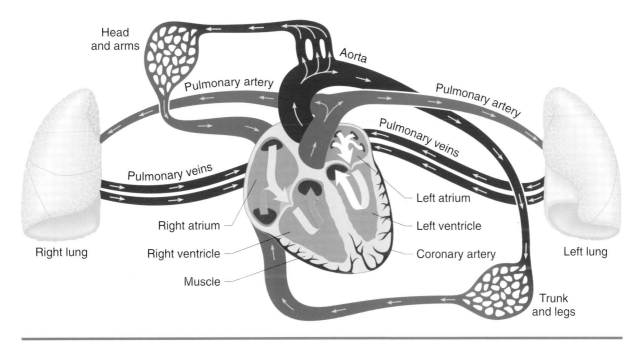

**FIGURE 7.1** Anatomy of the heart and circulatory system.

- rheumatic heart disease,
- congestive heart failure,
- bacterial endocarditis,
- aneurysms,
- hypertension, and
- stroke.

## Heart Attack

The classic heart attack is called *coronary thrombosis* or *myocardial infarction*. Coronary heart disease (CHD) is the most common form of cardiovascular disease leading to a heart attack. An attack occurs when blood flow to a portion of the heart is blocked in one of the coronary arteries. See figure 7.2 for three examples of blockage. The heart tissues below the point of blockage in the arterial blood flow will not receive blood and oxygen. The heart muscle cells can suffer irreversible damage if the blood supply is not quickly restored through treatment. Depending on the location and treatment of the blockage, damage to the heart can be relatively minor, major, or fatal. If a large area of the heart is deprived of oxygen, it may stop, resulting in death. Even if the blood supply is restored, the

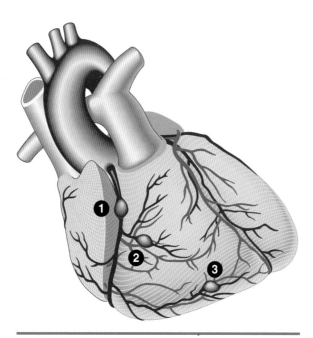

**FIGURE 7.2** Blood flow blockage in the coronary arteries leads to heart attacks.

**HEALTHCHECK**

**Look again at figure 7.2. Which of the three locations represents the most serious heart attack?**

The first location is the most serious, because blockage occurs further up the arterial tree and more heart tissue will be deprived of blood and oxygen.

heart has been damaged and the functional capacity will be lower.

Many people receive no signs of an impending heart attack, but some people are forewarned by

- uncomfortable pressure, fullness, squeezing, or pain in the center of the chest that lasts 2 minutes or longer;
- pain that spreads to the shoulders, neck, or arms; or
- severe pain, dizziness, fainting, sweating, nausea, or shortness of breath.

The person feeling any of these signs should get help immediately.

 **KEY POINT** Warning signs of a heart attack include uncomfortable pressure or pain in the center of the chest that lasts 2 minutes or longer; pain that spreads to the shoulders, neck, or arms; or severe pain, dizziness, fainting, sweating, nausea, or shortness of breath. If you experience any of these signs you should seek medical help immediately.

## Atherosclerosis

Coronary artery blockages, which, as just described, can lead to heart attacks, usually develop through a process called *atherosclerosis*. As plaque builds on the internal walls, or *intima*, of the arteries, the arterial opening gradually narrows and hardens (see figure 7.3). Plaque is made of fatty substances, cholesterol, cellular waste products, calcium, and fibrin (a clotting material in the blood). As these deposits form in the arteries, the arteries lose their elasticity and begin to restrict blood flow. As atherosclerosis develops, arteries become more vulnerable to being blocked by blood clots and pieces of the plaque that break loose.

Atherosclerosis is a slow-developing disease that may begin for many in childhood and continue through adulthood. Blockage of a coronary artery can lead to a heart attack; blockage of a cerebral artery can lead to a stroke.

## Angina Pectoris

Blockage of a coronary artery can also lead to *angina pectoris,* which is marked by chest pain due to lack of oxygen to the heart. The oxygen deficiency isn't enough to cause a heart attack; the heart is receiving some oxygen, but not enough, and this is what causes the pain. A person might experience *angina* before having a heart attack; angina certainly signals a high risk for a heart attack. Not all people who have angina pectoris go on to experience a heart attack, however. And not all heart attacks are preceded by an "angina attack."

## Arrhythmias

An *arrhythmia* is an abnormal heartbeat caused by a breakdown of the heart's electronic impulses. As with angina, an arrhythmia is another sign that a heart attack could occur, although not all arrhythmias are life-threatening. Sometimes an arrhythmia can be triggered by too much caffeine or nicotine consumption; cocaine usage can also trigger this condition. Arrhythmias are defined as *bradycardia* (heartbeat too slow); *tachycardia* (heartbeat too fast); or *fibrillation* (heartbeat fluttering sporadically). All arrhythmias cause the heart to pump blood inefficiently and at a low volume. If the blood flow becomes too low, tissues and organs throughout the body will not function correctly and death can result.

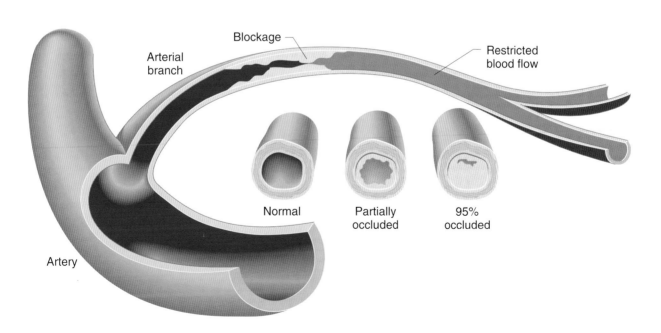

**FIGURE 7.3** Development of atherosclerosis.

Adapted from J. Wilmore, 1986, *Sensible fitness* (Champaign, IL: Human Kinetics), 6.

## Congenital Heart Defects

A *congenital heart defect* occurs when the heart or blood vessels near the heart weren't developed normally by the time a baby was born, and blood flow to the heart is abnormal. Congenital heart defects can range from slight heart murmurs caused by irregular valves to more serious dysfunctions that may require surgery.

## Rheumatic Heart Disease

*Rheumatic heart disease* is caused by a bacterial infection that produces high fever (rheumatic fever) and inflammation that damages the heart valves. This bacterial infection begins as strep throat and if untreated can lead to rheumatic fever. Anyone can contract this infection, but it is most common in children from ages 5 to 15, resulting in over 5,000 deaths per year in the United States. This disease can cause problems that are similar to those caused by congenital heart defects.

## Congestive Heart Failure

*Congestive heart failure* is a condition that occurs when other specific heart diseases have damaged the heart to such a degree that it can no longer properly function. Heart muscles weakened by rheumatic fever, pneumonia, or other cardiovascular problems don't respond well to stress, and blood begins to pool in the heart and in other body areas, such as the legs and ankles. The heart enlarges from the pooled blood, and the amount of blood that can be circulated decreases. Congestive heart failure can be fatal if not treated.

## Bacterial Endocarditis

*Bacterial endocarditis* comes from a direct bacterial infection of the heart valves or lining of the heart. It can cause permanent damage to the heart. This infection usually occurs in people with damaged or abnormal heart tissue; people with normal hearts rarely have this disease.

## Aneurysms

An *aneurysm* occurs when a coronary artery is weakened and begins to bulge. Aneurysms can also occur in the brain and other parts of the body. In extreme cases an aneurysm can burst, causing internal bleeding and a lack of blood flow to the heart or brain. High blood pressure increases the risk of an aneurysm.

## Hypertension

*Hypertension* is a condition that occurs when a person's blood pressure is continuously abnormally high. An occasional reading of high blood pressure doesn't indicate hypertension, but if an adult's blood pressure is continuously equal to or greater than 140 over 90, that person has hypertension. Both values are measured in millimeters of mercury (mm Hg). The 140 refers to the *systolic blood pressure* when the heart is contracting; the 90 refers to the *diastolic blood pressure* when the heart is relaxing. High blood pressure is often associated with excess weight and with hardening of the arteries (arteriosclerosis). High blood pressure speeds the process of arteriosclerosis, because the heart has to pump harder to get the blood through the arteries, placing the arteries under greater strain than normal. Hypertension can damage vital organs and increase the risk of failure of the heart and kidneys. It is also a primary risk factor for stroke.

 Blood pressure of 140/90 or higher indicates hypertension, which can damage vital organs and increase the risks of heart or kidney failure or stroke. People with hypertension need to seek medical assistance in treating the disease.

## Stroke

A *stroke* or "brain attack"—caused by a lack of blood flow to the brain—is the third leading cause of death in the United States. A *cerebral thrombosis* occurs when atherosclerosis blocks blood flow in the cerebral artery. A *cerebral hemorrhage* happens when an artery within the brain bursts because of a weak spot (an aneurysm) in the arterial wall or because of a head injury. About 500,000 Americans have strokes each year. Of these, about one-third die within a year. Those who survive may suffer a variety of impairments, including paralysis, lack of muscular control, and loss of speech or of short- and long-term memory.

The severity of a stroke depends on the amount of brain tissue that is deprived of blood flow. Brain cells can die after several minutes of being oxygen-deprived. These brain cells can't be replaced; the parts of the body that were controlled by the dead brain cells are permanently affected.

Warning signs for a stroke include

- sudden weakness or numbness of the face, arm, or leg on one side of the body;

- sudden dimness or loss of vision, particularly in one eye;

- loss of speech, or trouble talking or understanding speech;

- sudden severe headaches with no known cause; and

- unexplained dizziness, unsteadiness, or sudden falls, especially if experienced with any of the other symptoms.

Warning signs for a stroke include sudden weakness or numbness of the face, arm, or leg on one side of the body; sudden dimness or loss of vision, particularly in one eye; loss of speech, or trouble talking or understanding speech; sudden severe headaches with no known cause; and unexplained dizziness, unsteadiness, or sudden falls.

## RISK FACTORS FOR CORONARY HEART DISEASE AND STROKE

The American Heart Association has identified several risk factors for CHD and stroke. The following section provides an overview of those risk factors.

## Major Risk Factors for Coronary Heart Disease

*Epidemiology* is the study of the incidence and distribution of diseases, injuries, and accidents in human populations, and epidemiological research uncovers risk factors for specific diseases. *Risk factors* are variables that are associated with an increased risk or probability that someone may develop morbidity (illness) or incur mortality (death) from a specific disease. For example, if you smoke you have an elevated risk or probability of illness or death from CHD. Major risk factors are those that medical research has shown to definitely be associated with a significant increase in the risk of developing morbidity or incurring mortality from a specific disease. Major risk factors for CHD include factors that can't be altered and factors that can. We'll look first at unalterable factors.

### Unalterable Risk Factors for Coronary Heart Disease

There are three major risk factors for CHD that you *can't* do anything about: your heredity (including race), your gender, and your age. We'll take a brief look at each.

*Heredity.* Those with a family history of CHD are more likely to develop a cardiovascular disease than those with no such family history. A family history and increased risk are indicated by CHD in a father or brother who is less than 55 years old or in a mother or sister who is less than 65 years old. This genetic link to CHD includes racial differences. Distinct trends indicate that certain races are more predisposed to developing cardiovascular disease than others. African-Americans and Hispanics are more likely to have high blood pressure than Caucasians, leading to greater chances of heart disease. In fact, African-American men are 49% more likely to die from cardiovascular disease than Caucasian men. Asian-Americans have lower rates of CHD than Caucasians because they have lower prevalences for CHD risk factors.

*Gender.* Men are at greater risk of CHD than women, especially through middle age. Women's estrogen levels help prevent CHD; once estrogen levels drop (e.g., through menopause or a hysterectomy), their risk increases. Women under 35 have a very low risk of cardiovascular disease unless they have some complicating factors such as kidney problems or diabetes.

*Age.* The older we get, the more likely we are to develop CHD. The risk of heart attack increases dramatically after age 65 (three out of four people who have a heart attack are age 65 or older).

### Alterable Risk Factors for Coronary Heart Disease

There are six major risk factors for CHD that you *can* do something about. These factors include high blood pressure, high blood cholesterol, smoking, diabetes, obesity, and physical inactivity. These risk factors and the factors previously mentioned that we can't change (heredity, gender, and age) are grouped into two categories of risk: *major risk factors* and *contributing risk factors* (see table 7.1). As you read through the following sections, consider which factors are present in your life and how you can

take steps to make those factors less of a risk. In Lab 7 you'll be evaluating your own risk of heart attack.

*High Blood Pressure.* Blood pressure is the force exerted by the blood flow through the arteries and arterioles (small arteries) of the cardiovascular system. Blood pressure is a function of the force of the heart as it pumps blood and the resistance of the arteries to blood flow. Arteries have a muscular media that can be contracted (narrowing the artery) to increase resistance, increase blood pressure, and lower blood flow. The muscular media can also be relaxed (opening the artery) to decrease resistance and blood pressure and increase blood flow. When functioning well, the cardiovascular system maintains a normal blood pressure with appropriate blood flow to areas of the body as it is needed.

### Table 7.1  Risk Factors for Coronary Heart Disease

| Major alterable | Major unalterable | Contributing |
|---|---|---|
| Hypertension | Age | Stress |
| Tobacco smoking | Genetics | |
| Cholesterol | Gender | |
| Physical inactivity | | |
| Obesity | | |
| Diabetes | | |

### HEALTHCHECK

**My dad takes an aspirin every day to lower his risk for heart disease. Does this really work?**

Regular use of aspirin can help prevent CHD; people who have never had a heart attack can lower their risk of having one by taking aspirin regularly. Aspirin can also lower the risk of further heart attacks for those who have had one already. However, people with liver and kidney disease, ulcers, or bleeding problems should not take aspirin.

The American Heart Association defines optimal blood pressure as 120 or less (systolic) over 80 or less (diastolic). They classify other blood pressure readings as follows:

**Normal:** < 130/< 85

**High normal:** 130-139/85-89

**Stage 1 hypertension (mild):** 140-159/90-99

**Stage 2 hypertension (moderate):** 160-179/100-109

**Stage 3 hypertension (severe):** ≥180/≥110

*Hypotension,* or low blood pressure, is also a concern, but is much less common than hypertension. Even people with very low blood pressure readings, such as 90/50, are healthy so long as they aren't experiencing any hypotension symptoms such as dizziness or fainting.

According to the American Heart Association, nearly 50 million Americans have hypertension. Hypertension is known as the "silent killer" because people don't feel sick from it and many don't know they have it. High blood pressure can lead to a variety of cardiovascular diseases, including heart disease, congestive heart failure, and stroke. (It is a major risk factor for stroke.) It scars and hardens the arteries, hurrying the process of atherosclerosis, and can also lead to kidney failure.

Ways to reduce blood pressure include

- reducing sodium and fat in the diet;
- improving cardiovascular endurance by being more physically active;
- for people who are obese, losing excess weight; and
- undergoing "antihypertensive" drug therapy (especially when the other methods haven't produced the desired results).

Of special note: Women who use oral contraceptives have a higher risk for developing hypertension, and women with normal blood pressure may develop high blood pressure during pregnancy. Pregnant women may develop hypertension if they are overweight, have a family

## HEALTHCHECK

### I have a lot of sodium in my diet. Does that mean I'll develop high blood pressure?

Not necessarily. Some people can consume a lot of sodium but are not "salt sensitive" and do not retain excess fluids and develop high blood pressure. However, some people are sensitive to sodium, and a high intake will contribute to the development of high blood pressure while also negatively affecting those who are already hypertensive. Remember, many processed foods are high in sodium. The American Heart Association recommends that healthy adults consume a maximum of 2,400 milligrams of sodium per day. That's equivalent to 1 1/4 teaspoons of salt per day.

history of high blood pressure, or have kidney disease. (Typically this hypertension goes away after the woman gives birth.) Finally, African-Americans and Hispanics have a higher prevalence of high blood pressure than Caucasians and should be especially aware of their blood pressure and of methods to lower it if it is high.

Hypertension is known as the "silent killer" because many people don't know they have it. Have your blood pressure checked regularly by qualified professionals and take measures to lower it if it's high.

***High Blood Cholesterol.*** As described in chapter 5, blood *cholesterol* is a fatlike substance found in the body's cells and bloodstream. You need a certain amount of cholesterol in order for your body to function normally; it helps form cell membranes, hormones, and other substances. The human body produces about 1,000 milligrams of cholesterol a day, primarily through the liver; we also consume cholesterol through our diet (perhaps 400 to 500 milligrams a day). When cholesterol levels are too high, our risk for developing CHD increases.

The liver produces two types of *lipoproteins,* which transport cholesterol in the blood: *high density lipoproteins (HDL)* and *low density lipoproteins (LDL).* These lipoproteins combine with cholesterol to form HDL-C and LDL-C (the "C" stands for "cholesterol"); HDL-C and LDL-C, along with other cholesterol in our body, form our total cholesterol in the bloodstream. HDL-C is called the "good" cholesterol because it transports cholesterol through the bloodstream to the liver for further metabolism or excretion. LDL-C is the "bad" cholesterol because not all of it is transported and metabolized or excreted; high levels of LDL-C hasten the process of atherosclerosis. LDL-C is more likely than HDL-C to become part of the plaque deposits on arterial walls.

The American Heart Association and the National Heart, Lung, and Blood Institute have established these standards for total cholesterol and LDL-C levels:

### Total Cholesterol

*Desirable:* less than 200 milligrams per deciliter of blood

*Borderline high:* between 200 and 239 milligrams per deciliter

*High:* 240 milligrams per deciliter or higher

### Low Density Lipoprotein-Cholesterol

*Desirable:* less than 130 milligrams per deciliter of blood

*Borderline high:* between 130 and 159 milligrams per deciliter

*High:* 160 milligrams per deciliter or higher

An HDL-C level of 35 milligrams per deciliter or lower is considered low. A low level of HDL-C is also considered a risk because this is the "good" cholesterol.

As we age, our total cholesterol levels tend to increase. The American Heart Association recommends that Americans under age 19 have a total cholesterol level of less than 170 milligrams per deciliter. See figure 7.4 for an estimation of the number of Americans who have high total cholesterol levels.

The ratio of total cholesterol to HDL-C is important to note. A person with a total cholesterol

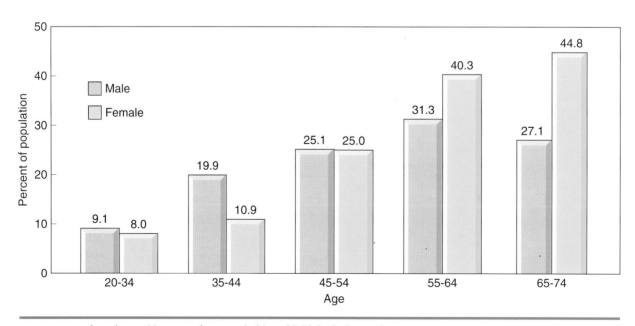

**FIGURE 7.4** Americans 20 years of age and older with high cholesterol.

Data from National Health and Nutrition Examination Survey (NHANES) III, National Centers for Health Statistics 1996.

count of 180 and an HDL-C count of 40 has a ratio of 4.5 (180/40). Average cholesterol ratios are about 4.5 for females and 5.0 for males. Males and females with ratios below 3.5 have only about half the risk of cardiovascular disease that people with the average ratio have. Figure 7.5 shows the risk of CHD in relation to differing cholesterol ratios. Again, your total cholesterol level might appear to be acceptable, but your HDL-C level is the critical figure used in the ratio formula to determine risk. The higher your HDL-C, the lower your cholesterol ratio.

Diet and physical activity are key factors in lowering total cholesterol and elevating HDL-C. People with dangerously high levels of total cholesterol or low levels of HDL-C may require drug therapy.

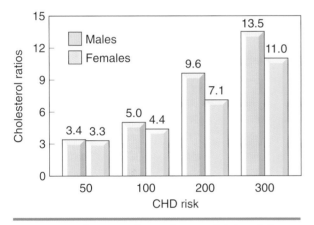

**FIGURE 7.5** Coronary heart disease risk in relation to cholesterol ratios.

Data from National Heart, Lung, and Blood Institute 1998.

 Your total cholesterol level should be below 200 milligrams per deciliter of blood. Your LDL-C count should be less than 130 milligrams per deciliter. It's desirable that your ratio of total cholesterol to HDL-C be 3.5 or less.

While not a major risk factor for CHD, *triglycerides* are another form of fat in the bloodstream. High triglyceride levels increase the risk of CHD, especially in women. The American Heart Association has established four standards for triglyceride levels:

**Normal:** < 200 milligrams per deciliter of blood

**Borderline high:** 200-400 milligrams per deciliter

**High:** 400-1,000 milligrams per deciliter

**Very high:** > 1,000 milligrams per deciliter

Physical activity and diets lower in saturated fat and alcohol are recommended to lower triglyceride levels.

*Smoking.* Smoking tobacco presents one of the most preventable lifestyle risks associated with morbidity and mortality in the United States. Smoking is the direct cause of more than 400,000 deaths in the United States each year. The risk for death due to heart attack is twice as high for pack-a-day smokers than for nonsmokers and is triple for those who smoke two packs a day or more. The good news, though, is that smokers who have quit for three years have nearly the same risk of CHD as lifetime nonsmokers—and by 10 years the risk is the same.

Smoking releases nicotine and some 1,200 other toxic compounds into the bloodstream and dramatically hastens the process of atherosclerosis. Smoking also increases the likelihood of blood clots within the arteries; when coupled with the effects of advancing atherosclerosis, this can completely block an artery and cause a stroke or heart attack.

Smoking also increases the heart rate, elevates blood pressure, and can cause arrhythmias. In

---

**HEALTHCHECK**

**A woman has a total cholesterol level of 240 and an HDL-C level of 30. What is her cholesterol ratio, and what is your interpretation of the ratio?**

The ratio is 8 (240/30), which is high and indicates an elevated risk of CHD.

## OF INTEREST

### The High Cost of Cardiovascular Disease

According to the American Heart Association, the cost of cardiovascular disease and stroke in 1998 was estimated at $274.2 billion. This figure includes direct costs, which represent the cost of physicians and other professionals, hospital and nursing home services, medications, and home health and other medical durables. It also includes lost productivity resulting from morbidity and mortality.

See the chart below for a breakdown of the costs of cardiovascular diseases and stroke. (Note that the totals may not add up because of rounding and overlap.)

Reproduced with permission. © *Heart and Stroke Facts: 1998 Statistical Supplement*, 1997. Copyright American Heart Association.

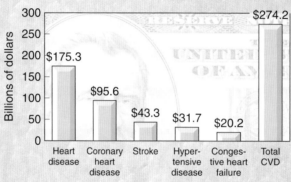

addition, it decreases the body's "good" cholesterol, HDL-C.

Environmental smoke, sometimes called secondhand smoke or passive smoking, increases the risk of death from heart attack by 30% if the exposure is consistent and long. And pipe and cigar smokers aren't immune: even if they don't inhale, they're absorbing toxins through the mouth, increasing their risk of cardiovascular disease and greatly increasing their risk of cancer.

 Smokers are more than twice as likely to die from a heart attack as are nonsmokers; however, smokers who have quit for three years lower their risk of CHD to nearly that of lifetime nonsmokers.

*Diabetes.* Diabetes mellitus is a metabolic disorder in which the body improperly controls blood sugar levels (see chapter 9 for more information). This affects cholesterol levels and thus

becomes a cardiovascular disease risk. In fact, the incidence of CHD among those who have diabetes is quite high. In type I diabetes (also called *juvenile diabetes* because it occurs mainly in young people), the pancreas produces little or no insulin. In type II diabetes (often called *adult-onset diabetes*), the pancreas produces too little insulin or the body doesn't use it correctly. Type II diabetes can often be overcome through weight control, proper nutrition, and exercise. Physical activity makes the body more sensitive to insulin. Aerobic exercise may also help in preventing diabetes among adults.

Physical activity makes the body more sensitive to insulin, which allows proper control of blood sugar levels. Being physically active can help prevent diabetes among adults.

*Obesity.* Excessive body fat is often accompanied by a host of cardiovascular problems: elevated cholesterol and triglyceride levels, high blood pressure, diabetes, and low levels of cardiovascular fitness. Even with none of these complicating factors in place, excessive fat alone presents a risk for developing cardiovascular disease. In chapter 4 we defined excessive fat (obesity) as 25% or greater body fat for men and 30% or greater body fat for women.

***Physical Inactivity.*** In 1992 the American Heart Association elevated physical inactivity from a contributing risk factor for cardiovascular disease to a major risk factor. Inactive people are twice as likely as active people to die from cardiovascular disease. In fact, Blair et al. (1996) found that people with low levels of cardiovascular endurance had risks of dying from CHD two to *four* times higher than did people who had moderate to high levels of cardiovascular endurance. Unfortunately, no matter which ethnic group you examine, more than half of the U.S. population is considered sedentary (see figure 7.6). Physical inactivity is the most prevalent risk factor for CHD.

Being physically active has a positive impact on a number of the risk factors we've just discussed. It can help lower blood pressure, reduce body fat, decrease cholesterol and triglyceride levels, improve HDL-C levels, control diabetes, manage stress, and maintain a healthy heart. The exercise and physical activity guidelines presented in chapter 2 provide you with the knowledge to design an exercise program to reduce your risk of CHD.

 There are a number of CHD risk factors that you can control: high blood pressure, high blood cholesterol, elevated triglycerides, smoking, diabetes, excessive fat, and physical inactivity. Inactive people are twice as likely as active people to die from cardiovascular disease.

## Contributing Risk Factors for Coronary Heart Disease

Contributing risk factors are those associated with increased risk of cardiovascular disease, but their significance and prevalence have yet to be precisely determined.

Excessive and prolonged stress can strain the heart (see chapter 11). Responses that don't effectively help manage the stress can lead to cardiovascular disease, especially when combined with other unhealthy habits such as overeating or smoking (two unhealthy ways to deal with stress).

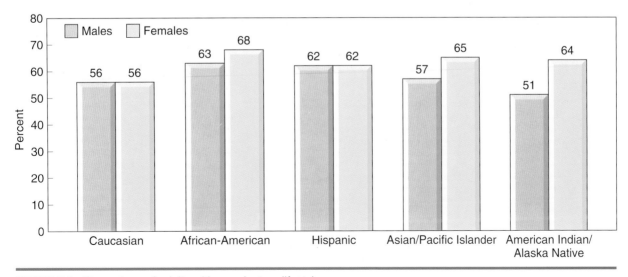

**FIGURE 7.6** Percentage of adults with a sedentary lifestyle.
Data from American Heart Association 1991-1992.

Responding to stress and to life in general with hostility and anger may also increase our chances of developing cardiovascular disease. Research shows that those who are hostile, quick-tempered, mistrusting, and cynical are more likely to develop CHD than people who are more trusting and calm and have a positive outlook. The physiological stress response, which in part triggers an elevation in blood pressure, puts those who are hostile and angry at greater risk than those who are not.

## Major Risk Factors for Stroke

As with CHD, some risk factors for stroke are genetic; others are a function of natural processes. Certain risk factors originate from a person's lifestyle and environment. Those that result from lifestyle and environment can be altered. Here we'll look at those risk factors for stroke that can be altered, those that can't, and other possible risk factors.

### Unalterable Risk Factors for Stroke

As with CHD, heredity, gender, and age are unalterable risk factors for stroke. Your chance of stroke is greater if you have a family history of stroke, and it's greater if you are male. Men have about a 19% greater chance of stroke than do women. And African-Americans have a much higher risk of stroke than do Caucasians (African-American men have a 97% increased risk of death due to stroke than Caucasian men), partly due to higher incidence of high blood pressure in African-Americans. As for age, the chance of stroke more than doubles for each decade of life after age 55.

Two other risk factors that can't be changed are diabetes mellitus (while this is treatable, having it still increases the risk of stroke) and having had a prior stroke.

### Alterable Risk Factors for Stroke

Several risk factors can be treated. Among these are high blood pressure (the most important controllable risk factor) and heart disease. Cigarette smoking is also a prime risk factor for stroke; the use of oral contraceptives combined with cigarette smoking greatly increases the risk.

In addition, a person who has had one or more transient ischemic attacks (a "mini stroke" in which the signs of a stroke only last for a few minutes) is nearly 10 times as likely to have a stroke as someone of the same age and sex who hasn't. Finally, a high red blood cell count increases the risk of a stroke. Even a moderate increase in the number of red blood cells thickens the blood and makes clots more likely.

### Other Risk Factors for Stroke

Contributing risk factors for stroke include high blood cholesterol and lipids, physical inactivity, and obesity. Other factors that may increase risk, although documentation is not as strong, are geographic location (strokes are more common in the southeastern United States), season and climate (extreme temperatures are correlated with strokes), socioeconomic factors (people with low incomes have higher rates of stroke than do more affluent people), excessive drinking of alcohol (more than two drinks a day raises blood pressure), and certain types of drug use (cocaine use has been closely related to strokes).

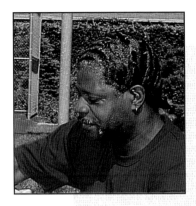

# Health Concepts

As we saw at the beginning of the chapter, Mark was concerned about the chest pains he felt and was wondering if they were evidence of heart disease. He wasn't sure whether his being physically active was healthy for him at that point or whether the activity actually might bring on a heart attack. Certainly, based on Mark's symptoms, concerns of this nature need to be addressed by a physician. Regular medical checkups are important for everyone, but even more important as we get older. However, in general, physical activity is instrumental in *lowering* the chances of heart disease, not increasing them.

## SUMMARY

▐ Cardiovascular disease is the leading cause of death in the United States, accounting for nearly half of the country's deaths. More than 58 million Americans have some form of heart disease.

▐ The death rate from cardiovascular disease has dropped by more than 25% in the last 10 years. This decline is attributable in part to changes in lifestyle behaviors: not smoking, getting regular exercise, eating well, maintaining a healthy body weight, and managing stress.

▐ Cardiovascular diseases include heart attacks, atherosclerosis, angina pectoris, arrhythmias, congenital heart defects, aneurysms, hypertension, and stroke.

▐ Coronary heart disease is the most common form of cardiovascular disease leading to a heart attack. An attack occurs when blood flow to a portion of the heart is blocked by one of the coronary arteries. Coronary artery blockages usually develop through a process called *atherosclerosis.* As plaque builds on the internal walls of the arteries, the arterial opening gradually narrows and hardens. As these deposits form in the arteries, the arteries lose their elasticity and begin to restrict blood flow.

▐ *Hypertension* is a disease that occurs when a person's blood pressure is continuously abnormally high. If an adult's blood pressure is continuously equal to or greater than 140 over 90, that person has hypertension. Hypertension is known as the "silent killer" because people don't feel sick from it and many don't know they have it. High blood pressure can lead to a variety of cardiovascular diseases, including heart disease, congestive heart failure, and stroke.

▐ A *stroke* is caused by a lack of blood flow to the brain. The severity of a stroke depends on the amount of brain tissue that is deprived of blood flow. Brain cells can die after several minutes of being oxygen deprived. These brain cells can't be replaced; the parts of the body that were controlled by the dead brain cells are permanently affected.

▌ There are three major risk factors for cardiovascular disease that you can't do anything about: your heredity, your gender, and your age.

▌ Major risk factors for coronary heart disease (CHD) that you *can* change include high blood pressure, high blood cholesterol, smoking, diabetes, obesity, and physical inactivity.

▌ High density lipoprotein-cholesterol (HDL-C) is called the "good" cholesterol because it transports cholesterol through the bloodstream to the liver for further metabolism or excretion. Low density lipoprotein-cholesterol (LDL-C) is the "bad" cholesterol because not all of it is transported and metabolized or excreted; high levels of LDL-C hasten the process of atherosclerosis.

▌ It's desirable to have less than 200 milligrams per deciliter of total cholesterol and less than 130 milligrams per deciliter of LDL-C. Your total cholesterol count is considered high if it is 240 or above; your LDL-C count is high if it is 160 or above.

▌ Smoking is the direct cause of more than 400,000 deaths in the United States each year. The risk for death due to heart attack is twice as high for pack-a-day smokers as for nonsmokers, and triple for those who smoke two packs a day or more.

▌ Physical inactivity is the most prevalent major risk factor for CHD. Inactive people are twice as likely as active people to die from CVD (CHD and stroke).

*We've discussed the major causes and risk factors for cardiovascular disease and looked at ways you can use physical activity to promote cardiovascular health. What are the most common health problems of the musculoskeletal system, and what can you do to enhance the health of your muscles and bones? In the next chapter we'll look at the overall effects of physical activity on musculoskeletal health—especially how it impacts osteoporosis, arthritis, and low back pain.*

## KEY TERMS

angina

arrhythmia

atherosclerosis

cerebral hemorrhage

cerebral thrombosis

cholesterol

coronary thrombosis

diastolic blood pressure

epidemiology

high density lipoproteins (HDL)

hypertension

hypotension

lipoproteins

low density lipoproteins (LDL)

myocardial infarction

risk factor

stroke

systolic blood pressure

triglycerides

# 7

# Evaluating Risks of Heart Attack

## THE PURPOSE OF THIS LAB EXPERIENCE IS TO

▌ evaluate your risk for experiencing a heart attack.

The American Heart Association developed a heart attack risk factor assessment in 1995. Complete the assessment, adapted here, by circling the number next to the statement that's most true for you. Once you've determined your risk, decide whether you should modify certain lifestyle behaviors to lower your risk.

**Cigarette Smoking**

| | |
|---|---|
| I never smoked or stopped smoking three or more years ago. | 1 |
| I don't smoke but I live and/or work with smokers. | 2 |
| I stopped smoking regularly within the last three years. | 3 |
| I smoke regularly. | 4 |
| I smoke regularly and live and/or work with other smokers. | 5 |

**Total Blood Cholesterol**

Use the number from your most recent blood cholesterol measurement.

| | |
|---|---|
| Less than 160 | 1 |
| 160 to 199 | 2 |
| Don't know | 3 |
| 200 to 239 | 4 |
| 240 or higher | 5 |

**High Density Lipoprotein ("Good")-Cholesterol**

Use the number from your most recent HDL-C measurement.

| | |
|---|---|
| Over 60 | 1 |
| 56 to 60 | 2 |
| Don't know | 3 |
| 35 to 55 | 4 |
| Less than 35 | 5 |

*(continued)*

*(continued)*

### Systolic Blood Pressure

Use the first (highest) number from your most recent blood pressure measurement.

| | |
|---|---|
| Less than 120 | 1 |
| 120 to 139 | 2 |
| Don't know | 3 |
| 140 to 159 | 4 |
| 160 or higher | 5 |

### Excess Body Weight

| | |
|---|---|
| I am within 10 pounds of my desirable weight. | 1 |
| I am 10 to 20 pounds above my desirable weight. | 2 |
| I am 21 to 30 pounds above my desirable weight. | 3 |
| I am 31 to 50 pounds above my desirable weight. | 4 |
| I am more than 50 pounds above my desirable weight. | 5 |

### Physical Activity

Choose the column (A, B, or C) that best describes your usual level of physical activity.

| A | B | C |
|---|---|---|
| *Highly active* | *Moderately active* | *Inactive* |
| My job requires very hard physical labor (such as digging or loading heavy objects) at least 4 hours a day **OR** I do vigorous activities (jogging, cycling, swimming, etc.) at least three times per week for 30 to 60 minutes or more **OR** I do at least 1 hour of moderate activity such as brisk walking at least four days a week | My job requires that I walk, lift, carry, or do other moderately hard work for several hours per day (day care worker, stock clerk, busboy/waitress) **OR** I spend much of my leisure time doing moderate activities (dancing, gardening, walking, or housework) | My job requires that I sit at a desk most of the day **AND** Much of my leisure time is spent in sedentary activities (watching TV, reading, etc.) **AND** I seldom work up a sweat and I cannot walk fast without having to stop to catch my breath |

**Rating Your Activity Level**

| | |
|---|---|
| Column A | 1 |
| Between Columns A and B | 2 |
| Column B | 3 |
| Between Columns B and C | 4 |
| Column C | 5 |

**Scoring**

Add your answers for each question to arrive at your total score.

| If your total score is: | Your heart attack risk is: |
|---|---|
| 6 to 13 | Low |
| 14 to 22 | Moderate |
| 23 to 30 | High |

Your score is simply an estimate of your possible risk. A high score doesn't mean you will surely have a heart attack, and a low score doesn't mean you're safe from heart disease. Check your individual category scores to see which factors are increasing your risk of heart attack most, and take steps to lower those risk factors.

# Chapter 8

# Musculoskeletal Health

*Elaine Trudelle-Jackson, M.S., P.T.*

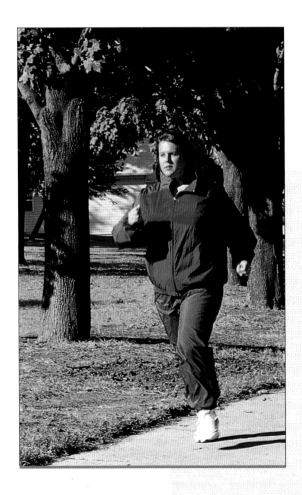

I saw a doctor a few days ago and I happened to mention that my mom has osteoporosis. The doctor suggested I start jogging to help prevent developing osteoporosis myself later on, and also to help lose weight. I've tried jogging before, but each time I do, I stop after about three or four weeks because I get these various aches and pains. Naturally I forgot to mention this to the doctor.

I suppose I can try jogging again—maybe the discomfort will go away once I get in better shape. I just wonder if I'm doing more harm than good, though. Am I just supposed to "gut it out" and fight through the pain? I look at the problems my mom has with osteoporosis and I certainly don't want to develop the same problems. So I guess I'll try jogging again. I'm just not sure what to do if I start hurting again.

—Staci, 21-year-old junior

## *What do you think?*

Many people are confused about the aches and pains that can occur when beginning an exercise program. Two responses are to stop the activity or, as Staci puts it, to "fight through the pain." But stopping physical activity altogether only harms your fitness and health, and ignoring or fighting through pain may lead to musculoskeletal injuries. Should Staci be jogging, given her history of discomfort? What activities might cause less pain? And can physical activity really help prevent osteoporosis?

It's easy to see how physical activity can directly impact the health of our muscles and bones. In previous chapters we've discussed the role physical activity plays in building muscular strength and endurance. To gain a fuller understanding of how physical activity impacts musculoskeletal health, however, we'll discuss the structure and function of healthy joints and look at the overall effects of physical activity on musculoskeletal health. Within that context we'll explore two joint diseases—rheumatoid arthritis and osteoarthritis—and consider the role of physical activity in preventing and treating osteoarthritis. We'll also look at the causes and management of soft tissue injuries such as sprains and strains and examine bone injuries as well, including the effects of aging on bones. And toward the end of the chapter we'll address osteoporosis, Staci's biggest concern, along with low back pain, which about 8 of 10 people will experience in their lives. We'll define who's at risk and how physical activity can be used to prevent and treat both conditions.

## EFFECTS OF PHYSICAL ACTIVITY ON MUSCLE AND BONE

In chapter 3 we examined the effects of physical activity on muscular strength and endurance and on flexibility. As we put tension on our muscles, we build muscular strength; we increase strength by taxing our muscles beyond their accustomed loads. Further, we learned that muscle develop-

ment is specific: only the fibers that are engaged in the activity can increase in strength.

We also learned of a certain type of muscle soreness—delayed onset muscle soreness—that affects untrained muscles 24 to 48 hours after exercise. Delayed onset muscle soreness is not an injury and usually goes away within four or five days. As your muscles become trained, you are less likely to experience delayed onset muscle soreness.

It's obvious, then, that physical activity has a direct effect on muscles. But what about its impact on bones? We all know that accidents can cause bones to fracture, but can physical activity have a positive impact on the health of our bones?

Physical activity provides bones with the stresses that they need in order to grow normally and become strong. In fact, when no physical activity to a body part is possible, such as when the part must be placed in a cast or when the muscles surrounding a bone are paralyzed, the bone's size and strength are substantially reduced, making the bone weak and easy to injure. We'll look at *how* physical activity helps to promote healthy bones later in this chapter.

This entire book is based on the evidence that physical activity improves health and fitness and enriches our lives in many ways. We have explored the benefits of physical activity from a variety of angles: how it improves our cardiorespiratory system, increases muscular strength and endurance, improves flexibility, helps achieve and maintain a healthful weight, lessens the chance of developing serious diseases, and so on. But physical activity isn't without its risks. In terms of musculoskeletal health, physical activity holds several risk factors that increase the likelihood of injury to muscle or bone. Knowing those risk factors in advance can help you minimize your chance of injury.

## RISK FACTORS FOR MUSCULOSKELETAL INJURIES

Researchers have identified these risk factors for sustaining musculoskeletal injuries while engaging in physical activity:

- **Aging:** As a person ages beyond 30 years, the size and quality of the collagen fibers that make up the musculoskeletal system begin to decrease, thus making tissues such as ligaments, tendons, and cartilage more susceptible to injury.

- **Structural faults in the musculoskeletal system:** Structural faults such as misalignment of bones in a joint result in abnormal forces exerted on the joint tissues. Ligaments may be overstretched and cartilage and bone excessively compressed. Certain types of physical activity may increase the abnormal forces already present and increase the likelihood of injury.

- **Excessive body weight:** Excessive body weight (being overweight or obese) causes abnormally high compressive forces in joints and can damage them. The more overweight you are, the higher the compressive forces during weight-bearing activity and the greater the risk for injury over time. Certain types of physical activity, such as jogging, can further increase the already excessive joint compressive forces and result in injury.

- **Previous musculoskeletal injuries:** People who have had previous musculoskeletal injuries sustain additional injuries (injuries to the same area or joint, as well as other injuries) more often than those who have not had previous musculoskeletal injuries. According to Pate and Macera (1994), it isn't clear whether this increased risk for further injury is due to incomplete healing of the original injury, an uncorrected structural malalignment, or a personal susceptibility to reinjury.

If you have one or more of these risk factors, you should choose your type and intensity of exercise carefully. For example, as related at the beginning of the chapter, Staci noted that she had various aches and pains when she jogged. We know for sure she has at least one of the four risk factors: being overweight. She may also have structural faults that contribute to her injuries; that's impossible for us to tell. But with at least one risk factor present, she should consider other modes of exercise—perhaps walking, supplemented by weight lifting. Weight-bearing exercises, as we'll learn in more detail later, can be effective in combating osteoporosis.

Some people may be inactive for years before deciding to become regularly physically active. They may jump into exercise with zeal and intensity, trying to get into shape quickly, making up for years of lost ground. Those who take this approach invite musculoskeletal injuries.

If you have one or more risk factors for musculoskeletal injury, choose your type and intensity of exercise carefully.

Although the next example of injury risk is specific to one type of training, distance running, it might apply to other types of physical activity that put similar stress on the body. Numerous studies have pointed to the strong relationship between injury and mileage per week; as runners increase their training to beyond 20 miles (32 kilometers) per week, they also increase their chances of injury. Whether increases in other types of physical activity bring with them increased risks of musculoskeletal injury probably depends on the activity itself; high-mileage distance running puts great strain on the feet and legs, and injuries in this activity are common. Walking provides many of the same benefits as running and presents a lower risk of musculoskeletal injury. Those who have one or more of the four risk factors just mentioned may be able to avoid injury by walking rather than jogging or running.

## STRUCTURE AND FUNCTION OF HEALTHY JOINTS

In general, a joint is a structure that connects two or more bones. The majority of joints in the body are classified as *diarthrodial,* or *synovial,* joints (see figure 8.1). Synovial joints have certain structures in common: a fibrous joint capsule lined with synovial membrane and joint cartilage.

Two types of cartilage contribute to joint function. The first is *hyaline,* or *articular,* cartilage. Articular cartilage lines the ends of the bones that form an articulation. (An articulation is the juncture between bones.) A layer of articular cartilage about 2 to 4 millimeters thick lines the

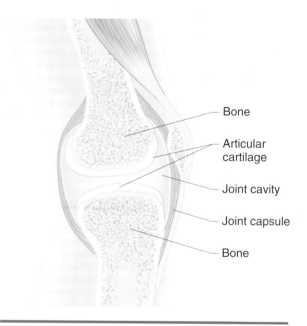

**FIGURE 8.1**    A typical synovial joint.

joint surfaces of all synovial joints. Synovia is the lubricating fluid secreted by the membranes of the joint capsule; it lubricates the joint surfaces. This articular cartilage minimizes the friction between the bony surfaces.

The second type of cartilage that contributes to joint function is *fibrocartilage,* which is lo-

---

### Tips for Preventing Musculoskeletal Injuries

Want to know how to be active and avoid injury? Here are a few tips:

▌ Warm up before exercise and cool down afterward. Include stretching as part of your warm-up and cool-down.

▌ If you're beginning an exercise program, begin slowly and progress carefully. Whether you're a beginner or a veteran, *slowly* extend your limits in muscular strength and endurance. Don't try for "big breakthroughs."

▌ During intense activity, don't hold your breath or strain beyond normal limits.

▌ Use proper form in completing weight-lifting exercises.

▌ Use quality equipment that is in good repair.

▌ Listen to your body. If it's telling you to stop or cut back on a particular activity or exercise, then stop or cut back. If you are injured during an activity, stop the activity and treat the injury.

cated in some, but not all, joints. It serves various functions. For instance, the discs located in the spine are a type of fibrocartilage whose function is to act as a shock absorber. In other places, fibrocartilage helps bones fit together better at their joints.

Typically the activities of daily living provide adequate stimulus to maintain healthy joint cartilage. This stimulus involves intermittent compression (pushing together) of joint surfaces, accomplished either by bearing weight through the joint or by contracting muscles surrounding the joint. Cycles of joint loading and unloading through either of these two mechanisms bring synovial fluid to the joint's surface, and thus aid in nourishing the joint and keeping it healthy.

Ligaments help stabilize joints, and a ligamentous sleeve called a *capsule* surrounds the joint, providing further support. Ligaments, muscles, and tendons all contribute to a joint's range of motion (ROM); these tissues must be flexible enough to allow the joint to move through its full ROM.

People tend to lose flexibility as they age. Changes in the structure of muscles, tendons, and ligaments make these tissues less extensible and contribute to the loss of joint ROM. These structural changes are similar to those experienced when a joint is immobilized for a long period of time. Older people become less flexible in part because they are less active—and less likely to move their joints through their full ranges of motion—than they once were. They tend to experience loss of flexibility equally throughout their bodies.

Younger people's loss of flexibility tends to be more restricted. Younger people often lose mobility in certain joints because of a sustained posture—for example, sitting in a chair for a long time, day after day. Doing this can limit flexibility in the knees and hips.

The common denominator in the loss of flexibility is *immobility*. A joint will lose its ability to move through full ROM unless it is *made* to move through that full range on a regular basis. Doing this ensures that the soft tissues surrounding the joint will maintain enough flexibility to allow full joint ROM.

 **KEY POINT** People tend to lose flexibility when they are less active. The key to remaining flexible is to be active and move your joints through their full ranges of motion.

## JOINT DISEASES

The most common condition directly affecting joints is *arthritis*, which means joint *(arthro)* inflammation *(itis)*. The Arthritis Foundation reports that nearly 40 million Americans are affected by some form of this disease, making it the number one cause of disability in the United States. There are as many as 100 forms of arthritis, but the two most prevalent are *osteoarthritis* and *rheumatoid arthritis.*

### Osteoarthritis

Osteoarthritis is the most common type of arthritis, affecting nearly 16 million Americans. Osteoarthritis is called *degenerative joint disease* because it is characterized by degenerating joint articular cartilage. Osteoarthritis can and often does affect more than one joint, but it is possible to have osteoarthritis in an isolated joint. Osteoarthritis affects middle-aged and older people and is often considered to be an inevitable part of aging.

Factors that contribute to the disease's development include age, obesity, previous injury to a joint, and faulty joint alignment. Genetics may play a role, but it isn't clear that it does. It's not known whether a person inherits a disposition to develop osteoarthritis or whether abnormal joint structure (also inherited) leads to developing the disease. For example, someone who is bowlegged is more likely to develop osteoarthritis in the knees, perhaps because of having inherited this particular structural problem rather than osteoarthritis itself.

Physical activity may also play a role in development of the disease. Repeated movements during an occupation or through sport can lead to osteoarthritis. However, physical activity—when incorporated correctly in terms of frequency, intensity, time, and type—can be helpful for those who have this disease. The goal is to restore health to the degenerating cartilage; cycles of compression and decompression, accomplished by bearing weight through the joint or by contracting muscles surrounding the joint, can help restore health or at least decrease the rate of degeneration.

 Physical activity can help prevent or treat osteoarthritis by developing healthy articular cartilage.

## Rheumatoid Arthritis

Rheumatoid arthritis is a systemic disease—that is, it affects multiple systems in the body, including multiple joints. Rheumatoid arthritis affects 2.1 million Americans, 1.5 million of them women. The onset is normally in middle age, though the disease can begin at any age. Rheu-

### Exercising With Osteoarthritis

A goal with osteoarthritis is to develop healthy articular cartilage by putting the joint surfaces through cycles of compression and decompression. The surfaces of a joint are compressed when a muscle that crosses the joint contracts; the surfaces are decompressed when the muscle relaxes.

So what type of exercise is appropriate for people who have osteoarthritis? Here are three types.

- *Calisthenic exercises* are exercises performed without added resistance in which joints are moved rhythmically and repeatedly through their ranges of motion; the term covers a wide variety of exercises such as sit-ups, push-ups, and jumping jacks. Calisthenic exercises that take the joint through its full ROM are appropriate. The drawback here is that performing the same joint movements for 20 to 30 minutes can become quite boring.
- *Stationary cycling* with little or no resistance is excellent exercise for the knees and hips.
- *Walking* and *jogging* are also good ways to put the joint surfaces through cycles of compression and decompression. Jogging results in much higher magnitudes of compression than does walking. Research shows that jogging or running is fine in moderation, provided the person has no joint structural abnormalities or malalignments. If walking or jogging causes increased pain or swelling, however, you should go to a non-weight-bearing activity such as cycling or a decreased weight-bearing activity such as underwater walking or jogging.

Joint pain or swelling is the body's way of telling you that you're doing too much of an activity or are doing an inappropriate activity. If you're having difficulty finding an activity that doesn't make your joints feel worse, ask your physician to refer you to a physical therapist. You may need to start with lower levels of activity or a different type of activity altogether.

## HEALTHCHECK

### How might repeated movements lead to osteoarthritis?

Repeated movements can lead to osteoarthritis especially when the movement involves high forces. A baseball pitcher, for example, can develop osteoarthritis in the elbow because the high compressive forces that are concentrated in one area of the joint surface can cause irritation. When this irritation occurs repeatedly over a long enough time, osteoarthritis can develop. However, physical activity, when incorporated correctly, should provide the stimulus to nourish rather than irritate joints.

matoid arthritis is an autoimmune disease; for some unknown reason, the body's natural immune system begins to attack its own healthy joint tissue, resulting in inflammation and subsequent damage to the joint cartilage and bone. The effects of this joint inflammation are pain, warmth, redness, and swelling.

We don't know what causes the immune system to suddenly malfunction, but we know that genetics plays a role. Most people who have rheumatoid arthritis have a genetic marker called HLA-DR4. People with this marker don't always develop rheumatoid arthritis; in fact, most people with this marker don't develop the disease, but they are predisposed to it. Researchers believe that a virus may trigger rheumatoid arthritis in people who have this inherited tendency to develop the disease.

Because of the involvement of multiple systems and joints, people with rheumatoid arthritis should be under the care of a medical doctor. (Chiropractic doctors can offer temporary pain relief for certain musculoskeletal conditions, but they aren't medical doctors.) Although medical doctors can't stop or reverse the effects of rheumatoid arthritis, they can help relieve the symptoms and preserve normal joint function by prescribing medication that controls the inflammation leading to joint destruction.

Physical activity can benefit people with rheumatoid arthritis, but their exercise programs should be developed and monitored by qualified medical personnel such as physical or occupational therapists who have a good understanding of the disease process. Inappropriate exercise can have a very detrimental effect on rheumatoid arthritic joints, including increased destruction of joint surfaces.

## SOFT TISSUE INJURIES

Musculoskeletal injuries that involve tissues such as ligaments, muscles, tendons, and bursa are known as *soft tissue injuries.* These injuries can be painful and can restrict a person's ability to perform a task or exercise. Here we'll describe injuries to the tissues just mentioned. We'll also describe a type of injury called *overuse injury.*

### Ligament Injuries

Ligaments hold bones together at a joint. When a ligament is overstretched and some of its fibers are damaged, the resulting injury is a *sprain.* The damaged ligament becomes inflamed and painful. A more serious ligament injury can result in a *tear.*

Because ligament injuries can result in a joint's becoming unstable, it is important that they are properly diagnosed and treated. Many ligament injuries involve contact (e.g., a blow to the knee in football). However, ligament injuries can also occur without contact: when a person turns an ankle while walking on an uneven surface, for example. In either case, the joint is forced to move beyond the range it was designed to move in, stretching or tearing the ligaments. The pain from a ligament injury is immediate and severe. Swelling always occurs but may be less noticeable in some ligaments due to their location. Sprains (and strains, which are described in the next section) can be classified as grade I (minimal disruption), II (significant tearing), or III (complete tear) in severity through a clinical assessment by a medical caregiver.

## Soft Tissue Injuries by Their Common Names

Following are the signs and causes of common injuries that are often associated with physical activity.

■ **Charlie horse:** This refers to a muscle contusion or deep bruise to the quadriceps resulting from a direct blow to the front or outer front of the thigh. The thigh becomes discolored from bleeding within the injured tissue; the injured muscle becomes swollen and tender. The pain becomes worse when the injured muscle is contracted or stretched. If this injury isn't allowed to heal, it can be reinjured and calcium deposits can form within the injured tissue. Stretching the muscle before it's healed should be avoided for this reason.

■ **Groin pull:** This is a strain of the adductor muscles on the inner thigh. It occurs when the muscles are forcefully contracted or overstretched. A groin pull is susceptible to reinjury until fully healed, so adequate warm-up and cooldown, as well as adequate stretching before and after physical activity, are recommended.

■ **Jumper's knee:** This injury occurs when the patellar tendon, which runs from the kneecap to the tibia (lower leg bone), becomes inflamed. The patellar tendon attaches the quadriceps muscle to the tibia. Jumper's knee is a tendinitis occurring from overuse of the quadriceps and tendon unit in repetitive knee movements such as occur in jumping. Pain is felt below the kneecap when the quadriceps contract, and is most severe when the contraction occurs with the knee flexed. The medical name for jumper's knee is *patellar tendinitis.*

■ **Shin splints:** This injury is an inflammation at the attachment of the tibialis posterior muscle to the tibia; thus, it is another form of tendinitis that results in pain over the front of the lower leg. It has many causes, perhaps the most common being posterior tibial syndrome. The pain associated with posterior tibial syndrome occurs on the inside of the tibia (shinbone). Typically a person feels this pain when beginning to exercise; it eases during exercise, but returns in greater intensity after exercise.

■ **Tennis elbow:** Another tendinitis, this involves inflammation of one or more of the tendons connecting the muscles that extend from the wrist and fingers to the outer part of the arm just above the elbow. Pain, felt at the attachment above the elbow, occurs with forceful wrist extension. Tennis players who have a faulty backhand stroke or an improper grip size or string tension in their racket often get tennis elbow. So do many people who don't play racket sports—gardeners, for example, because of the repeated wrist extension that weeding requires. The medical name for tennis elbow is *lateral epicondylitis.*

■ **Golfer's elbow:** This is similar to tennis elbow but involves tendinitis of the tendon(s) of the muscles that flex the wrist and fingers. Pain is felt at the attachment to the inner part of the arm just above the elbow. Golfers and racquetball players most frequently get this injury, but anyone who performs repeated forceful wrist flexion is at risk. The medical name for golfer's elbow is *medial epicondylitis.*

▌ **Shoulder impingement syndrome:** This is an inflammation of the bursa and/or the tendons located under the tip of the shoulder. It results from repeated impingement of these structures when the arm is repeatedly raised overhead. Shoulder impingement syndrome is a bursitis and/or tendinitis that may or may not be caused by overuse. It can result from weakness of the muscles responsible for assisting in raising the arm overhead. Participating in physical activity that calls for repeated forceful arm movements overhead—such as swimming—can cause this condition, especially if the activity is begun too aggressively.

## Muscle Injuries

Overstretching, or contracting a muscle very strongly when it is stretched, can result in a muscle *strain*. (*Strains* affect muscles; *sprains* affect ligaments. People often confuse these two terms. See figure 8.2 for examples of a sprain and a strain.) A more serious injury to a muscle can result in its being torn. Another type of muscle injury is a *contusion*, which is a deep muscle bruise. Contusions occur when a muscle receives a direct blow—for example, when a person's knee is driven into another person's thigh during a football tackle.

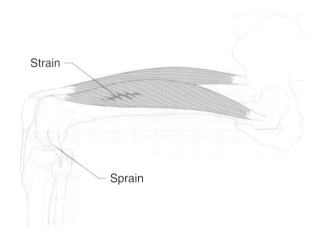

**FIGURE 8.2**    Ligament sprain vs. muscle strain.

## Tendon Injuries

Tendons attach muscle to bone. They are exceptionally strong and thus are not often torn through

trauma, but they can become inflamed from rubbing against surrounding bone or another tendon. This inflammation is referred to as *tendinitis*.

Tendinitis can also occur as a result of continual tension in the tendon from excessive repetition of the same motion. Minor injuries to some tendon fibers cause a low level of inflammation and pain that often are unnoticed except when the repetitive motion is performed. Thus, in most cases tendinitis is an overuse injury, but it can lead to a tear if it is ignored.

## Bursa Injuries

A *bursa* is a fluid-filled sac whose function is to decrease friction between tendons or between tendon and bone. In providing this function, the bursa itself sometimes becomes inflamed; this inflammation is referred to as *bursitis* (see figure 8.3 for a comparison of tendinitis and bursitis). Bursitis also often occurs as a result of excessive repetition of a motion and thus is usually an overuse injury. Decreased flexibility of a tendon overlying a bursa can also lead to bursitis.

## Overuse Injuries

Another type of injury is classified as an *overuse injury* (also referred to as *cumulative trauma disorder* or a *repetitive strain injury*). Although sprains, strains, tears, and contusions are often the result of a specific incident, many other soft

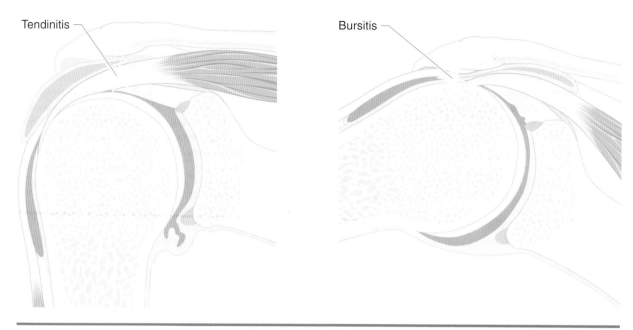

Tendinitis

Bursitis

**FIGURE 8.3** Tendinitis vs. bursitis.

tissue injuries—including tendinitis and bursitis—occur gradually, brought on by the cumulative effects of repeating the same motion or motions over and over. These types of injuries are called overuse injuries. Overuse injuries often occur to soft tissues, but can involve other structures as well. For example, a marathon runner who logs 50 miles per week and who sustains a stress fracture in the foot has suffered an overuse injury. A postal worker who performs the same wrist motion for hours at a time and who develops tendinitis in her wrist as a result also has an overuse injury.

Overuse injuries are the fastest growing medical problem in the workplace today. According to the National Institute for Occupational Safety and Health (1997), repeated trauma disorders account for 62% of all occupational illnesses. In

 Overuse injuries are the fastest growing medical problem in the workplace today. The best ways to avoid them are to decrease the number of repetitions of the motion that is causing the problem or to correct the movement itself.

combating this problem, companies have frequently sought the professional help of ergonomists, physical therapists, and occupational therapists. Sometimes the companies need to redesign tools used by the worker.

## Treatment of Soft Tissue Injuries

Although the soft tissues we've just described serve different functions in the musculoskeletal system, their responses to injury are quite similar. The initial response to a soft tissue injury is *inflammation*. This is what makes the tissue hot, red, painful, and swollen.

Inflammation is a normal tissue response; it is the first step that the tissue takes to heal itself. This phase of healing usually lasts 24 to 48 hours, but it can last four to five days. People experience the greatest pain and discomfort at this stage.

Although you can't do anything to prevent injured tissue from becoming inflamed, you can take steps to minimize the *effects* of inflammation. The *RICE* treatment—rest, ice, compression, and elevation—effectively limits the swelling and pain. These four elements of treatment

## Carpal Tunnel Syndrome

Carpal tunnel syndrome (CTS) is the most frequently reported of all cumulative trauma disorders. CTS is an inflammation of the tendons of the wrist as they pass through a "tunnel" formed by the bones of the wrist known as carpals. The inflammation causes swelling in the tendons, which puts pressure on the median nerve, which is also located in the carpal tunnel. The result is a painful tingling in the hand and fingers and subsequent loss of strength in the muscles of the thumb and fingers if pressure on the nerve is not relieved. The most common cause of CTS is repetitive forceful bending movements of the wrist or sustaining awkward wrist positions for long periods of time. The repetition could come from a number of activities: typing, using hand tools, playing a musical instrument, knitting, and so on. CTS can also be caused by a trauma to the lower arm or wrist. In addition, some people seem more predisposed to CTS, perhaps because of differences in the amount of lubrication of the wrist's flexor tendons.

The first line of defense usually involves using a wrist rest (for keyboard users) and an ergonomic glove (which keeps the wrist straight). Other treatment options include cortisone injections and nonsteroidal anti-inflammatory drugs. The last option is outpatient surgery.

Preventive measures focus on using proper ergonomics in the environment that is causing the CTS: using correct wrist and elbow angles, correct waist and back angles, and proper positioning of the feet.

Transverse carpal ligament

Carpal bones

Median nerve

Flexor tendons

---

are done simultaneously, not sequentially. Here's a brief description of how RICE works.

• **Rest.** Resting an injured body part gives it a chance to heal. Putting further stress on it can result in exacerbating the injury or prolonging the healing process. Although the amount of rest needed will vary depending in part on the injury's severity, most minor injuries can begin to be rehabilitated after 72 hours of rest—with avoidance of any activities that stress the injured tissue.

• **Ice.** Placing ice on the injured area will reduce the swelling, pain, and heat associated with inflammation. Ice the injured body part for 10 to 15 minutes at a time (with about 1 hour between icings). Generally ice is most effective for the first three days, but you should use it as long as you have inflammation. Your first inclination might be to apply heat to a soft tissue injury. However, although the heat may feel soothing at first, it will soon make the pain worse by leading to more inflammation, which is what causes the tissues to become hot, red, swollen, and painful in the first place. After 72 hours, most of the inflammation is usually gone, and it is then appropriate to use heat if you prefer. Ice is still an excellent choice to relieve pain when inflammation is gone; in addition, the effects of ice last longer than those of heat.

• **Compression.** Compressing the injured area with an elastic wrap reduces the amount of space available for swelling. The pressure should be applied firmly and evenly around the injury. As with rest and ice, compression is typically used for the first 72 hours after injury (minor injuries may not require this long a treatment).

• **Elevation.** Elevating the injured area reduces swelling by not allowing blood to pool in the extremities. Elevate the injured part as much as possible during the first 72 hours.

If your pain and swelling haven't substantially subsided within four or five days, you should see a physician.

---

**HEALTHCHECK**

**If 10 to 15 minutes of ice helps reduce soft tissue inflammation and pain, why shouldn't I leave ice on all the time for the first two or three days after an injury?**

The reason is that leaving ice on for too long reduces blood flow to the injured area and interferes with the body's healing process. You're using ice to temporarily reduce the *effects* of the inflammation; 10 to 15 minutes is sufficient for this. You can, of course, reapply ice every hour or so as needed for pain. Once the inflammation is gone, you can apply ice for 20 minutes at a time to relieve pain.

---

## Physical Activity and Soft Tissue Injuries

If you sustain a soft tissue injury, exercises that are specific to the injury can facilitate the healing process and maybe even help heal it in such a way that you are less likely to reinjure the same tissue. If you have difficulty recovering from an injury, a physical therapist can help you develop an exercise program specific to your injury.

Appropriate exercise can

• facilitate healing by increasing circulation to the injured area, thereby bringing more nutrients and oxygen to the tissue;
• prevent the injured area from getting stiff and losing ROM while the tissue heals itself; and
• prevent or minimize development of muscle weakness.

If your ROM is decreasing or your muscles are getting weak, see your physician. The injury may be taking too long to heal, or something is preventing it from healing properly. If you wait too long, it is more difficult to restore function to the injured part.

There is no set timeline for returning to activity following an injury. The timing depends on the type and severity of the injury and your body's response to the injury (how well your body heals itself). You should not return to your usual physical activity if you still have swelling or if you do not have full, pain-free ROM to the injured part.

When you do return to physical activity, always start at a lower level than where you left off and progress gradually. If pain and swelling develop in the injured part during or after the activity, stop. This usually is a sign that healing is not complete, and you risk making the injury worse. That will increase the time needed to heal and the time spent away from physical activity.

## BONE INJURIES

If you have a healthy skeletal system, your bones are capable of resisting most forces exerted on them during exercise. Because of this, exercise-associated injuries to the skeletal system are less frequent than soft tissue injuries. People with healthy bones don't sustain *fractures* (broken bones) unless they experience substantial trauma to a bone. Fractures can occur in contact sports such as football, but are uncommon in noncontact sports or in health-related exercise programs.

A *stress fracture* is a type of fracture that comes from overtraining rather than acute trauma. Stress fractures occur from repetitive force on a bone. Runners can be prone to such fractures in their feet or legs. When a stress fracture first develops, the area involved is painful with exercise, but the pain eases off after exercise. As the stress fracture progresses, however, the pain becomes worse after the activity is stopped.

Stress fractures are hard to diagnose initially because they don't show up on x-rays until the bone-producing cells produce bone that appears as a small white line on the x-ray, which indicates that the bone is already healing. Usually, with rest, the bone heals itself in four to six weeks, often without needing to be in a cast. Some stress fractures, however, depending on location, can take longer to heal. Stress fractures of the pelvis, for example, can take up to a year to heal.

Only a physician can diagnose bone injuries, using an x-ray or bone scan. If you are injured, you'll need to temporarily stop or modify your physical activity until the bone is completely healed. If the fracture must be casted or immobilized by some other method, you'll need to stop physical activity involving that body part. Once the bone is healed and your cast is removed, resume physical activity at a lower level than where you left off before the injury, and progress gradually. Even though the injury is healed, the rest of the bone and the soft tissues surrounding it will be weaker because of the reduced activity during the healing process.

If the fracture is not casted, you may modify your physical activity to one that is less stress-ful to the affected bone. For example, if you normally jog and you sustain a stress fracture to a bone in your leg, you may modify your activity to jogging or walking underwater (but you should first check with your physician).

With any bone injury, your physician should decide when it is safe to return to physical activity, on the basis of the results of an x-ray or bone scan. Once you are cleared to return, remember to start slowly and progress gradually.

## OSTEOPOROSIS

*Osteoporosis* means bone *(osteo)* that is porous *(porosis)*. Osteoporosis is a pathological condition in which the loss of bone mineral density accelerates beyond the loss expected with normal aging (see figure 8.4a-b). The diagnosis of osteoporosis is established or confirmed through measurements of bone mineral density. The Osteoporosis and Related Bone Diseases-National Resource Center estimates that about 25 million Americans—80% of them women—have osteoporosis. In spite of the associated bone loss, there are often no symptoms associated with osteoporosis.

The Osteoporosis and Related Bone Diseases-National Resource Center also reports that osteoporosis is responsible for 1.5 million fractures annually. This includes more than 500,000 vertebral fractures, 300,000 hip fractures, and 200,000 wrist fractures. Osteoporosis is the primary underlying cause of fractures in the elderly. It's easy to see why there is a great need for research to develop ways to prevent and treat osteoporosis *before* fractures occur.

### Risk Factors for Osteoporosis

You are at risk for developing osteoporosis if you

- are Caucasian or Asian,
- are female,
- are older than 45,

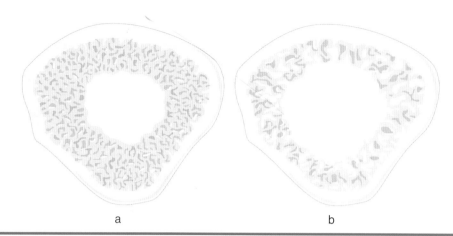

**FIGURE 8.4** *(a)* Normal and *(b)* osteoporotic bone.

- have experienced early menopause (either naturally or through the removal of your uterus or ovaries),
- have a family history of osteoporosis,
- are underweight or have a small frame,
- have amenorrhea,
- have an inadequate calcium intake (premenopausal women and women who take estrogen supplements require about 1,000 milligrams daily; postmenopausal women who do not take estrogen supplements need about 1,500 milligrams daily),
- exercise less than two to three times per week,
- smoke cigarettes,
- use medications such as corticosteroids or anticonvulsants for a prolonged period of time, or
- are male and have low testosterone levels.

The largest at-risk group is Caucasian postmenopausal females. After menopause, a woman produces less estrogen; the hormone estrogen slows the resorption of bone, and a *lack* of estrogen is a major cause of osteoporosis in

### The Effect of Aging on Bone

Bone is a dynamic tissue that undergoes continuous turnover, or *remodeling*. *Osteoclasts* are cells that resorb (break down and assimilate) bone; *osteoblasts* are bone-forming cells that lay down new bone. This breaking down of old bone and laying down of new bone continues throughout life, although the balance between the opposing cellular functions changes with age. For the first 35 years of life, the resorption and new formation of bone go on at similar rates, but after that the rate of resorption exceeds that of bone formation. This results in a decline in **bone mineral density**. This imbalance is minor at first but becomes significant throughout the years. Though it may sound ominous, this loss of bone density is a normal part of aging and doesn't represent a disease process. It is only pathological (altered or caused by disease) when bone loss occurs at a higher rate than it does during normal aging.

women. Early menopause—before the age of 45—is an especially strong predictor of osteoporosis. This is true whether early menopause begins naturally or results from surgical procedures such as a hysterectomy (removal of the uterus) or oophorectomy (removal of the ovaries). Women with very low body fat as a result of overtraining or poor eating habits may become amenorrheic (without menses). These women are also at risk due to diminished estrogen levels.

Cigarette smoking is also believed to play a role in the development of osteoporosis because it lowers women's estrogen levels. This encourages an early menopause, which is a significant risk factor.

Calcium deficiency has been shown to cause osteoporosis in animals and is thus labeled a risk for humans. Calcium in the blood sustains various physiological functions, such as the ability to produce muscle contractions. When your blood calcium drops to inadequate levels, then calcium is removed from your bones to maintain these functions. According to the National Institutes of Health, the usual daily intake of calcium in the United States is 450 to 550 milligrams. Postmenopausal women who don't take estrogen supplements need about 1,500 milligrams a day, while premenopausal women and women who take estrogen supplements require about 1,000 milligrams daily.

Understanding these risk factors is particularly important because early osteoporosis presents no signs or symptoms. Blood and urine samples typically taken during annual physical exams do not diagnose osteoporosis. The National Osteoporosis Foundation reports that bone density loss doesn't show up on x-rays until a person experiences 30% loss. The lab at the end of this chapter will help you determine your risk of developing osteoporosis. If you do have risk factors such as family history or amenorrhea, you may want to ask your physician to conduct a bone densitometry. Imaging techniques to measure bone density are more expensive than regular x-rays, but densitometry can detect osteoporosis at an early stage, allowing you to treat the disease and prevent fractures.

## Physical Activity and Osteoporosis

Preventing and treating osteoporosis center on estrogen replacement therapy, increased calcium intake, and exercise. We'll focus here on the role of physical activity in preventing and treating osteoporosis.

Physical activity can help prevent osteoporosis by increasing bone mass. This understanding came about, in part, from learning what happened to bone in the *absence of* physical activity. Astronauts, who are in an environment with no gravitational forces, have shown marked bone loss. Bedridden people have evidenced similar bone losses.

Bones must be "mechanically loaded" to promote optimal bone mass. "Mechanically loaded" means that the bone must be compressed or pushed upon. This can be accomplished in two ways: in a weight-bearing position (e.g., standing compresses the bones in your legs; sitting compresses the bones in your spine) or through muscle contraction. When you contract the muscles that cross a joint, the two surfaces of the bones in the joint are compressed against each other. So it's clear that physical activity plays a key role in the development and maintenance of healthy bone.

It's also clear that the type of physical activity should be weight bearing; non-weight-bearing activities such as swimming or riding a bike (though you do get some weight-bearing effect through the spine if you're sitting upright) are less effective in stimulating bone mass. Walking and jogging are examples of weight-bearing physical activity that is most effective in preventing and treating osteoporosis.

 Weight-bearing physical activity helps prevent osteoporosis by increasing bone mass.

Bassey and Ramsdale (1994) conducted a study of bone mineral density in young women who participated in six months of either high-impact exercise or low-impact exercise. The women who participated in high-impact exercise showed greater improvements in bone mineral density than those who participated in low-impact exercise. The risk of injury, however, is considerably higher with high-impact exercise.

There's sometimes a fine line involved in choosing an exercise program that will provide optimal benefits without undue risk of injury. Considering other factors such as age and fitness level can help. For older people, walking stimulates the bones well enough and has a low risk of injury. Krall and Dawson-Hughes (1994) demonstrated that walking about 1 mile (1.6 kilometers) a day had beneficial effects on bone mineral density in healthy, postmenopausal women. For younger, more active people, however, walking doesn't provide enough stimulus to produce positive changes in bone mineral density (Uusi-Rasi et al. 1994). According to a publication by the President's Council on Physical Fitness and Sports (1995), the selected exercise should provide forces that are *greater* than those experienced on a day-to-day basis. Thus jogging or another weight-bearing exercise may be a better choice for younger, more active people who feel they are at risk for developing osteoporosis.

Weight training can also be used to prevent or treat osteoporosis. The compressive forces generated by muscle contractions on a bone can produce positive changes in bone mineral density. Exercises performed while standing are especially beneficial because they add weight bearing through the legs and spine and require postural control. In the elderly, declines in postural control and muscle strength of the legs are linked to increased incidence of falls. Weight training can be especially helpful for the elderly. Weight training is also a good form of exercise for younger people who don't want to jog but want positive changes in bone mineral density.

Two notes on physical training and the prevention or treatment of osteoporosis: people must exercise regularly for at least six months before changes in their bone density can be detected, and the benefits gained are specific to the body

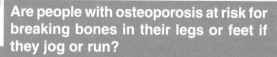

**HEALTHCHECK**

**Are people with osteoporosis at risk for breaking bones in their legs or feet if they jog or run?**

Yes. Female distance runners who become amenorrheic and exhibit decreased bone density have a higher incidence of stress fractures than distance runners with normal bone density.

areas that sustain the highest loads. Walking and jogging will most affect the spine and lower extremities; grip strength exercises will affect the wrist and forearm bones.

## LOW BACK PAIN

One of the most prevalent afflictions that can affect the musculoskeletal system is low back pain. About 8 of 10 people experience some back pain in their lives, and nearly 6 in 10 lose work time because of low back pain. Even though about 6 in 10 people will recover on their own within one week, and about 95% will recover within three months regardless of treatment, the costs associated with low back pain are staggering. In 1990, $24 billion was spent directly on treating low back pain, pointing to two facts: the sheer numbers of people incurring low back injuries are high, and the treatments are expensive. Webster and Snook (1994) found that while low back pain claims in 1989 accounted for only 16% of all workers' compensation claims, they accounted for 33% of the total cost of all claims. Low back pain is also extremely costly in terms of lost wages and disability.

### Structure and Function of the Back

Thirty-three vertebrae stacked one on top of the other compose the spine. The vertebral column is divided into five regions: the *cervical, thoracic, lumbar, sacral,* and *coccygeal* regions (see figure 8.5). Low back pain generally affects the lumbar region but can also affect the sacral region.

In between each vertebral bone is a vertebral *disc*. The fibrocartilaginous disc is a form of specialized cartilage whose primary function is shock absorption. When viewed from behind, the vertebral column should be straight up and down with no lateral deviations. *Scoliosis* is a condition in which lateral curvatures are seen when the vertebral column is viewed from behind.

When viewed from the side, the vertebral column should present four distinct anterior-posterior curves (see figure 8.5). Curves that are convex (curving outward) are ***kyphotic curves***. The thoracic and sacral regions present kyphotic curves. Curves that are concave (curving inward) are ***lordotic curves***. This type of curve is seen in the cervical and lumbar regions.

These curves assist in absorbing shock and give the back its normal posture. In standing, for example, the lordotic curve forms a hollow in the lower back. Some curvature in the lumbar region *(lumbar lordosis)* is essential for a healthy back, but excessive or decreased curvature can cause problems (see figure 8.6).

In addition to forming the normal postural curves, the vertebral column houses the spinal cord. The spinal cord runs down through the spinal canal and gives off spinal nerves (nerve roots) that come out at each vertebral level behind the disc (see figure 8.7). In order to function properly, these nerves must have a clear passageway out.

Each vertebra is joined to the vertebra above and the one below by pairs of synovial joints called *zygapophyseal* or *facet joints*. Ligaments surround and stabilize these joints as well as the joints formed by the vertebrae and discs. Finally

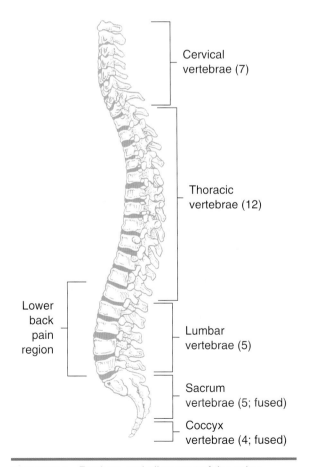

**FIGURE 8.5** Regions and alignment of the spine.

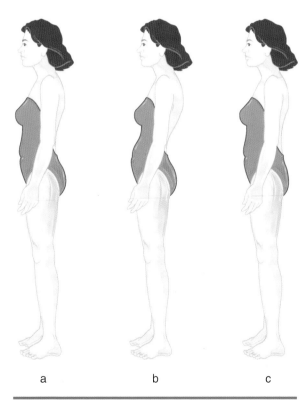

**FIGURE 8.6** *(a)* Correct standing posture, *(b)* excessive lordosis, and *(c)* decreased lordosis.

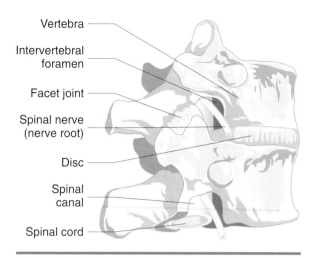

Vertebra

Intervertebral
foramen

Facet joint

Spinal nerve
(nerve root)

Disc

Spinal
canal

Spinal cord

**FIGURE 8.7** Spine segment with exiting nerve root.

there are several layers of muscle that produce and control back movements.

## Causes of Back Pain

The leading causes of low back pain are soft tissue injuries, disc problems, and facet joint problems. Most often the exact cause of a low back pain episode is unknown. According to Nachemson et al. (1987), the cause of the pain can be established for only about 2% of people who seek treatment for low back pain. If the condition persists for six weeks, the cause can be established in 15% of the cases; if it continues for three months, the cause is understood in 30% of the cases.

Nachemson et al. (1987) hypothesize that injury to muscle or its tendinous attachment to the bone accounts for many cases of low back pain. Minor injuries to muscle or tendon generally heal quickly without treatment, as do most cases of acute low back pain. Back pain caused by a disc usually doesn't resolve as quickly. A disc can put pressure on and irritate spinal nerves, causing pain, weakness, and tingling in one or both legs.

Facet joint problems involve the articular cartilage in these joints. Osteoarthritis of the spine, for example, causes pain and swelling in the facet joints. This condition is often chronic—meaning it never goes completely away—and the degenerative changes in the facet joints can cause the spinal canal to narrow. If the narrowing is severe, the spinal cord can be compressed, producing a number of symptoms, such as tingling and muscle weakness, in the legs. This condition is known as *spinal stenosis*.

### HEALTHCHECK

**My father has had a history of back pain. Does that mean I'm more likely to develop back pain?**

No, not unless your father's back pain is caused by a structural abnormality in his spine that you have inherited. In general, low back pain is not an inherited condition, but one that develops as a result of lifestyle, occupation, and habits.

## Preventing Back Pain

The first step in preventing low back pain is to understand the associated risk factors. (The laboratory at the end of this chapter will help you assess your risk for developing back pain.) The primary risk factors for low back pain are related to occupation. The highest incidence of back pain is associated with jobs on the two extremes of physical activity: those that are very physically demanding and those that are sedentary.

### Physically Demanding Jobs

Strength and endurance of back and abdomen muscles are related to the incidence of low back pain in physically demanding jobs (Keyserling, Herrin, and Chaffin 1980; Suzuki and Endo 1983). Snook, Campanelli, and Hart (1978), in a major study of American workers, found that 49% of all low back injuries were caused by lifting tasks. These lifting injuries may occur as a result of heavy lifting that a worker performs infrequently or as a result of lifting submaximal loads repeatedly. Workers need to build the muscle strength and endurance required for the job.

Proper lifting techniques are also critical in preventing low back injuries. When lifting an object from the ground or floor, first straddle the object. Then lower your body toward the object by bending your knees rather than leaning forward at the waist. Keep your back straight, grasp the object, and bring it as close to you as possible before attempting to lift it. Then raise the object by straightening your knees (see figure 8.8). Lifting objects with your back rounded (see figure 8.9) increases the risk of injury.

### Sedentary Jobs

Workers (and students!) who sit for long periods of time need to be especially careful to use correct sitting posture to avoid back pain. Correct posture maintains the normal lordotic curve in the low back (see figure 8.10a). Slouching or slumping down puts great strain on back muscles. Slouching causes the soft tissues that are anterior to your spine to become tight, resulting in loss of the normal lordotic curve. In addition, the posture of the low back during sitting strongly influences the posture of your neck. Sitting in a slouched position puts you in a for-

ward head posture (see figure 8.10b), which causes the muscles in your neck to work harder to keep your head supported over the vertebral column. After a while, the muscles become tired and cause you to have neck pain or headaches. Chairs with properly adjusted backrests can help you achieve and maintain good sitting posture. Even when you do sit correctly, it's important to stand up frequently and stretch or move around.

 Keys to keeping a healthy back are using correct posture and lifting techniques and maintaining strong back and abdominal muscles.

### Treating Back Pain

Most people who have an episode of low back pain don't need to see a health care provider. Typically the symptoms go away within a week, without treatment. However, using ice can help relieve some of the discomfort when the injury first occurs. As described earlier, soft tissues respond to injury by becoming inflamed, swollen, and hot. Ice helps to keep these responses under control.

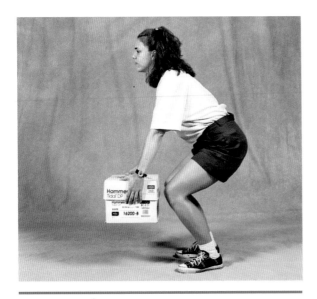

**FIGURE 8.8**  Correct lifting technique: notice the straight back and bent knees.

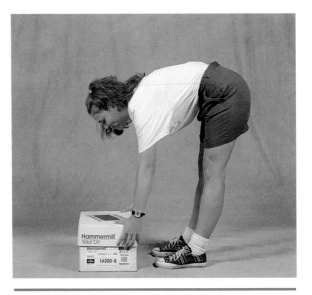

**FIGURE 8.9**  Poor lifting technique: notice the rounded back and straight legs.

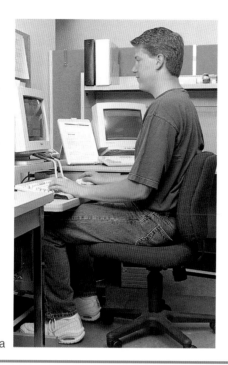 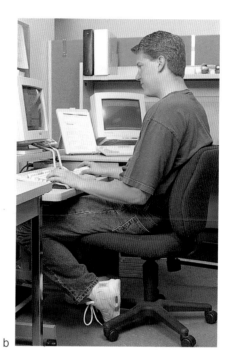

a        b

**FIGURE 8.10** *(a)* Correct and *(b)* incorrect sitting postures.

Health care providers used to routinely prescribe bed rest for back injuries. Today, in certain cases bed rest might be recommended for a day or two, but health care providers are now encouraging physical activity to accelerate the healing process. There are differing opinions on what type of exercise is best, but there is consensus that any movement is better than no movement. The exercises in the lab at the end of this chapter present gentle ways to begin moving your back after an injury.

Of course, you need to be cautious about how you move your back shortly after an injury. Even a day or two after an injury, many people can

### Tips for Preventing Back Pain

Do you want to be among the 2 in 10 people who *don't* experience back pain in their lives? Try incorporating the following tips:
- Use correct sitting and standing postures.
- Use correct lifting techniques, letting your legs, and not your back, do the work. If an object is too heavy, get some help.
- Balance heavy loads and carry them as close to you as possible.
- Strengthen your back and abdominal muscles.
- Don't wear high-heeled shoes; these increase the curvature in your lower back.
- When sitting for a long period of time, choose a chair with good lower back support.
- If you carry a backpack or book bag on one shoulder, switch sides regularly.
- Don't sleep on soft mattresses; these offer little support to the back.

exercise safely so long as their back movements are in a *pain-free range*. Avoid any movement that increases pain. The key is to move as much as you can without pain. Movements that cause pain prolong the inflammatory response and delay the healing. Such movements may also encourage abnormal healing and lead to chronic back problems. If your pain becomes worse or doesn't improve within 7 to 10 days, you should see a health care provider.

You should also consult with a health care provider before beginning exercise if your back pain resulted from a trauma such as an automobile accident or a severe fall. Numbness, tingling, weakness, or severe pain in one or both legs in-

Physical activity can speed the healing process for an injured back. Even a day or two after an injury, many people can exercise safely so long as their back movements are in a *pain-free range*.

dicates that your back pain could be caused by something other than a soft tissue injury; you should see a health care provider if you experience these sensations.

Most importantly, if you experience numbness or tingling in the groin or rectal region, or if you have difficulty controlling your bladder or bowel, you should see a physician immediately.

## ⚪ OF INTEREST

**POINT**

### Musculoskeletal Injuries and the Economy

Musculoskeletal injuries don't just hurt our bodies; they hurt our pocketbooks. Here's a breakdown of how people pay the price for musculoskeletal injuries:

- According to the Osteoporosis and Related Bone Diseases-National Resource Center, Americans spend $10 billion annually in hospital and nursing home expenses for osteoporosis and associated fractures. That works out to about $27 million each day!

- The Arthritis Foundation reports that musculoskeletal conditions such as osteoarthritis and rheumatoid arthritis cost the U.S. economy about $24.6 billion annually in direct health care costs and lost wages and productivity.

- In 1990, people treated for low back pain spent $24 billion on direct medical costs for that treatment.

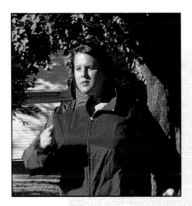

## Health Concepts

As related at the beginning of the chapter, Staci was in a quandary: her mother has osteoporosis and her doctor recommended that Staci jog to help prevent developing it herself. (As you now know, heredity plays a role in the development of osteoporosis.) But jogging causes Staci discomfort. She wasn't sure if she should "fight through the pain."

Well, Staci's on the right track: physical activity can help prevent osteoporosis by increasing bone mass. And weight-bearing activities such as jogging or walking are more helpful than non-weight-bearing activities. In Staci's case, however, walking may be better for her. And weight training would also be helpful, because it can produce positive changes in bone mineral density.

## SUMMARY

▌ Risk factors for sustaining musculoskeletal injuries while engaging in physical activity include older age, structural faults in the musculoskeletal system, too much body weight, and previous musculoskeletal injuries.

▌ A healthy joint's surfaces are covered with 2 to 4 millimeters of smooth *articular cartilage* that is kept lubricated with *synovial fluid.* Synovial fluid is the articular cartilage's primary source of nutrition and thus is critical to the joint's health.

▌ Arthritis affects nearly 40 million Americans, making it the number one cause of disability in this country. *Osteoarthritis* is the most common type of arthritis, affecting nearly 16 million Americans. Osteoarthritis is called a *degenerative joint disease* because it is characterized by degenerating joint articular cartilage. Factors that contribute to osteoarthritis include age, obesity, previous injury to a joint, and faulty joint alignment.

▌ Physical activity can help prevent and treat osteoarthritis because it can help develop healthy articular cartilage by putting the joint surfaces through cycles of compression and decompression.

▌ *Rheumatoid arthritis* affects multiple systems in the body. It is an autoimmune disease in which the body's natural immune system attacks its own healthy joint tissue, resulting in inflammation and damage to the joint cartilage and bone.

▌ Musculoskeletal injuries that involve tissues such as ligaments, muscles, tendons, and bursa are known as *soft tissue injuries.* Many soft tissue injuries occur gradually, brought on by the cumulative effects of repeating the same motion or motions over and over. These types of injuries are called *overuse injuries.*

▌ An effective treatment approach to soft tissue injuries is *RICE:* rest, ice, compression, and elevation. This approach minimizes the effects of inflammation and speeds the healing process.

▌ A *fracture* occurs when a bone is broken; a *stress fracture* occurs from repetitive force on a bone that initially causes pain with exercise but then eases off with rest. As a stress fracture progresses, the pain becomes worse after the activity is stopped.

▌ *Osteoporosis* is a pathological condition in which the loss of bone mineral density accelerates beyond the loss expected with normal aging. The diagnosis of osteoporosis is established or confirmed through measurements of bone mineral density.

▌ It's estimated that about 25 million Americans—80% of them women—have osteoporosis. Risk factors include age, gender, race, heredity, hormonal changes, diet (i.e., calcium deficiency), and low body weight. The largest at-risk group is Caucasian postmenopausal females.

▌ Weight-bearing physical activity can help prevent osteoporosis by increasing bone mass. Weight training can also help prevent osteoporosis by improving bone mineral density.

▌ About 8 in 10 people experience back pain at some time in their lives. Leading causes include soft tissue injuries, disc problems, and facet joint problems. Proper posture and correct lifting techniques can help prevent back pain.

▌ Physical activity can help a person recover more swiftly from back pain, so long as the activity does not increase the pain.

*We've just explored how physical activity impacts a number of musculoskeletal health problems, including osteoporosis, arthritis, soft tissue injuries, and back pain. In the next chapter we'll look at the number two cause of death: cancer. We'll also examine diabetes mellitus, a disease that affects millions of Americans every year.*

## KEY TERMS

| | |
|---|---|
| arthritis | lumbar lordosis |
| bone mineral density | osteoporosis |
| bursitis | overuse injury |
| contusion | soft tissue injuries |
| cumulative trauma disorder | sprain |
| inflammation | strain |
| kyphotic curves | stress fracture |
| lordotic curves | tendinitis |

8

# Determining Risks of Developing Osteoporosis and Back Pain, and Learning Back Exercises

8

### THE PURPOSES OF THIS LAB EXPERIENCE ARE TO

▌ determine your risk of developing osteoporosis,

▌ assess your risk of developing back pain, and

▌ learn and perform back exercises that can strengthen the back and prevent back pain.

### Determine Your Risk of Developing Osteoporosis

The National Osteoporosis Foundation has identified a variety of risk factors for osteoporosis. Complete the following evaluation related to those risk factors. The more questions you answer yes, the higher your risk for developing osteoporosis.

| | YES | NO |
|---|---|---|
| 1. Are you female? | ❑ | ❑ |
| 2. If you are female: | | |
|     Have you gone through menopause? | ❑ | ❑ |
|     Have you had a history of abnormal menstrual cycles? | ❑ | ❑ |
|     Have your ovaries been removed through surgery? | ❑ | ❑ |
| 3. Are you over 50 years of age? | ❑ | ❑ |
| 4. Are you Caucasian or Asian? | ❑ | ❑ |
| 5. Are you thin and small boned? | ❑ | ❑ |
| 6. Are you a regular smoker? | ❑ | ❑ |
| 7. Do you drink more than one beer or other alcoholic drink on a daily basis? | ❑ | ❑ |
| 8. Does your normal diet lack calcium rich foods (dairy products)? | ❑ | ❑ |
| 9. Does your lifestyle include regular weight-bearing physical activity? | ❑ | ❑ |
| 10. Do you have arthritis? | ❑ | ❑ |
| 11. Have you had to take anti-inflammatory drugs or thyroid medication for extended periods of time? | ❑ | ❑ |
| 12. Do you have a family history of osteoporosis? | ❑ | ❑ |

## Assess Your Risk of Developing Back Pain

Take the following quiz to see how many of the risk factors apply to you. Note that each factor is controllable—you can take action to lessen that risk. Answering "yes" indicates that you are at risk for that particular factor.

|  |  | YES | NO |
|---|---|:---:|:---:|
| 1. | Am I overweight? | ❏ | ❏ |
| 2. | Does my stomach stick out? | ❏ | ❏ |
| 3. | Do I smoke, especially heavily? | ❏ | ❏ |
| 4. | Do I sit for prolonged periods of time, especially without breaks? | ❏ | ❏ |
| 5. | Is my chair at work comfortable? | ❏ | ❏ |
| 6. | Do I do repetitive pushing and pulling or lifting while bending or twisting (whether working at home, in an office, in a warehouse, or outdoors)? | ❏ | ❏ |
| 7. | Does my work require me to use power tools or heavy moving equipment or to drive a lot? | ❏ | ❏ |
| 8. | Is my bed comfortable? | ❏ | ❏ |
| 9. | Do I stand in one place a lot? | ❏ | ❏ |
| 10. | Do I slouch most of the time? | ❏ | ❏ |
| 11. | Is my car seat comfortable for me? | ❏ | ❏ |
| 12. | Do I engage in any kind of exercise or sport regularly? | ❏ | ❏ |
| 13. | Does stress in my daily life make my back pain worse? | ❏ | ❏ |
| 14. | Do I get enough calcium in my diet, especially if I'm over 50? | ❏ | ❏ |

Now that you've checked your own personal risk factors with help from the YMCA's *Healthy Back Book*, use the following adapted descriptions of what each factor is and determine how to change them.

### Overweight (Questions 1 and 2)

If you're overweight, you probably aren't physically fit, and fitness has been shown to be related to back health. If some of that weight is a potbelly, it may be adding even more stress to your lower back muscles.

### Risky Movements (Questions 6, 7, 11, and 12)

Whether you're on the job, in class, at home, or playing sports, there are certain movements that increase stress on your spine. Lifting is one; lifting as you bend or twist is even worse. Repetitive back movements, such as pitching a softball or working on an assembly line, can also tire muscles and cause pain. Using correct posture for lifting, driving, and other work tasks can offer you some protection.

### Smoking (Question 3)

The connection between smoking and back pain is not obvious, but a number of studies have shown a strong relationship between the two. Some speculate that smoking causes coughing, which in turn stresses the back muscles. Recent studies indicate that smoking accelerates the blood flow around the discs, depriving them of nutrients. Because smoking puts you at risk for cancer, heart disease, and many other serious illnesses, as well as for back pain, we suggest you quit if you now smoke.

### Being Sedentary (Questions 4 and 12)

Studies have shown that people who are the most fit are the ones least likely to have back pain (not counting sport injuries). This probably is the case in part because the muscles that support your back are conditioned by exercise; regular aerobic exercise may also more directly help the discs in the back by increasing blood flow around them, supplying more nutrients. In addition, weight-bearing exercise helps maintain or increase your bone mass, which helps prevent osteoporosis.

Besides getting regular aerobic exercise, you can improve the strength and flexibility of the muscles that support your back with exercises that focus on those particular muscles (see the next section).

### Bad Posture (Questions 4, 5, 8-11)

Slouching or slumping won't necessarily do permanent damage to your back, but it can cause pain. Like the other muscles in your body, those in your neck and back can become fatigued if held in one position too long. The obvious solution is to sit and stand in ways that relieve stress on muscles and also to move and stretch more often. Having a comfortable bed and chair can help ease back pain as well.

### Pain and Stress (Question 13)

Back pain, like any pain, is likely to feel worse when you're under stress. Conscious relaxation may help you reduce your pain by relaxing tense muscles and lowering your stress level.

### Lack of Calcium (Question 14)

An adequate supply of calcium throughout your life can provide some protection against developing osteoporosis. You don't have to drink milk if you hate it; other foods can supply calcium.

## Perform Back Exercises

The following exercises are reprinted from the *YMCA Healthy Back Book* (1994). Perform the exercises according to the instructions, and have a partner check you for correct form. Do the same for your partner. The Level 1 exercises are a good place to start if you are just beginning an exercise program for your back or if you are recovering from a back injury. When you can consistently perform the exercises in Level 1 for the maximum number of repetitions, you can then move to Level 2.

Perform these exercises daily, or at least as often as you do your regular exercise program. Since the exercises are best done after you've warmed up your muscles, a good way to incorporate them into your regular program is to perform them after your exercise. For example, if you walk five times per week, make a habit of doing these back exercises at the end of the walk when your muscles are warm.

**Level 1 Exercises**

*Pelvic Tilt (Standing)*

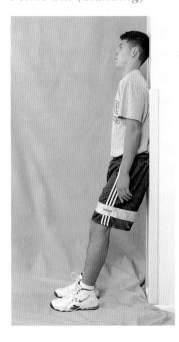

- Stand with your back against a wall, feet shoulder-width apart, and heels 12 to 18 inches (30 to 46 centimeters) from the wall. Slightly bend your knees.
- Rotate your pelvis so your lower back contacts the wall. Tighten your lower abdominal muscles and hold this "pelvic brace" for 5 seconds.
- Repeat 15 to 20 times.

*Pelvic Tilt (On Your Back)*

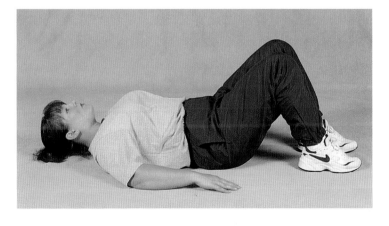

- Lie on your back with both knees bent, feet flat on the floor, and arms at your sides. (You might want to place a small pillow under your head or neck.)
- Exhale and rotate your pelvis so your lower back contacts the floor. Tighten your lower abdominal muscles and hold this pelvic brace for 5 seconds.
- Repeat 15 to 20 times.

## Back Arch

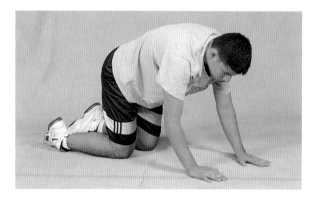

- Get on all fours on the floor and pull in your abdominal muscles.
- Drop your head forward and round your back as you tilt your pelvis. Hold for 5 seconds.
- Repeat 5 to 10 times.

## Leg Raise

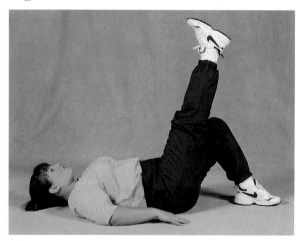

- Lie on your back with both knees bent, feet flat on the floor, and arms at your sides. (You might want to place a small pillow under your head or neck.) Do a pelvic tilt and hold; your abdominal muscles should be tight.
- Exhale and straighten one knee, slowly raising your leg as high as possible without pain. Don't allow your pelvis to rock or to roll upward. Try to keep your leg straight without locking your knee. Hold this position for 5 seconds, then slowly return your leg to the floor.
- Repeat 5 to 10 times per leg.

## Prone on Elbows

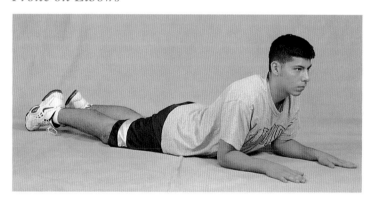

- Lie facedown on the floor with your arms at your sides and your head turned to one side. Take deep breaths and try to relax for 3 to 5 minutes.
- Place your elbows under your shoulders as you ease your trunk up, then rest your weight on your forearms. Use your shoulders and arms to push your head and upper trunk up; don't use your back muscles to lift. Look straight ahead. Hold this position for 15 to 30 seconds.
- Do once per exercise session.

## *Prone Extension*

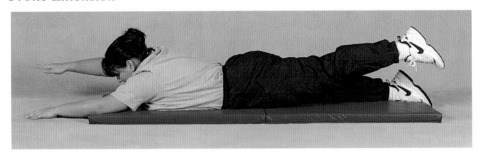

- Lie facedown with your arms extended over your head.
- Exhale, slowly lifting your left arm and right leg 6 to 12 inches (15 to 30 centimeters) off the floor, and hold for 5 seconds. Keep your eyes to the floor, and don't hold your breath. Lower your arm and leg, and repeat using your right arm and left leg.
- Repeat 10 to 15 times per pair.

## *Wall Slide*

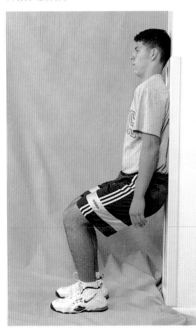

- Stand with your back against a wall, feet shoulder-width apart, knees slightly bent, and heels 12 to 18 inches (30 to 46 centimeters) from the wall.
- Exhale, and rotate your pelvis so your lower back comes in contact with the wall. Tighten your lower abdominal muscles and hold.
- Bend your knees while sliding your back down the wall. Don't ever bend your knees more than 90 degrees. If your knees hurt, try bending them only slightly. Hold the bottom position for 10 to 20 seconds.
- Repeat 5 to 10 times. Try to build up so you can hold the bottom position for 2 minutes. Reduce the number of repetitions as you increase the length of time you hold at the bottom position.

*Quadruped*

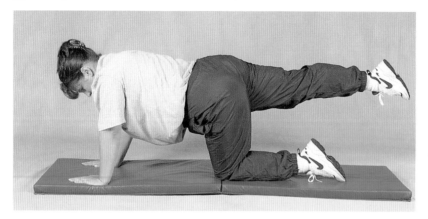

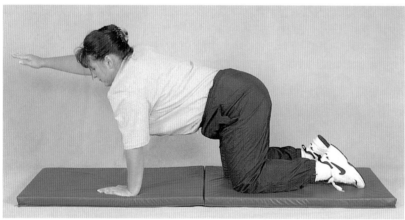

- Get on all fours. Brace your pelvis by pulling in your abdominals and holding your back in a pain-free position.
- Slowly raise each arm and leg, one at a time, to a horizontal position and hold for 5 seconds; then lower the limb. Keep your trunk from sagging by maintaining your pelvic brace, and keep your eyes on the floor.
- Repeat 5 to 10 times per limb.

*Trunk Curl*

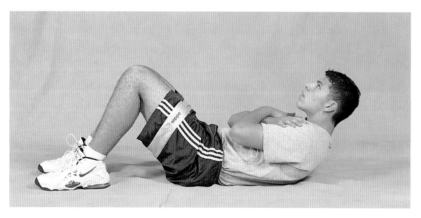

- Lie on your back with both knees bent and feet flat on the floor. Cross your arms across your chest, do a pelvic tilt, and hold.
- Keeping your lower back in contact with the floor, exhale and slowly raise your shoulder blades off the floor; then lower them, inhaling as you return to the starting position. Keep your eyes on the ceiling; try not to bend your neck forward.
- Repeat 15 to 30 times.

## Hip Flexor Stretch

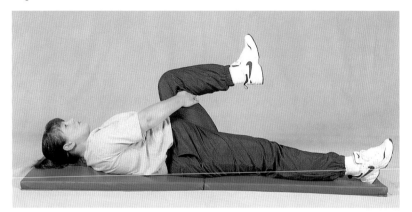

- Lie on your back with your legs straight and arms at your sides.
- Grasp one thigh behind your knee and pull it toward your chest until your lower back is in contact with the floor. Keep the opposite leg straight.
- If your extended leg does not stay on the floor, hold this position for 5 to 10 seconds, and repeat 5 to 10 times per leg.
- If you are doing this exercise correctly and your extended leg is in contact with the floor, you can eliminate this exercise from your routine—your hip flexors are flexible. Try this exercise periodically to make sure they remain flexible.

## Single Leg Raise

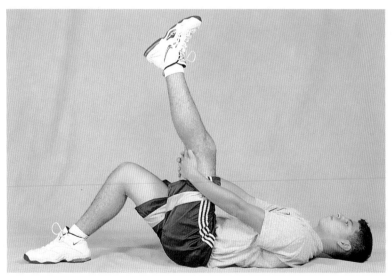

- Lie on your back with both knees bent, feet flat on the floor and arms at your sides. (You might want to place a small pillow under your head or neck.) Exhale, do a pelvic tilt, and hold.
- Straighten one knee and slowly raise your leg as high as possible without pain (don't point or flex your foot). After you have lifted your leg as far as you can, keeping your knee straight but not locked, gently pull your leg closer to you as you contract the front of your thigh. Hold for 10 seconds.
- Repeat 5 to 10 times per leg.

*Press-Up*

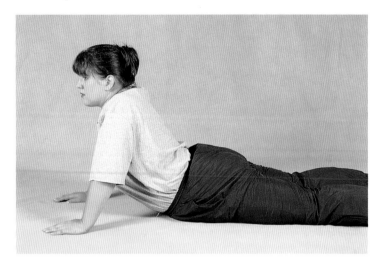

- Lie facedown with your hands near your shoulders.
- Keeping your weight on your hands, use your shoulders and arms to push your head and upper trunk up; try to keep the rest of your body relaxed. Don't use your back muscles to lift, and keep your pelvis on the floor. Hold the upper position for 2 seconds, keeping your eyes straight ahead.
- Repeat 5 to 10 times. Each time you repeat, extend your arms a bit farther.

# Chapter 9

# Cancer and Diabetes

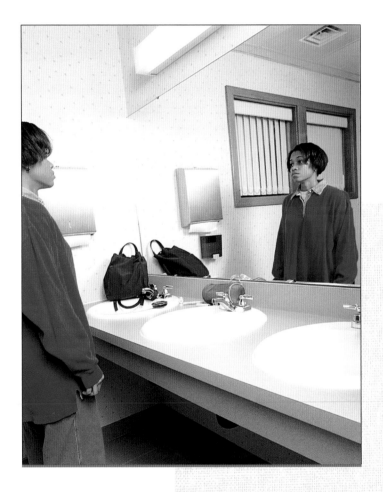

I found a lump in one of my breasts today. My roommate told me I should get it checked out, but I don't know. I'm pretty sure it's nothing—there's never been any breast cancer in my family. It'll probably go away in a few days. And besides, we're heading into finals week and I don't have an hour or two to waste going to the clinic and just sitting. It does bother me a little bit but I can get it checked after finals, if it's still there. I think I'll probably give it a week or so and see if it goes away.

—Natalie, 19-year-old freshman

## *W*hat do you think*?*

Two risk factors in Natalie's favor are her family history and her age: women over 50 years old are more susceptible to breast cancer than younger women. But there are other risk factors for breast cancer. Do you know what they are? Is there any danger in Natalie's waiting to see if the lump goes away?

In this chapter we'll look at two major diseases: cancer and diabetes mellitus. Cancer is the second leading cause of death in the United States, and diabetes mellitus is a serious disease that afflicts about 15.7 million Americans.

We'll look at several types of cancer, exploring their causes and risk factors. Some risk factors we can't change (such as age and heredity); others we can. We'll look at ways to prevent cancer by working on the factors that we can change. And within those risk factors, we'll examine how physical activity affects cancer and diabetes.

## CANCER

The word "cancer" evokes a response of dread and fear. Cancer is a disease that is associated with pain, suffering, and high financial costs. As we've already mentioned, it is the number two cause of death in the United States, behind cardiovascular disease—and it is projected to overtake cardiovascular disease as the leading cause of death early in the twenty-first century. The American Cancer Society reports that 1,228,600 new cases were diagnosed and 564,800 people died of cancer in 1998. These statistics don't include the more than 1 million cases of skin cancer expected to be reported for that year. Eight million Americans are alive with a history of cancer, past or active. The lifetime risk of developing some type of cancer is one in two for men and one in three for women (American Cancer Society 1998). The good news is that the cancer death rates have dropped in the 1990s, by 2.6% between 1990 and 1995.

The effects of physical activity on cancer are not as clear-cut as they are for cardiovascular disease, but physical activity does have benefits both for preventing certain types of cancer and for surviving the disease. With that in mind, we'll briefly describe what cancer is and how it develops, define some of the more common cancers, and outline the risk factors and the lifestyle behaviors that minimize those risks.

## Cancer: The Development of Mutant Cells

*Cancer* is a complex group of diseases characterized by the uncontrolled growth and spread of abnormal cells. A cell with normal genes or genetic control produces normal cell growth or division. But some genes or genetic control of cells become abnormal, and cancer begins to develop (see figure 9.1). *Genes* are the microscopic structures in every cell that contain the genetic codes that determine to a large degree our appearance, personality, body composition, intelligence, natural resistance to disease, and fitness level. These genetic or inherited traits, along with our environment, make us the persons we are. Genes contain instructions that control when our cells grow and divide. Certain genes called *oncogenes* promote cell division, while tumor suppressor genes slow down cell division or cause cells to die at the appropriate time. Cancers can be caused by gene mutations (defects) that activate oncogenes or deactivate tumor suppressor genes; these defects in gene control of cell division can then lead to cancer. These abnormal cells form masses called *tumors.* Some tumors are not cancerous; these are called *benign* tumors. Benign tumors remain localized and usually are treated with little risk of death. *Cancerous* tumors, however, spread, or *metastasize,* to other areas of the body. As these tumors spread, they interfere with the normal functioning of the body; this is how cancer kills.

**KEY POINT** *Cancer* is a complex group of diseases characterized by the uncontrolled growth and spread of abnormal cells. Cancers can be caused by gene mutations (defects) that activate oncogenes or deactivate tumor suppressor genes; these defects in gene control of cell division can then lead to cancer.

Some cancers develop very quickly (e.g., lung cancer); others develop slowly (e.g., basal cell skin cancer). Cells become abnormal for a variety of reasons. Most adults have cancerous or precancerous cells in their bodies; these cells are normally destroyed by a person's immune system. But as we age the immune system may become weakened and may not destroy all the cancerous cells. In addition, some diseases may weaken the immune system; for example, AIDS patients have high rates of cancer because of their weakened immune system. External agents such as tobacco smoke, chemicals, ultraviolet light, radiation, and viruses can also cause cancer. As these agents come into contact with the body's cells they can cause gene mutations that lead to cancer.

As a cancer develops, it is classified as follows:

- Carcinoma: cancer of the soft tissues and organs (e.g., skin, lung, stomach, ovaries)
- Sarcoma: cancer of the bones, muscles, and connective tissue

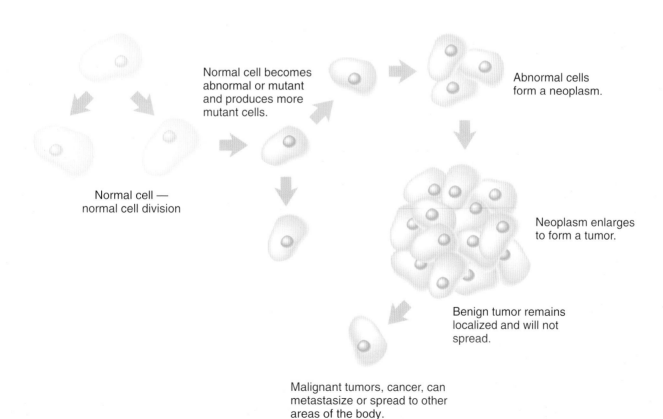

**FIGURE 9.1** Development of mutant cancer cells.

- Lymphoma: cancer of the lymphatic system, which is part of the immune system
- Leukemia: cancer of the blood-forming tissue (bone marrow)

Lung cancer, breast cancer, and colon and rectal cancer are the top three cancer killers for women; lung cancer, prostate cancer, and colon and rectal cancer are the top three killers for men (see figure 9.2).

## Signs and Risk Factors

We've already alluded to a number of general risk factors for cancer: aging, heredity, tobacco, chemicals, ultraviolet light, radiation, and viruses. However, it is becoming clear that simple lifestyle behaviors such as not using tobacco, eating a healthy balanced diet, and being physically active will cause the greatest reductions in morbidity and mortality rates due to cancer. This is certainly true for these lifestyle changes in relation to the major cancer killers we'll discuss here. In the following sections we'll take a look at specific signs and symptoms and risk factors for the four cancers just mentioned as the leading causes of cancer deaths: lung, breast, prostate, and colon and rectal cancers. (In the lab at the end of the chapter you'll be evaluating your own risk for these diseases.)

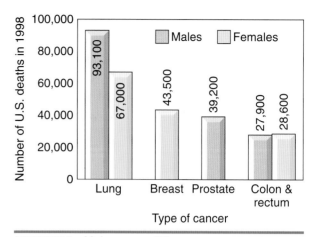

**FIGURE 9.2** Major cancer killers.
Adapted from American Cancer Society, 1998, *1998 Cancer Facts & Figures*.

### Lung Cancer

As shown in figure 9.2, lung cancer is the leading cause of cancer deaths in both men and women, with men at a higher risk of developing lung cancer than women. Older people are more likely than younger people to develop lung cancer; lung cancer is relatively rare in people under 40, but the number of cases goes up after age 50 and even more so after age 65. Signs of lung cancer include a persistent cough, blood-streaked sputum (spit or phlegm), chest pain, and recurring pneumonia or bronchitis. Unfortunately, these signs become apparent after the disease has progressed significantly; that's why lung cancer is so deadly. Smoking tobacco presents

## The Seven Danger Signs of Cancer

According to the American Cancer Society, these are the seven danger signs of cancer. If you have any of these symptoms, you should immediately see your physician.
1. A change in bowel movements or urination
2. A sore that won't heal
3. Sudden bleeding or discharge
4. A lump or hardening in the breasts or anywhere else
5. Frequent and prolonged indigestion or difficulty swallowing
6. Changes in the color or size of moles or warts
7. Hoarseness and persistent cough

the most severe risk for lung cancer—smokers are *10 to 20 times* more likely to develop this cancer than nonsmokers. Other risks include exposure to industrial or organic chemicals, radon, and asbestos; radiation from occupational, medical, or environmental sources; air pollution; tuberculosis; and environmental tobacco smoke.

 Cigarette smokers are *10 to 20 times* more likely to develop lung cancer than nonsmokers.

**Table 9.1 Chances of Developing Breast Cancer With Age**

| Age | Chances |
| --- | --- |
| By age 25 | 1 in 19,608 |
| By age 30 | 1 in 2,525 |
| By age 35 | 1 in 622 |
| By age 40 | 1 in 217 |
| By age 45 | 1 in 93 |
| By age 50 | 1 in 50 |
| By age 55 | 1 in 33 |
| By age 60 | 1 in 24 |
| By age 65 | 1 in 17 |
| By age 70 | 1 in 14 |
| By age 75 | 1 in 11 |
| By age 80 | 1 in 10 |
| By age 85 | 1 in 9 |
| Ever | 1 in 8 |

### HEALTHCHECK

**If a regular smoker was also regularly physically active, would that person's risk of early mortality decrease?**

Most regular smokers aren't regularly physically active. But smokers who are physically active have lower death rates than smokers who are sedentary. Of course, exercising doesn't eliminate the risks incurred through smoking.

## Breast Cancer

Breast cancer is the most common cancer among women, excluding skin cancers; women have a one in eight lifetime chance of developing breast cancer. Men can also develop breast cancer, but the risk is very low. Any noticeable change in the breast may be a sign of breast cancer (see page 233 for the American Cancer Society's recommendations regarding breast self-examinations). There are many risk factors for breast cancer—the biggest are family history (a grandmother, mother, or sister with breast cancer), including specific gene susceptibility; aging (see table 9.1); obesity; physical inactivity; and menstrual irregularities. The risk is also greater for women who bear children for the first time when past the age of 30 and for women who have never borne children.

## Prostate Cancer

Prostate cancer, which affects only men, is the most common cancer (excluding skin cancer) among American men. Prostate cancer is the second leading cause of cancer death in men, surpassed only by lung cancer. Warning signs of prostate cancer include changes in urination patterns, blood in urine, pain during urination, and constant pain in the lower trunk or upper thighs. Age, race, obesity, family history (father or brother with prostate cancer), and high-fat diets are all associated with an increased risk for prostate cancer. The chance of having prostate cancer increases rapidly after age 50—more than 80% of all cases are diagnosed in men over the age of 65. In addition, prostate cancer is about twice as common among African-American men as it is among Caucasian American men.

## Colon and Rectal Cancer

Colon and rectal cancers accounted for about 11% of new cases of cancer in 1998. The main signs of these cancers are rectal bleeding, blood in the stool, and a change in bowel habits. Risk factors for colon and rectal cancer include a

## Tobacco and Your Health

In 1998, over 430,000 Americans (3 million people worldwide) will die because of tobacco use. Tobacco smoking is a major risk factor for lung cancer and coronary heart disease (tobacco use accounts for one in three cancer deaths in the United States). It is also associated with a variety of other cancers—including cancer of the mouth, pharynx, larynx, esophagus, pancreas, uterus, cervix, kidney, and bladder—as well as other diseases such as colds, gastric ulcers, chronic bronchitis, emphysema, and stroke. Tobacco use is the most preventable cause of death in the United States.

Tobacco smoke contains over 40 chemicals that are considered to be cancer causing. In addition, the 1998 Surgeon General's Report on Nicotine Addiction indicated that nicotine in tobacco is extremely addictive. Although the vast majority of smokers are interested in quitting, their addiction to nicotine makes this a difficult process. However, by 1994, 46 million Americans who smoked regularly quit successfully, and with the advent of nonprescription aids such as gum and patches that gradually wean smokers off nicotine, there is even more hope for those who wish to stop.

Environmental smoke and smokeless tobacco have also been related to a variety of health problems. Environmental tobacco smoke, also called "secondhand" or "sidestream" smoke, has all of the damaging chemicals of tobacco smoke that is directly inhaled. Individuals exposed to constant large doses of secondhand smoke develop many of the same health problems as smokers. Children and unborn babies exposed to smoke at home or in the mother's womb have high frequencies of respiratory illness, ear infections, and limited lung function. Smokeless chewing tobacco is associated with very high risks for oral cancers.

Trends in tobacco smoking are generally positive in the United States. Over 50% of adults smoked tobacco regularly in the early 1960s; this figure had dropped to about 25% in 1998. This reduction was initiated by aggressive education on the dangers of smoking and public health efforts to reduce tobacco use and social acceptance of smokers. However, 47 million adults (and 16% of high school students) in the United States still smoke, with minorities, men, and people with lower education levels showing the highest rates.

Tobacco generates billions of dollars of economic activity in the United States; however, because of the health consequences, the health costs associated with tobacco use are estimated at $100 billion a year—$3.90 for each pack of cigarettes sold.

personal or family history of colorectal cancer or polyps; inflammatory bowel disease; physical inactivity; age (about 90% of people found to have colorectal cancer are older than 50); a high-fat or low-fiber diet; and an inadequate intake of fruits and vegetables.

## Preventing, Detecting, and Treating Cancer

Some cancers can be prevented through lifestyle behaviors. Eliminating tobacco use, consuming alcohol in moderation, having a healthy diet

# Breast Self-Examinations

The American Cancer Society recommends that women examine their breasts monthly, using the following three-step method. The best time to examine your breasts is about a week after the start of your period, when breasts are usually not tender or swollen. (Adapted from *How To Do Breast Self-Examination* pamphlet, 1992.)

## Step 1: Before a Mirror

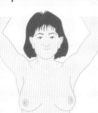

Inspect your breasts with your arms at your sides. Then raise your arms overhead, checking for changes in shape or contour and for swelling or dimpling of skin. Check for any changes in the skin or nipples.

Then place your palms on your hips and press down firmly to flex your chest muscles. Don't look for the left and right breasts to exactly match; few women's do.

## Step 2: Lying Down

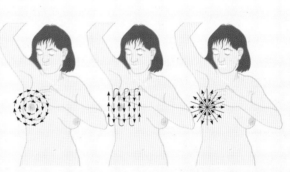

Place a pillow under your right shoulder. Keep the middle three fingers of your left hand flat and feel for lumps or changes in your right breast using rubbing motions like the three shown here. Press firmly enough to feel the different breast tissues. Feel all of the breast and chest area from the collarbone to the base of a properly fitted bra, and from the breastbone to the underarm. Repeat on the other breast. Squeeze the nipple of each breast to look for any discharge. Report any discharge to your physician.

## Step 3: In the Shower

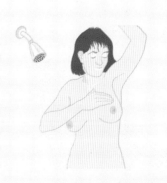

Examine your breasts during a bath or shower; hands glide easier over wet skin. Keep your fingers flat and move them gently over every part of each breast. Check for lumps, hardening, or thickening.

If you find a lump or discharge you should see your physician as soon as possible. However, don't be frightened; most breast lumps or changes are not cancer. But only your doctor can make the diagnosis.

(based on the principles explained in chapter 5), limiting sun exposure, engaging in prudent sexual behavior, and maintaining sufficient physical activity levels are lifestyle behaviors that lower the risk of cancer. For example, about 175,000 of the 564,800 estimated cancer deaths in 1998 were caused by tobacco use. The cure for a diagnosed cancer is related to early detection and effective treatment. Table 9.2 summarizes the diagnostic tests recommended by the American Cancer Society for early detection of cancer. Regular medical checkups with a primary care physician and/or gynecologist for women are the first step.

Cancer can be treated by

- surgery (surgical removal of the malignant tumors),
- radiation (x-ray or radiotherapy to kill cancer cells),
- chemotherapy (drug therapy to kill cancer cells),
- hormone therapy (controlling hormones to retard the growth of malignant tumors), and
- immunotherapy (activating the body's immune system to destroy cancer cells and retard tumor growth).

## The Most Common Cancer: Skin Cancer

Skin cancer in its various forms is the most frequently diagnosed cancer in the United States. In 1998, there were about 1 million cases of basal cell carcinoma and squamous cell carcinoma. *Melanoma*, the most serious type of skin cancer, was diagnosed in 41,600 new cases in 1998. More than 7,300 people died from melanoma in 1998; all other skin cancers accounted for slightly more than 1,900 deaths.

The principal sign of melanoma is any noticeable change in a mole or dark-pigmented area of the skin. The American Cancer Society has devised an "ABCD rule" for detecting melanoma:

A = Asymmetry. One half of the mole or pigmentation does not match the other half.

B = Border irregularity. The edges are ragged, notched, or blurred.

C = Color. The color is not the same across the entire mole or pigmentation.

D = Diameter. The diameter is greater than 6 millimeters. Any sudden or progressive increase in size should be examined.

Primary risks for skin cancer are light or fair complexion; exposure to ultraviolet radiation (sunlight), coal tar, pitch, creosote, arsenic, and radium; and family history. Most skin cancers in the United States are caused by exposure to sunlight. These are the best ways to prevent cancers from the sun's rays:

▮ Avoid sun exposure from 10 A.M. to 3 P.M.; ultraviolet radiation is strongest during these times.

▮ Wear protective clothing and sunscreen with a skin protection factor (SPF) of at least 15.

▮ Avoid getting sunburns that cause your skin to peel. This is especially damaging to babies and young children. Sunburns in childhood greatly increase the risk of adult skin cancer.

## Table 9.2 American Cancer Society Recommendations for the Early Detection of Cancer

| Site | Recommendation |
|------|----------------|
| Breast | Women 40 years of age and older should have an annual mammogram, should have an annual clinic breast exam (CBE) performed by a health care professional, and should perform monthly self-examination. The CBE should be conducted close to the scheduled mammogram.<br><br>Women ages 20-39 should have a CBE performed by a health care professional every three years and should perform monthly breast self-examination. |
| Prostate | Both the prostate-specific antigen blood test and the digital rectal examination should be offered annually, beginning at age 50, to men who have a life expectancy of at least 10 years and to younger men who are at high risk.<br><br>Men in high-risk groups, such as those with a strong family history (two or more affected first-degree relatives) or African-Americans, may begin at a younger age (e.g., 45 years). |
| Colon and rectum | Men and women age 50 or older should follow *one* of these examination schedules:<br>• A fecal occult blood test every year and a flexible sigmoidoscopy every 5 years[1]<br>• A colonoscopy every 10 years[1]<br>• A double-contrast barium enema every 5 to 10 years[1] |
| Uterus | Cervix: All women who are or who have been sexually active or who are 18 and older should have an annual pap test and pelvic examination. After three or more consecutive satisfactory examinations with normal findings, the pap test may be performed less frequently. Discuss the matter with your physician.<br><br>Endometrium: Women at high risk for cancer of the uterus should have a sample of endometrial tissue examined when menopause begins. |

[1]A digital rectal exam should be done at the same time as sigmoidoscopy, colonoscopy, or double-contrast barium enema. People who are at moderate or high risk for colon or rectal cancer should talk with a doctor about a different testing schedule.

Adapted from American Cancer Society, 1998, *1998 Graphical Data: Summary of ACS Recommendations for the Early Detection of Cancer in Asymptomatic People.*

### HEALTHCHECK

**Hormones play an important role in diabetes and cancer. What are hormones and where do they originate?**

Hormones are chemical messengers secreted by glands of the endocrine and/or exocrine system that are needed for normal control of the body's functions. The pancreas secretes the hormone insulin for the proper control of blood sugar levels. Diabetes is the inability to produce or utilize insulin properly. Gender related hormones such as estrogen and testosterone have a role in certain types of cancer.

Treatment strategy depends on the type and location of cancer; one or more types of treatment may be involved in the strategy. Cancer is a complex disease with a variety of malignant cell types that respond to different treatments in different ways. Early diagnosis is critical to the successful treatment and cure for cancer. A cure is hard to define, but people are usually considered cured after they have had no further symptoms for five years after receiving the last treatment.

Generally, five-year survival rates after initial diagnosis have been used to study the interaction between detection stage and treatment. Figure 9.3 summarizes five-year survival rates by stage of diagnosis for the major cancer killers. Lung cancer, the number one cancer killer, has very low survival rates. It is difficult to detect early and tends to spread quickly. Breast, prostate, and colon cancer have survival rates greater than 90% when detected early at the local stage of the disease. The rates of survival drop to very low levels when the disease is detected later and has spread to distant areas of the body. Prevention, detection, and treatment of cancer have improved in the 1990s; the rate of cancer deaths in the United States has dropped by 2.6%. This is due in part to lower numbers of adults who smoke, better diagnostic tests, and improved treatments for all cancers.

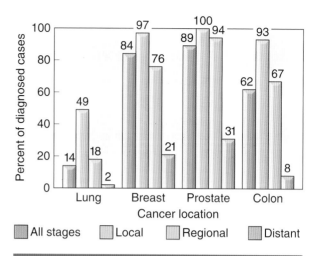

**FIGURE 9.3**   Five-year survival rates for cancer patients.
Adapted from American Cancer Society, 1998, *1998 Graphical Data 5 Year Relative Survival Rate by Stage at Diagnosis.*

Among the ways to reduce your risks of developing cancer are to eat healthy foods, exercise regularly, refrain from smoking, and maintain a healthy body weight.

## Nutrition and Food Supplements

The Food Guide Pyramid presented in chapter 5 emphasizes the importance of a diet high in breads, grains, fruits, and vegetables. The Ameri-

### Minimizing the Risk Factors

To minimize the risk of cancer, the American Cancer Society recommends the following:

∎ Don't smoke. Avoid environmental (secondhand) smoke. Don't use smokeless tobacco.

∎ Use a sunscreen with an SPF rating of 15 or higher to protect your skin against excessive sun exposure. Also wear protective clothing.

∎ Achieve and maintain a healthy weight. Obesity is a risk factor for some cancers.

∎ Exercise regularly.

∎ Eat foods high in fiber and low in fat; maintain a healthy diet. Avoid salt-cured, nitrite-cured, and smoked foods.

∎ Drink alcohol moderately if at all.

∎ Avoid excessive radiation exposure. Have medical x-rays taken only when absolutely necessary. Have your house checked for radon exposure.

∎ Avoid occupational exposure to carcinogens.

∎ Follow the cancer-screening test recommendations of the American Cancer Society and watch for warning signs of cancer (see "The Seven Danger Signs of Cancer" on page 230).

can Cancer Society supports this type of diet for lowering the risk of several types of cancer. You have probably heard or read that dietary supplements of vitamins and minerals called antioxidants may be important in reducing the risk of coronary heart disease and cancer. Antioxidant nutrients include vitamin C, vitamin E, selenium, and carotenoids. Antioxidants are found in fruits and vegetables. They are believed to protect the body against oxygen-induced damage to tissues that occurs with normal metabolism. Because such damage is associated with increased cancer risk, these nutrients are also thought to protect against cancer. However, clinical studies of antioxidant supplements don't demonstrate a reduction in cancer risk.

Similarly, scientific research hasn't found that beta carotene (another antioxidant) reduces cancer risk. In fact, in three major studies, people were given high doses of synthetic beta carotene supplements in an effort to prevent lung and other cancers. In two of the studies, beta carotene was linked to *higher* risk of lung cancer in cigarette smokers; in the third study, the results were neutral.

It would certainly be advisable to take a multiple-vitamin supplement if you don't have a balanced diet, but spending money on supplements appears not to be warranted now.

### Physical Activity and Cancer

The American Cancer Society recommends a lifetime of regular physical activity, focusing on the vital role that physical activity and good nutrition play in maintaining a healthy body weight and preventing obesity. Physical activity is also important in maintaining a neutral energy balance, which lowers the risk of colon, prostate, endometrium, breast, and kidney cancers. Physical activity may also have positive effects on hormone levels that will reduce the risk of breast and prostate cancer. In addition, physical activity stimulates the bowel and decreases digestion time; this lowers the time that cancer-causing substances produced during digestion are present in the colon, which in turn lowers the risk of

## POINT OF INTEREST

### The High Cost of Cancer

The highest cost of cancer, of course, is in terms of human lives and suffering. But this deadly disease is the source of substantial financial burdens on individuals and on our nation as well: in 1998, for example, the American Cancer Society estimated that cancer would cost Americans $107 billion. (This represented about 1/10 of the total 1998 estimated U.S. health care cost of over $1 trillion.)

See the chart for a breakdown of the estimated costs of cancer in 1998 in terms of lost productivity, medical services, and mortality. Improved treatments, therapies, and detection procedures relieve suffering and save lives, but at a high health care expense for our nation. Preventing cancer through healthful lifestyle choices will save not only lives, but dollars.

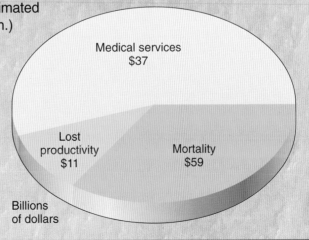

Medical services
$37

Lost productivity
$11

Mortality
$59

Billions of dollars

colon cancer. Blair et al. (1989) demonstrated a strong reduction in cancer deaths as cardiovascular endurance increased (see figure 9.4). However, compared to research on the role of physical activity in reducing coronary heart disease risk, the overall research is not as supportive for the causal role of physical activity in helping to prevent or increase survival of all types of cancers.

 **KEY POINT** Physical activity is important in maintaining a neutral energy balance, which lowers the risk of colon, prostate, endometrium, breast, and kidney cancers. Physical activity may also have positive effects on hormone levels that will reduce the risk of breast and prostate cancer. In addition, physical activity stimulates the bowel and decreases digestion time, which in turn lowers the risk of colon cancer.

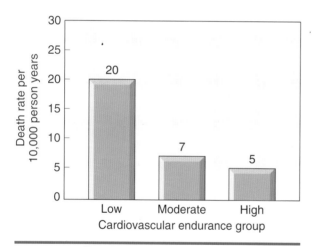

**FIGURE 9.4** Relationship of fitness to cancer deaths.

**HEALTHCHECK**

**Physical inactivity is a major risk factor for coronary heart disease. It is also a major risk factor for developing cancer?**

No. Physical inactivity is a risk factor associated with a few (not all) types of cancer (for example, breast, prostate, and colon). Physical inactivity has not been as strongly related to cancer development as it has to coronary heart disease.

## DIABETES MELLITUS

*Diabetes mellitus* is a metabolic disorder resulting in the inability to properly metabolize carbohydrates and control blood sugar levels because the normal insulin mechanism is ineffective. In healthy people the pancreas produces the hormone insulin, which regulates carbohydrate, fat, and protein metabolism. When insulin is not properly regulated in the body, people have to modify their diet and sometimes take medication to control their carbohydrate metabolism. In advanced cases, people must inject insulin every day to control their blood sugar (glucose) levels. About 15.7 million Americans have diabetes; of these, about 5.4 million have not been diagnosed. About 800,000 new cases of diabetes are reported each year. The economic cost of diabetes was estimated at $98 billion in 1997.

Diabetes may lead to kidney failure, circulation problems, gangrene and amputation, blindness or retinal damage, heart attack, or stroke. It is a major risk factor for coronary heart disease, and it is the seventh leading cause of death from disease in the United States.

There are two main types of diabetes: *type I diabetes* (sometimes referred to as *juvenile diabetes* because it often occurs in young children) and *type II diabetes* (sometimes called *adult-onset diabetes* because it develops in adulthood). A third type, *gestational diabetes,* can develop during pregnancy; it typically disappears after the baby is delivered, although it does leave women more prone to developing type II diabetes later in life.

Type I diabetes is an immune-response disorder that requires daily injections of insulin because the pancreas produces little or no insulin on its own. Type I diabetes is also referred to as insulin-dependent diabetes mellitus. People of all ages—not just youngsters—can contract this disease. An estimated 500,000 to 1,000,000 Americans have type I diabetes.

Type II diabetes is the more common type, affecting more than 14 million Americans. Type

II diabetes is also called non-insulin-dependent diabetes mellitus. The pancreas produces an insufficient amount of insulin in type II diabetes also, but type II diabetes can often be managed through diet, exercise, and weight control. About 8 of 10 people with type II diabetes are overweight.

 Type II diabetes can often be managed through diet, exercise, and weight control.

Warning signs of the two types of diabetes include the following:

## Type I

- High levels of sugar in the blood or urine
- Frequent urination (including bed-wetting in children)
- Extreme hunger or thirst
- Extreme weight loss
- Weakness and tiredness
- Feeling edgy and having mood changes
- Feeling nauseous, vomiting

## Type II

- Any type I symptoms
- Repeated or hard-to-heal infections of the skin, gums, vagina, or bladder
- Blurred vision
- Tingling or loss of feeling in the hands and feet

## Risk Factors

The primary risk factor for developing type I diabetes is heredity. People who have parents or siblings with type I diabetes are at the greatest risk. Risk factors for type II diabetes that can be controlled include obesity, smoking, physical inactivity, hypertension, low HDL (high density lipoprotein)-cholesterol, and high triglycerides. Risk factors for type II diabetes that you can't

control are aging (type II diabetes usually occurs in people over 45), heredity (including ethnicity—Hispanics, African-Americans, and Native Americans have an increased risk for developing type II diabetes) and family history, gestational diabetes, and having had a high birth weight baby. The lab at the end of the chapter will give you a chance to assess your risk for diabetes.

### HEALTHCHECK

**Why do some pregnant women develop diabetes?**

Several of the hormones produced during pregnancy have a "locking effect" on insulin that decreases the body's ability to transmit glucose to the cells, which leads to increased glucose levels in the blood—diabetes. In most women the pancreas simply produces more insulin to counteract this effect, but for some women this extra insulin isn't enough and they develop gestational diabetes.

Understanding the risk factors and paying attention to the warning signs can help in preventing diabetes or detecting it early on to begin proper management of the disease.

 Heredity is the primary risk factor for type I diabetes. There are a variety of risk factors for type II diabetes. Obesity, smoking, physical inactivity, hypertension, low HDL-cholesterol, and high triglycerides are the risk factors that you can alter through lifestyle choices to lower your risk of developing the disease.

## Physical Activity and Diabetes Mellitus

People with type II diabetes can reduce their risk of becoming insulin dependent by maintaining their weight in a healthy range, getting the proper nutrition, and being physically active. Helmrich et al. (1991) found that increased physical activity helps prevent type II diabetes and is especially important for those with the highest risks. Physical activity burns calories and helps maintain or reduce weight, and it also can improve the body's response to insulin. Helmrich et al. also reported a decreased risk of developing type II diabetes for each weekly caloric expenditure increase of 500 (from a range of 500 to 3,500 calories expended per week). In addition, Manson et al. (1991) found that women between the ages of 34 and 59 reduced their risk of developing diabetes by about 33% when they engaged in vigorous physical activity at least once a week.

 Increased physical activity helps prevent type II diabetes and is especially important for those with more risk factors. Physical activity helps maintain or reduce weight, and it also can improve the body's response to insulin.

Engaging in moderate-intensity aerobic exercise at least three days per week for 20 to 60 minutes at a time is even more beneficial in preventing type II diabetes. Doing so significantly affects weight and glucose control. People over 35 years old who have type II diabetes should receive their physician's permission before beginning an exercise program. The American Diabetes Association also recommends regular cardiorespiratory exercise for people with type I diabetes; however, exercise alone will not improve glucose control. Regular exercise will help people with type I diabetes control their body weight, but they need to watch carefully for hypoglycemia (too little blood sugar) when their exercise and insulin levels interact to decrease blood sugar levels below a healthy range. People with type I diabetes should work closely with their health care team to determine a careful balance of food, insulin, and physical activity that will maintain good glucose control and promote health-related fitness. See "Exercise Prescription for People With Diabetes" for more specific information on appropriate exercise.

## Exercise Prescription for People With Diabetes

What type of exercise should people with diabetes engage in, and how long and intensely should they exercise? Here's a brief look at an exercise prescription for those with diabetes, based on the FITT model described in chapter 2:

*Frequency*
- Three to seven days per week for glucose control (for type II diabetes)
- Five to seven days per week for weight control

*Intensity*
- 50% to 80% maximal oxygen consumption ($\dot{V}O_2$max; see chapter 2)
- 55% to 80% of maximal heart rate

*Time*
- 30 to 60 minutes per session:
  - 5 to 10 minutes of warm-up
  - 20 to 40 minutes of aerobic activity
  - 5 to 10 minutes of cool-down

*Type*
- Aerobic exercise: walking, jogging, cycling, swimming, and so on

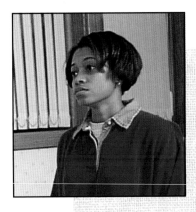

# Health Concepts

You'll recall from the beginning of the chapter that Natalie had discovered a lump in one of her breasts. She wondered whether she should get it checked immediately or wait to see if it went away. The wise decision is to *always* immediately check such a sign; it may turn out to not be cancerous, but if it is, the earlier the detection and treatment the better. Even though Natalie's family doesn't have a history of breast cancer, she should do a self-examination monthly.

## SUMMARY

▮ Cancer is the second leading cause of death in the United States and is projected to overtake cardiovascular disease as the leading cause early in the twenty-first century. In 1998, 1,228,600 new cases of cancer were diagnosed. However, the good news is that cancer death rates in the 1990s are declining for the first time.

▮ Cancer is characterized by the uncontrolled growth and spread of abnormal cells, which form *tumors*. Not all tumors are cancerous. Those that are, however, spread to other areas of the body and interfere with normal body function. This is how cancer kills.

▮ Danger signs for cancer include changes in bowel movements or urination; sores that won't heal; sudden bleeding or discharge; lumps or hardening; frequent and prolonged indigestion or difficulty swallowing; changes in the color or size of moles and warts; and hoarseness and persistent coughs.

▮ Skin cancer is the most frequently diagnosed cancer in the United States, and melanoma is the most serious type. The "ABCD rule" for detecting melanoma is

A = *Asymmetry* in a mole or pigmentation

B = *Border* irregularity (ragged, notched, or blurred edges)

C = *Color* variation across the mole or pigmentation

D = *Diameter* greater than 6 millimeters

▮ Physical activity can reduce the risk for colon cancer. Some research has shown that physical activity may lower the risk of other types of cancer, but further research is needed.

▮ About 15.7 million Americans have diabetes mellitus, which can lead to kidney failure, circulation problems, gangrene and amputation, blindness or retinal damage, heart attack, and stroke. Diabetes is the seventh leading cause of death from disease in the United States.

▌ There are two main types of diabetes. Type I requires daily injections of insulin to regulate blood sugar levels; type II in most cases can be controlled through diet, exercise, and maintenance of an appropriate weight.

▌ Risk factors for diabetes include smoking, obesity, hypertension, ethnicity, heredity, and age. Physical activity can help burn calories, maintain or reduce weight, and improve the body's response to insulin. People who are more physically active have a reduced risk of becoming diabetic, and those who have type II diabetes are less likely to become insulin dependent if they are regularly physically active.

*In the next chapter we're going to consider the impact physical activity has on pregnant women. Pregnancy brings with it special health needs—we'll explore the role physical activity plays in helping to meet those needs.*

## KEY TERMS

| | |
|---|---|
| benign | metastasize |
| cancer | oncogenes |
| diabetes mellitus | tumor |
| genes | type I diabetes |
| gestational diabetes | type II diabetes |
| melanoma | |

**9**

# Evaluating Risks of Cancer and Diabetes

**9**

## THE PURPOSES OF THIS LAB EXPERIENCE ARE TO

▌ evaluate your risk for developing some types of cancer and

▌ evaluate your risk for developing diabetes.

### Evaluate Your Cancer Risk

Cancer is a complex set of diseases with a variety of risk factors for various types of cancer. Complete the following risk factor assessment, developed by the American Cancer Society (1981), for the most common types of cancer discussed in this chapter. This will help you evaluate your risk. From the numbers in parentheses, select the one that corresponds to your answer and enter it in the space to the right. For example, for question #2 on lung cancer, if you are 20 years old (39 or less), enter 1 as your score. Men obviously don't need to respond to the questions regarding breast, cervical, or endometrial cancer. You may check your own risks with the answers contained in this questionnaire. *You are advised to discuss this questionnaire with your physician if you are at higher risk.*

**IMPORTANT: REACT TO EACH STATEMENT**
Individual numbers for specific questions are not to be interpreted as a precise measure of relative risk, but the totals for a given site should give a general indication of your risk.

| Lung Cancer |
| --- |

1. SEX:  a. Male (2)  b. Female (1)                                     1._____

2. AGE GROUP:  a. 39 or less (1)  b. 40-49 (2)  c. 50-59 (5)  d. 60 and over (7)     2._____

3. EXPOSURE TO ANY OF THESE:  a. Mining (3)  b. Asbestos (7)     3._____
   c. Uranium and radioactive products (5)  d. None (0)

4. HABITS:  a. Smoker (10)*  b. Nonsmoker (0)*                         4._____

5. TYPE OF SMOKING:  a. Cigarettes or little cigars (10)             5._____
   b. Pipe and/or cigar, but not cigarettes (3)  c. Nonsmoker (0)

6. NUMBER OF CIGARETTES SMOKED PER DAY:  a. 0 (1)  b. Less than     6._____
   1/2 pack per day (5)  c. 1/2-1 pack (9)  d. 1-2 packs (15)  e. 2+ packs (20)

7. TYPE OF CIGARETTE: a. High tar/nicotine (10)** b. Medium      7. _____
tar/nicotine (9)** c. Low tar/nicotine (7)** d. Nonsmoker (1)

8. LENGTH OF TIME SMOKING: a. Nonsmoker (1) b. Up to 15 years (5)    8. _____
c. 15-25 years (10) d. 25+ years (20)

SUBTOTAL _____

**Reducing Your Risk**

*If you stopped smoking more than 10 years ago, count yourself as a nonsmoker. If you have stopped smoking in the past 10 years, you are an ex-smoker. Ex-smokers should answer questions 5 through 8 according to how they previously smoked. Then ex-smokers may reduce their point total on questions 5 through 8 by 10% for each year they have not smoked. Current smokers should also answer questions 5 through 8.

**High tar/nicotine: 20 milligrams or more tar/1.3 milligrams or more nicotine;
medium tar/nicotine: 16-19 milligrams tar/1.1-1.2 milligrams nicotine;
low tar/nicotine: 15 milligrams or less tar/1.0 milligrams or less nicotine.

I am stopping smoking today. (Subtract 2 points.)      TOTAL _____

## Colon and Rectal Cancer

### I. Risk Factors

1. AGE GROUP: a. 40 or less (2) b. 40-49 (7) c. 50 and over (12)    1. _____

2. HAS ANYONE IN YOUR FAMILY EVER HAD: a. Colon cancer (18)    2. _____
b. Colon polyps (18) c. Neither (1)

3. HAVE YOU EVER HAD: a. Colon cancer (25) b. Colon polyps (25)    3. _____
c. Ulcerative colitis for more than seven years (18) d. Cancer of the
breast, ovary, uterus, or stomach (13) e. None of the above (1)

TOTAL _____

### II. Symptoms

1. Do you have bleeding from the rectum?      Yes _____ No _____

2. Have you had a change in bowel habits (such as
altered frequency, size, consistency, or color of stool)?    Yes _____ No _____

### III. Reducing Your Risk and Detecting Cancer Early

1. I have altered my diet to include less fat and more fruits, fiber, and cruciferous
vegetables (broccoli, cabbage, cauliflower, Brussels sprouts).    Yes _____ No _____

2. I have had a negative test for blood in my stool within the past year.    Yes _____ No _____

3. I have had a negative examination for colon cancer and polyps    Yes _____ No _____
within the past year (proctosigmoidoscopy, colonoscopy,
barium enema x-rays).

## Breast Cancer

1.  AGE GROUP:  a. Under 35 (10)  b. 35-39 (20)  c. 40-49 (50)
    d. 50 and over (90)                                              1. _____

2.  RACE:  a. Oriental (10)  b. Hispanic (10)  c. Black (20)  d. White (25)    2. _____

3.  FAMILY HISTORY:  a. None (10)  b. Mother, sister, or daughter with    3. _____
    breast cancer (30)

4.  YOUR HISTORY:  a. No breast disease (10)  b. Previous lumps or cysts (15)    4. _____
    c. Previous breast cancer (100)

5.  MATERNITY:  a. First pregnancy before 30 (10)  b. First pregnancy at 30    5. _____
    or older (15)  c. No pregnancies (20)

SUBTOTAL _____

### Reducing Your Risk

6.  I practice breast self-examination monthly. (Subtract 10 points.)

7.  I have had a negative mammogram and examination by a physician within
    the past year. (Subtract 25 points.)

TOTAL _____

## Skin Cancer

1.  Live in the southern part of the United States:                   Yes _____ No _____

2.  Frequently work or play in the sun:                               Yes _____ No _____

3.  Have a fair complexion or freckles (natural hair color of blond, red,
    or light brown; or eye color of gray, green, blue, or hazel):     Yes _____ No _____

4.  Work in mines, around coal tars, or around radioactivity:         Yes _____ No _____

5.  Experienced a severe, blistering sunburn before the age of 18:    Yes _____ No _____

6.  Have any family members with skin cancer or history of melanoma:  Yes _____ No _____

7.  Had skin cancer or melanoma in the past:                          Yes _____ No _____

8.  Use or have used tanning beds or sunlamps:                        Yes _____ No _____

9.  Have large, many, or changing moles:                              Yes _____ No _____

### Reducing Your Risk

10. I cover up with a wide-brimmed hat and wear long-sleeved
    shirts and pants:                                                 Yes _____ No _____

11. I use sunscreens with an SPF rating of 15 or higher when going
    out in the sun:                                                   Yes _____ No _____

12. I examine my skin once a month for changes in warts or moles:     Yes _____ No _____

## Lung Answers

1. Men have a higher risk of lung cancer than women. Since women are now smoking more, their incidence of lung and upper respiratory tract (mouth, tongue, and voice box) cancer is increasing.

2. The occurrence of lung and upper respiratory tract cancer increases with age.

3. Exposure to materials used in these and other industries has been shown to be associated with lung cancer, especially in smokers.

4. Cigarette smokers may have up to 20 times or even greater risk than nonsmokers. However, the rates for ex-smokers who have not smoked for 10 years approach those of nonsmokers.

5. Pipe and cigar smokers are at higher risk for lung cancer than nonsmokers. Cigarette smokers are also at a much higher risk for lung cancer than nonsmokers or than pipe and cigar smokers. All forms of tobacco, including chewing or dipping, markedly increase the user's risk of developing cancer of the mouth.

6. Male smokers of less than 1/2 pack per day have a lung cancer rate 5 times higher than nonsmokers. Male smokers of 1-2 packs per day have a lung cancer rate 15 times higher than nonsmokers. Smokers of more than 2 packs per day are 20 times more likely to develop lung cancer than nonsmokers.

7. Smokers of low tar/nicotine cigarettes have slightly lower lung cancer rates. Please note, however, that smokers of low tar/nicotine cigarettes may unconsciously smoke in a manner that increases their exposure to these chemicals.

8. The frequency of lung and upper respiratory tract cancer increases with the duration of smoking.

**If your total is:**

| | |
|---|---|
| 24 or less | You have a low risk for lung cancer. |
| 25-49 | You may be a light smoker and would have a good chance of kicking the habit. |
| 50-74 | As a moderate smoker, your risks of lung and upper respiratory tract cancer are increased. The time to stop is now! |
| 75 and over | As a heavy cigarette smoker, your chances of getting lung cancer and cancer of the upper respiratory or digestive tract are greatly increased. |

**Reducing Your Risk**

Make a decision to quit today. Join a smoking-cessation program. If you are a heavy drinker of alcohol, your risks for cancer of the head and neck and esophagus are further increased. Use of smokeless tobacco increases your risks of cancer of the mouth. Your best bet is not to use tobacco in any form. See your doctor if you have a nagging cough, hoarseness, persistent pain or sore in the mouth or throat, or lumps in the neck.

## Colon and Rectal Answers

1. Colon cancer occurs more often after the age of 50.

2. Colon cancer is more common in families with a previous history of this disease.

3. Polyps and bowel diseases are associated with colon cancer. Cancer of the breast, ovaries, uterus, or stomach may also be associated with an increased risk of colon cancer.

4. Bleeding may be a sign of colon or rectal cancer.

**I. Risk Factors\*—If your total is:**

5 or less    You are currently at low risk for colon or rectal cancer. Eat a diet high in fiber and low in fat and follow cancer checkup guidelines.

6-15    You are currently at moderate risk for colon or rectal cancer. Follow the American Cancer Society guidelines for early detection of colorectal cancer. These are (a) a digital rectal exam every year after age 40 and (b) a stool blood test every year and a sigmoidoscopic exam every three to five years after age 50.

16 or greater    You are in the high-risk group for colon or rectal cancer. This rating requires a lifetime, ongoing screening program that includes periodic evaluation of your entire colon. See your doctor for more information.

\*If your answers to any of the questions change, you should reassess your risk.

**II. Symptoms**—The presence of rectal bleeding or a change in bowel habits may indicate colon or rectal cancer. See your physician right away if you have either of these symptoms.

**III. Reducing Your Risk and Detecting Cancer Early**—Regular tests for hidden blood in the stool and appropriate examinations of the colon will increase the likelihood that colon polyps are discovered and removed early and that cancers are found in an early, curable state. Modifying your diet to include more fiber, cruciferous vegetables, and foods rich in vitamin A; and less fat and salt-cured foods may result in a reduction of cancer risk.

## Breast Answers

**If your total is:**

Under 100    Low-risk women (and all others). You should practice monthly breast self-examinations, have your breasts examined by a doctor as part of a regular cancer-related checkup, and have a mammography in accordance with American Cancer Society guidelines.

100-199    Moderate-risk women. You should practice monthly breast self-examination, have your breasts examined by a doctor as part of a cancer-related checkup, and have a periodic mammography in accordance with American Cancer Society guidelines or more frequently as your physician advises.

200 or higher    High-risk women. You should practice monthly breast self-examination; you should have your breasts examined by a doctor and have a mammography more often

than women who are at lower risk. See your doctor for the recommended frequency of breast physical examinations and mammography.

## Reducing Your Risk

One in eight American women will get breast cancer in her lifetime. Being a woman is a risk factor! Most women (75%) who get breast cancer don't have other risk factors. Breast self-examination and a mammography may diagnose a breast cancer in its earliest stage with a greatly increased chance of cure. When the disease is detected at this stage, cure is more likely and breast-saving surgery may be an option.

## Skin Answers

1. The sun's rays are more intense the closer one lives to the equator.

2. Excessive ultraviolet light from the sun causes cancer of the skin.

3. Persons with light complexions are at greater risk for skin cancer.

4. These materials can cause cancer of the skin.

5. A severe sunburn that occurs during childhood may increase one's risk for melanoma.

6. A tendency to have precancerous moles or melanomas may occur in certain families.

7. Persons with a previous skin cancer or melanoma are at increased risk for developing further skin cancer or melanoma.

8. Tanning beds use a type of ultraviolet ray that adds to the skin damage caused by the sun, contributing to skin cancer formation.

9. Any change in a mole may be a sign of melanoma.

The key is that if you answered "yes" to any of the first nine items you need to use protective clothing and use a sunscreen with an SPF rating of 15 or higher whenever you are out in the sun, and to check yourself monthly for any changes in warts or moles. A "yes" answer to items 10, 11, and 12 can help reduce your risk of skin cancer.

## Reducing Your Risk

Numerical risks for skin cancer are difficult to state. For instance, a person with a dark complexion can work longer in the sun and be less likely to develop cancer than a person with a light complexion. Furthermore, a person wearing a long-sleeved shirt and wide-brimmed hat may work for longer durations in the sun and be at less risk than a person who wears a bathing suit and works in the sun for only a short time. The risk for skin cancer goes up greatly with age.

Melanoma, the most serious type of skin cancer, can be cured when it is detected and treated at a very early stage. Changes in warts or moles are important and should be checked by your doctor. For more information, ask for the American Cancer Society pamphlet, *Melanoma/Skin Cancer, You Can Recognize the Signs.*

## Evaluate Your Diabetes Risk

The effects of diabetes can be severe, and complications can lead to heart disease, kidney disease, and blindness. About one-third of the people who have diabetes in the United States have not been diagnosed. Completing the following test (reprinted from the American Diabetes Association 1998) will help you evaluate your potential for developing the disease. Write down the points indicated for each statement that is *true* for you. If a statement is *not true* for you, enter a zero. Add your total score.

| At-Risk Weight Chart | |
|---|---|
| **Height**<br>**(without shoes)** | **Weight**<br>**(pounds without clothing)** |
| 4 ft 10 in | 129 |
| 4 ft 11 in | 133 |
| 5 ft 0 in | 138 |
| 5 ft 1 in | 143 |
| 5 ft 2 in | 147 |
| 5 ft 3 in | 152 |
| 5 ft 4 in | 157 |
| 5 ft 5 in | 162 |
| 5 ft 6 in | 167 |
| 5 ft 7 in | 172 |
| 5 ft 8 in | 177 |
| 5 ft 9 in | 182 |
| 5 ft 10 in | 188 |
| 5 ft 11 in | 193 |
| 6 ft 0 in | 199 |
| 6 ft 1 in | 204 |
| 6 ft 2 in | 210 |
| 6 ft 3 in | 216 |
| 6 ft 4 in | 221 |

If you weigh the same or more than the amount listed for your height, you may be at risk for diabetes. This chart is based on a measure called the Body Mass Index (BMI). The chart shows unhealthy weights for men and women age 35 or older at the listed heights. At-risk weights are lower for individuals under age 35.

1. My weight is equal to or above that listed in the chart.          **Yes 5** _____

2. I am under 65 years of age *and* I get little or no exercise during a usual day.          **Yes 5** _____

3. I am between 45 and 64 years of age.          **Yes 5** _____

4. I am 65 years old or older.          **Yes 9** _____

5. I am a woman who has had a baby weighing more than nine pounds at birth.     **Yes 1** _____

6. I have a sister or brother with diabetes.     **Yes 1** _____

7. I have a parent with diabetes.     **Yes 1** _____

        **TOTAL** _____

## Scoring 3-9 points

If you scored 3-9 points, you are probably at low risk for having diabetes now. But don't just forget about it—especially if you are Hispanic/Latino, African American, American Indian, Asian American, or Pacific Islander. You may be at higher risk in the future. Maintaining a healthy weight and performing regular exercise can help you reduce your risk. *New guidelines recommend everyone age 45 and over consider being tested for the disease every three years. However, people at high risk should consider being tested at a younger age.*

## Scoring 10 or more points

If you scored 10 or more points, you are at high risk for having diabetes. Only a doctor can determine if you have diabetes. See a doctor and find out for sure.

# Chapter 10

# Pregnancy

*Elaine Trudelle-Jackson, M.S., P.T.*

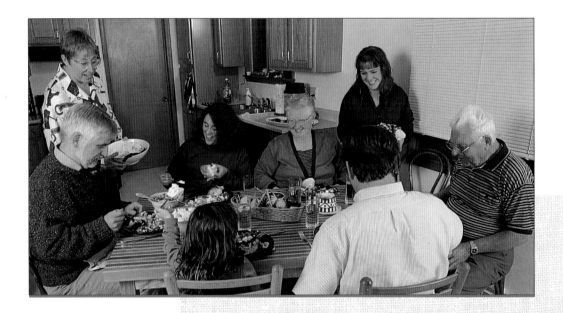

At dinner last weekend my sister Terri, who's four months pregnant, announced that she planned on jogging all the way through her pregnancy—she even joked that she'd jog to the hospital to have her baby. She's always been very active and doesn't want to gain too much weight or lose her shape. My grandmother said that all that jogging wouldn't be good for the baby—that in her day, women were told to take it easy during their pregnancy.

Terri may have been kidding about jogging to the hospital, but her comments—and grandma's warning—made me wonder: just how safe is it to exercise when you're pregnant? What activities are okay, and for how long?

—Megan, 21-year-old senior

*W*hat do you think *?*

Terri's used to being active and doesn't want to stop during her pregnancy. This is commendable, but Megan raises a good point: how long and how hard *can* you exercise while maintaining a healthy pregnancy? What activities are unsafe? For activities that *are* safe, what are the limits on those activities? Are there special benefits to exercising during pregnancy?

In this chapter we'll look at the benefits—and risks—of physical activity during pregnancy. We'll consider the body changes that occur during pregnancy and their implications for physical activity. And we'll also supply guidelines regarding physical activity for pregnant women.

## PHYSICAL ACTIVITY AND PREGNANCY

Megan's grandmother was right: doctors used to discourage physical activity during pregnancy. They told women to stay off their feet as much as possible and encouraged them to live a sedentary lifestyle. Now, however, the medical profession encourages women to take part in moderate physical activity so long as they have no preexisting conditions or medical complications. As a result, more women than ever before are realizing the benefits of physical activity during pregnancy. How active a woman is before becoming pregnant has implications for how active she can safely be during pregnancy.

Of course, pregnant women should first be cleared by their medical caregiver before taking part in regular physical activity. Conditions such as pregnancy-induced hypertension, preterm rupture of membranes, preterm labor during the current pregnancy or a prior pregnancy, incompetent cervix, persistent second- or third-trimester bleeding, or intrauterine growth retardation would contraindicate physical activity during pregnancy. For more information on contraindications, see "Warning Signs to Stop Exercising" on page 256.

Women who have achieved cardiorespiratory fitness before pregnancy should be able to safely maintain that level of fitness throughout pregnancy and the postpartum period, though they may have to modify their exercise regimens. In general, women note a progressive decline in exercise performance (i.e., a decreased ability to maintain prepregnancy intensity levels) in early pregnancy. In a study of women who performed regular *weight-bearing exercise* (e.g., running, aerobic dance, etc.) before and during pregnancy, about half of pregnant women voluntarily discontinued their regular physical activity by the third trimester (Collings, Curet, and Mullin 1983).

In addition, studies suggest that women who begin *non-weight-bearing exercise* (e.g., stationary cycling or swimming) early during their pregnancy can continue to exercise at a high intensity for a moderate duration into the third trimester. Despite findings suggesting that women who continue to exercise vigorously during pregnancy have lower birth weight babies, there are no data confirming that exercising within safe limits during pregnancy has any deleterious effects on the fetus. There *is,* however, evidence that physical activity during pregnancy has many benefits.

 Women who have achieved cardiorespiratory fitness before pregnancy should be able to safely maintain that level of fitness throughout pregnancy and the postpartum period, though they may have to modify their exercise regimens.

## BENEFITS OF PHYSICAL ACTIVITY

Women who are physically active during their pregnancy don't have easier deliveries. But they can experience a number of benefits that will help them feel better during their pregnancy and provide additional stamina and strength so that they can recover from childbirth more quickly than women who aren't active. Being physically active during pregnancy can

- improve circulation (which reduces the effects of varicose veins, a common malady of pregnant women);

- improve balance (which is difficult, because the center of gravity changes);

- reduce swelling;

- ease gastrointestinal discomforts, including constipation;

- reduce leg cramps;

- strengthen abdominal muscles;

- improve posture (which is affected by additional weight and redistribution of body mass);

- alleviate various discomforts of pregnancy, such as backaches and muscle and joint soreness;

- improve the sense of well-being, control, and body image;

- build endurance and cause labor to be perceived as less painful; and

- ease the postpartum recovery.

Varrassi, Bazzanno, and Edwards (1989) showed that women who exercised moderately and regularly during the last trimester perceived their labor as less painful than women who did not exercise. A possible explanation could lie in part in the increased level of endorphins in the bodies of the women who exercised regularly; endorphins act as a natural pain reliever.

### Activity, Smoking, and Birth Weight

Studies of the relationship between physical activity and weight of the baby at birth show mixed results. Current evidence indicates that moderate physical activity may increase birth weight but that more severe exercise regimens may cause lower birth weight (Pivarnik 1998). Brody (1993) showed that women who worked out for 30 minutes, five days a week, had bigger, healthier babies than sedentary mothers.

The results are not mixed for cigarette smoking. The National Center for Health Statistics (1996) reports that women who smoke are twice as likely to have low birth weight babies as mothers who don't smoke.

Women who are physically active during their pregnancy can experience a number of benefits that will help them feel better and provide additional stamina and strength so that they can recover from childbirth more quickly than women who aren't active.

## PHYSIOLOGICAL CONCERNS REGARDING PHYSICAL ACTIVITY

Wilmore and Costill (1999) outlined four major physiological concerns associated with being physically active during pregnancy: reduced uterine blood flow, hyperthermia, carbohydrate availability, and miscarriage and pregnancy outcome.

• **Reduced uterine blood flow.** The concern here is that blood will be diverted to the mother's active muscles, thus reducing the flow to the uterus. This potentially could lead to *hypoxia,* which is insufficient oxygen to the fetus. Studies show that uterine blood flow in sheep is reduced by about 25% during exercise, although it isn't clear whether this leads to fetal hypoxia (animal research has shown that a 50% or greater reduction is needed before the well-being of the fetus is affected). Increases in fetal heart rate have been interpreted as an index of hypoxia, but they more likely represent the fetal heart's response to increased hormone levels in the blood that result from the mother's exercise.

• **Hyperthermia.** *Hyperthermia* means exceptionally high temperature, which can result if the mother's core temperature substantially elevates during and following physical activity. Abnormal fetal development (e.g., central nervous system defects) has been documented in animals exposed to chronic thermal stress; in humans, this has been documented with high fever. Studies of animals have shown that fetal temperatures do increase with exercise, but it's not clear whether these increases are great enough to cause abnormal fetal development. To avoid the risk of hyperthermia, don't exercise in hot, humid weather.

• **Carbohydrate availability.** Here the concern is that if the mother uses more carbohydrate to fuel her body, less carbohydrate will be available to the fetus. Again, this potential is not well understood. Endurance athletes such as runners or triathletes who train or compete for long durations have reduced glycogen stores in the muscles and liver and reduced blood glucose concentrations. The effect of this on the fetus is not clear; however, the implication is. Pregnant women who exercise must take in additional carbohydrate calories.

• **Miscarriage and pregnancy outcome.** Some people have expressed concern that women who exercise might induce a miscarriage during the first trimester. Other fears are that exercise during pregnancy might induce early labor or cause abnormal fetal development. Fortunately, research shows no consistent evidence to support these fears. On the contrary, most studies show favorable outcomes for women who exercise during pregnancy. These outcomes include reduced maternal weight gain, shorter hospital stays, and fewer cesarean sections.

## PHYSICAL CHANGES AND IMPLICATIONS

The body undergoes many changes during pregnancy that have implications for physical activity. For example, the uterus pushes on the diaphragm, which can alter breathing; the heart enlarges; veins become softer to allow for greater blood flow; ligaments loosen; and breasts enlarge. All these changes are ways in which the body prepares for childbirth, but they impact the approach to physical activity as well.

### Breathing Changes

The diaphragm is a muscle that separates the lungs from the abdominal cavity and aids in breathing. As the uterus expands it presses on and moves the diaphragm upward, making it difficult to fully inhale (see figure 10.1a and b). Because of this, some women may feel breathless when they exercise vigorously, or they may hyperventilate, becoming light-headed or dizzy.

Oxygen consumption actually increases by 15% to 20% during pregnancy, although the oxygen reserve—the extra oxygen available in the blood and muscles—decreases. Because a pregnant woman's body supplies oxygen both to herself and the fetus, that reserve supply is tapped into, increasing oxygen consumption. Though these changes are most apparent in the third trimester, the feeling of being "winded" with even mild exercise can begin as early as 20 weeks.

Increased progesterone levels during pregnancy raise the normal breathing rate by 45%. Women can increase their aerobic capacity during pregnancy, but if they don't exercise it will likely decrease.

## Physical Activity Implications

- Don't overexert; overexertion can contribute to breathlessness and hyperventilation.
- Don't hold your breath when exerting yourself (see page 59 in chapter 3 for more information

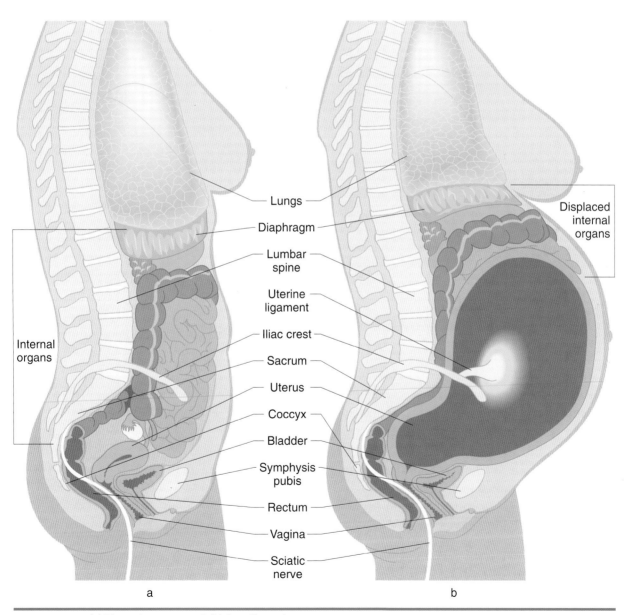

**FIGURE 10.1** *(a)* Normal organs and *(b)* the effect of pregnancy on organs.

## Warning Signs to Stop Exercising

A pregnant woman who experiences any of the following signs should not exercise (or should stop exercising immediately if she experiences them while exercising) and should contact her medical caregiver:

▍ Vaginal bleeding
▍ Abdominal or chest pain
▍ Leaking or gushing from vagina
▍ Sudden swelling of hands, face, or feet
▍ Severe, persistent headache
▍ Dizziness or light-headedness
▍ Noticeable reduction in fetal activity
▍ Painful, reddened area in the leg

▍ Severe pain in pubic area or hips
▍ Pain or burning sensation when urinating
▍ Irritating vaginal discharge
▍ Oral temperature over 100°F (38°C)
▍ Persistent nausea or vomiting
▍ Uterine contractions
▍ Heart palpitations
▍ Shortness of breath

### HEALTHCHECK

#### What are the signs of hyperventilation?

Hyperventilation occurs when you breathe too rapidly and deeply. Signs include dizziness or tingling in the lips or fingers. If you experience any of these signs, immediately stop what you're doing and consciously try to slow down your breathing.

on the Valsalva maneuver). This can cause dizziness or fainting.

- Lift your arms up and out to ease breathing. This relieves the pressure the uterus places on the diaphragm and allows the rib cage to expand.
- If you get side stitches (cramps that occur in the rib cage muscles), massage the sore muscles, blow out forcefully, and lift your knees while lying on your back.

## Heart and Circulatory Changes

During pregnancy, the heart wall thickens and the heart enlarges and moves upward because of pressure from the diaphragm. Blood volume progressively increases 30% to 50% throughout pregnancy; the resting heart rate may increase by up to 20% (10 to 20 beats per minute by full term). Cardiac output (the amount of blood pumped by the heart) increases by 40% to 50% to meet the needs of the growing uterus and fetus. Yet the cardiac reserve (the capacity of the heart to meet the body's demands) diminishes. This causes pregnant women to tire more quickly, especially during vigorous activity.

Strenuous exertion can cause an irregular or excessively pounding heartbeat; the woman should stop exercising if this happens.

Blood vessels soften and stretch to accommodate the increase in blood volume. This stretching may result in hemorrhoids, varicose veins, and swelling. In some cases the vessels don't stretch; instead they constrict and cause blood pressure to rise. This is known as pregnancy-induced hypertension, and it can be serious, even potentially fatal. Symptoms include fluid retention, sudden swelling, blurred vision, and severe headaches.

### Physical Activity Implications

- Exercise comfortably, not intensely.
- Do not hold your breath or perform activities that encourage the Valsalva maneuver (see chapter 3), which can cause excessive blood pressure and create undesirable forces on the uterus.
- Stop exercising when you become fatigued; don't exercise to exhaustion.
- Exercise can help varicose veins because it increases circulation.
- Rise and change directions slowly to avoid dizziness.
- After 20 weeks of pregnancy, avoid exercises that require you to lie flat on your back; this position can decrease cardiac output even further.

 A pregnant woman's cardiac output (the amount of blood pumped by the heart) increases by 40% to 50% to meet the needs of the growing uterus and fetus. Yet her cardiac reserve (the capacity of the heart to meet the body's demands) diminishes. This causes her to tire more quickly, especially during vigorous activity.

### HEALTHCHECK

#### Why are pregnant women susceptible to varicose veins?

Varicose veins are enlarged veins that can occur in any part of the body but are most common in the legs. This condition results in pain and swelling in the feet and ankles. In pregnant women the veins soften to accommodate the increased blood volume, and this softening occurs to a greater extent in the legs. Prolonged sitting or standing makes the condition worse, because the blood pools in the legs. Exercise, as well as elevating the legs, not standing or sitting too long at one time, and wearing support panty hose, helps ease the condition. Although varicose veins are often associated with pregnancy, this condition can also occur in occupations that require prolonged standing.

## Stomach and Intestinal Changes

Hormonal changes cause stomach and intestine activity to slow. The stomach and intestines are moved upward by the enlarged uterus (see figure 10.1b); this can cause heartburn and indigestion. Many pregnant women have problems with constipation because the digestive process slows. Nausea and vomiting—commonly known as "morning sickness," though it can occur at any time of the day—often occur, usually during the first trimester, because of hormonal changes.

### Physical Activity Implications

- Eat a healthy snack an hour or so before physical activity—fruit or crackers.
- To lessen the effects of nausea, don't let your stomach get empty.
- Exercise at the same time each day.
- Drink six to eight glasses of fluids per day. Be especially careful to drink enough fluids if you're vomiting. Avoid coffee, tea, colas, and other drinks that contain caffeine—these will cause you to lose even more fluid.

## Kidney and Bladder Changes

As the growing uterus presses on the bladder, women feel the need to urinate more frequently. Many women leak urine late in the pregnancy and retain fluids in the legs and ankles. Exercise can help reduce swelling by increasing circulation.

### Physical Activity Implications

- Doing pelvic floor exercises helps control the bladder muscles and prevent leaking urine.
- Make sure there's a bathroom nearby for frequent stops!

## Muscular, Joint, and Postural Changes

As a pregnant woman's uterus and breasts enlarge (as a result of increased *estrogen* levels), her center of gravity moves forward and upward.

As a result, women must make changes in their posture to maintain good balance and stability. Some common postural changes include walking with the feet further apart to create a wider base of support; rounding the upper back and shoulders because of increased breast weight; and increased lumbar lordosis, or swayback, to keep the center of gravity from moving too far forward. Some of these postural changes understandably cause muscle fatigue and soreness.

In addition, the hormone *relaxin* causes ligaments to relax and joints to become looser and more mobile in preparation for delivery. Looser joints and a shifted center of gravity make women more prone to injury in the third trimester. Weight-bearing joints, such as the back and pelvis, are prone to soreness and injury.

By the third trimester, abdominal muscles are stretched to their limit. One of these muscles, the rectus abdominis, can separate down the center of the abdomen, creating a condition known as *diastasis recti* (see figure 10.2a and b). The exact cause of this separation is not well understood, but contributing factors include pressure from the growing uterus, hormonal changes, and overstraining of the muscles. Regardless of the cause, the condition seems to be less common in women who have good abdominal muscle tone before pregnancy (Boissonnault and Blaschak 1988). Diastasis recti isn't painful, and women can continue to exercise when their stomach muscles separate. However, the exercises must be modified if the separation is greater than 1 inch (2.5 centimeters)—your medical caregiver

### Self-Test for Diastasis Recti

To check for separation of the abdominal muscles, a woman should lie on her back with her knees bent and her feet flat on the floor. She should lift her head and shoulders off the floor and pull her chin toward her chest. Placing her fingertips horizontally at navel level, she should press firmly on her stomach, feeling for separation between the bands of vertical muscles. If more than two fingers (greater than 1 inch) can be placed between the two bands, diastasis recti is present. She should then repeat the test to check for separation above and below the navel; separation can occur at any of these three places. Performing abdominal strengthening exercises with diastasis recti can make the separation worse, but a medical caregiver can provide corrective exercises. Women should stop all other abdominal exercises until the separation is two fingerwidths or less.

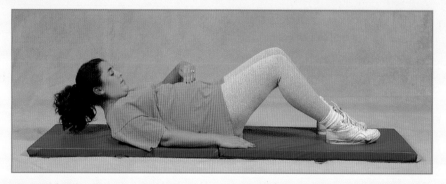

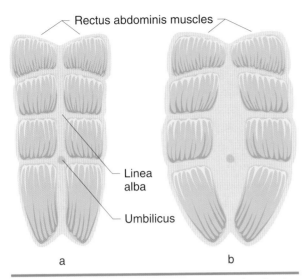

**FIGURE 10.2** *(a)* Normal abdominal muscles (rectus abdominis) and *(b)* separated abdominal muscles (diastasis recti).

can provide special exercises designed to help correct the condition.

### Physical Activity Implications

- Change directions slowly and avoid complicated foot patterns as the center of gravity shifts.
- Perform only mild stretching, and never stretch by bouncing—you can injure loosened joints.
- Do the self-test for diastasis recti before doing any exercises to strengthen the abdominal muscles (see "Self-Test for Diastasis Recti"). If the separation is greater than 1 inch (2.5 centimeters), check with your medical caregiver.
- Begin abdominal strengthening before pregnancy or early in pregnancy to reduce your chances of diastasis recti.
- Strengthen the abdominals, back muscles, and buttocks to achieve a healthy posture.

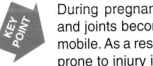 During pregnancy, ligaments relax and joints become looser and more mobile. As a result, women are more prone to injury in the third trimester. The joints of the pelvis and back are particularly prone to soreness.

## Metabolic Changes

*Insulin* levels increase during pregnancy, resulting in lower blood sugar in many women. Since exercise causes blood sugar levels to drop even more, *hypoglycemia* (abnormally low blood sugar) is more likely to occur during pregnancy if a woman exercises. This is why it's so important for pregnant women who exercise to eat an adequate amount of carbohydrates. Conversely, some pregnant women will experience *hyperglycemia* (abnormally high blood sugar). Hyperglycemia is a characteristic of *gestational diabetes* and usually goes away after the baby is born. Approximately 1 of 300 women contract gestational diabetes mellitus; the extent to which physical activity is affected depends on the severity of the condition. You'll evaluate your or your partner's risk for gestational diabetes in the lab at the end of this chapter.

### Physical Activity Implications

- Exercise may help treat or prevent gestational diabetes; this theory is currently under investigation.
- Pay attention to the warning signs of diabetes mellitus (see chapter 9, page 239).

## Breast Changes

The breasts enlarge and become sensitive; the nipples and areolas (the dark skin around the nipples) grow and become darker. Colostrum, a mixture of water, protein, minerals, and antibodies that the baby will feed on for the first few days, usually develops by 12 to 14 weeks.

### Physical Activity Implications

- Wear a supportive, comfortable sport bra when you work out.

## Pelvic Floor Changes

The pelvic floor muscles act as a sling to support the pelvic organs (bladder, uterus, and bowel). These muscles form a figure eight around the urethra, vagina, and anus—one end at the front and the other at the back of the pelvis. Ideally, this suspended sling forms a straight line between the two points of attachment (see figure 10.3a). During pregnancy, the pelvic floor stretches from the weight of the baby, and during birth these muscles are stretched even further to allow the baby to come out. It's easy to understand how pregnancy and childbirth can cause the pelvic floor muscles to sag, much like a loose hammock (see figure 10.3b). Pelvic floor exercises (see Lab 10) are important during pregnancy to maintain strength in these muscles and after delivery to restore the stretched muscles to their normal length. When these muscles are toned and strong, they are better able to support the enlarged uterus and to relax and allow the baby to be born. Strong pelvic floor muscles also alleviate the common postnatal problem of leaking urine when you laugh, sneeze, or run, because these muscles control the bladder.

## Physical Activity Implications

- Pelvic floor exercises tone and maintain the pelvic floor muscles. Perform them throughout your pregnancy.
- Perform pelvic floor exercises after delivery to avoid the lingering problem of urine leakage.

## PHYSICAL ACTIVITY GUIDELINES

Pregnant women should gain medical clearance to exercise. The benefits of exercise far outweigh the potential risks if caution is taken in following appropriate guidelines. The American College of Obstetricians and Gynecologists established the following guidelines in 1994.

- **Exercise at least three times per week.** Exercising less won't produce cardiorespiratory benefits; exercising at least three times per week will help women maintain or improve their fitness.

- **Don't exercise on your back after the first trimester.** Doing so may put pressure on the inferior vena cava, the vein that returns blood from the legs and torso to the heart. Too much pressure on the inferior vena cava can result in dizziness, nausea, and hypotension (abnormally low blood pressure).

- **Modify the intensity; listen to your body.** Less oxygen is available for aerobic exercise during pregnancy because of increased oxygen requirements and breathing difficulties. While no studies have shown that women need to lower their target heart range during pregnancy, they should modify the intensity of exercise according to how they feel.

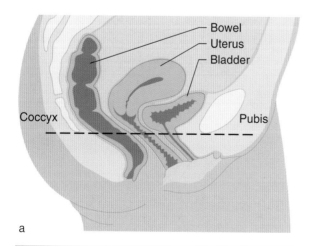

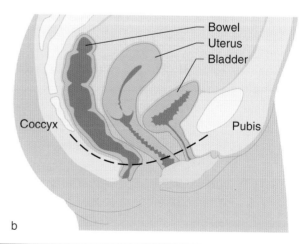

**FIGURE 10.3** *(a)* Good pelvic floor support has a firm base and keeps organs in place. *(b)* Poor pelvic floor support causes the organs to sag and contents to descend.

Women shouldn't exercise to exhaustion; they should stop when they get fatigued.

• **Don't jeopardize your balance.** As mentioned before, the center of gravity shifts during pregnancy; sudden changes in direction can cause pregnant women to lose their balance and risk a fall and injury.

• **Avoid activities that can cause abdominal trauma.** See "Safe—and Unsafe—Exercise for Pregnant Women" for activities to avoid.

• **Be careful not to overheat, especially in the first trimester.** Body core temperature shouldn't exceed 100°F (38°C). Pregnant women have more trouble keeping their body temperature down while exercising. They should drink plenty of water and avoid exercising vigorously in hot, humid conditions.

• **Warm up and cool down every time you exercise.** Light activity followed by stretching prepares muscles for exercise and gets the blood circulating; cooling down helps the heart rate return to normal, prevents blood from pooling in the legs and feet, and helps loosen tight muscles.

• **Eat enough calories for the extra energy you need for both your pregnancy and ex-**

### Safe—and Unsafe—Exercise for Pregnant Women

Women can safely take part in a number of physical activities throughout their pregnancy. The following are safe ways to exercise:

▌ **Walking**—Many call this the ideal exercise for pregnant women. Walking is recommended for women who have been sedentary.

▌ **Swimming**—Swimming is also ideal because it's non-weight-bearing and involves no ballistic movements or dangerous twists and turns.

▌ **Bicycling**—Biking is also good because it's non-weight-bearing, although once a woman's center of gravity shifts, she may want to switch to stationary biking.

▌ **Jogging**—Jogging is safe, but most physicians don't recommend it to women who haven't already been jogging. However, many women jog safely throughout their pregnancy.

▌ **Aerobic exercise class**—Low-impact aerobics is fine; high-impact aerobics is not, because of issues of balance and strain on the knees and back.

▌ **Racket sports**—Tennis, badminton, and racquetball are generally okay through the first two trimesters, but as balance and lateral movement become issues, these sports can become more difficult and risky.

▌ **Strength training**—Light weights are okay, but heavy weights can cause problems with blood flow to the fetus.

▌ **Aerobic equipment**—Pregnant women can safely use a number of pieces of equipment, such as stair climbers, treadmills, rowers, and stationary bikes.

▌ **Other activities**—Activities such as golf, bowling, step exercise, and cross-country skiing are generally safe during the first two trimesters but can cause balance problems in the third trimester.

▌ **Unsafe activities**—Activities that put the mother or the fetus at risk include skydiving, hang gliding, high diving, deep-sea diving, soccer, rugby, other contact sports, jumping feet first in water, downhill skiing, water skiing, horseback riding, field hockey, and basketball.

**ercise.** An additional 300 calories a day are usually required during pregnancy. Pregnant women who exercise probably need more than this, depending on how much they exercise.

While no studies have shown that women need to lower their target heart range during pregnancy, they should modify the intensity of exercise according to how they feel. Women shouldn't exercise to exhaustion; they should stop when they get fatigued.

In addition, pregnant women should

- rise slowly from the floor to avoid dizziness,
- begin an exercise program slowly and advance gradually if they've been sedentary,
- stop exercising and consult their medical caregiver if unusual symptoms appear (see

"Warning Signs to Stop Exercising" on page 256),

- not hold their breath while exercising, and
- return to their prepregnancy exercise routine slowly once they've given birth.

## HEALTHCHECK

**If the joints of pregnant women are so much looser because of hormonal changes, do women who are pregnant need to stretch before and after exercise?**

While it's true that the hormone relaxin loosens the joints, it's still wise for pregnant women to safely warm up and stretch before activity and to stretch easily afterward. This will help loosen tight muscles that are affected by postural changes, such as the back muscles. However, women should take caution in not stretching too far—especially in hip and knee joints.

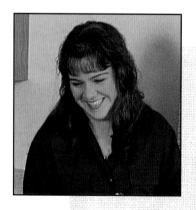

## Health Concepts

As you'll remember, Megan's sister, Terri, was planning on continuing to jog throughout her pregnancy. She had already attained a certain level of cardiorespiratory fitness before pregnancy; she should be able to safely maintain that level of fitness throughout pregnancy and the postpartum period, though she may have to modify her exercise intensity.

Terri's plan to preserve her fitness during her pregnancy should serve her well—women who are physically active during their pregnancy tend to feel better during their pregnancy and gain additional stamina and strength so that they can recover from childbirth more quickly than women who aren't active.

## SUMMARY

▌ The medical profession encourages pregnant women to take part in moderate physical activity so long as they have no preexisting conditions or medical complications. As a result, more women than ever before are realizing the benefits of physical activity during pregnancy.

▌ Women who are physically active during their pregnancy don't have easier deliveries—but they can experience a number of benefits that will help them feel better during their pregnancy and provide additional stamina and strength to recover from childbirth more quickly than women who aren't active.

▌ The body undergoes many changes during pregnancy that have implications for physical activity: breathing changes; heart and circulatory changes; stomach and intestinal changes; kidney and bladder changes; muscular, joint, and postural changes; metabolic and hormonal changes; breast changes; and pelvic floor changes.

▌ Women can safely take part in a number of physical activities throughout their pregnancy, including walking, jogging, bicycling, swimming, aerobic exercise, and strength training.

*Physical activity can have positive effects on women who are pregnant. It can also have a good impact on people's mental health. In the next chapter we'll look at how physical activity can enhance your mental health now and in the future.*

## KEY TERMS

| | |
|---|---|
| diastasis recti | hypoglycemia |
| estrogen | hypoxia |
| gestational diabetes | insulin |
| hyperthermia | relaxin |

**10**

**10**

# Estimating Risk for Gestational Diabetes and Exercising During Pregnancy

### THE PURPOSES OF THIS LAB EXPERIENCE ARE TO

▌ estimate your risk for developing gestational diabetes during pregnancy and

▌ learn appropriate exercises to improve abdominal strength, posture, and pelvic floor strength during pregnancy.

*Obviously, the lab exercises in this chapter are designed for women. If you're a man, you may want to go through this lab with a woman.*

### Evaluate Your Risk for Gestational Diabetes

As we've mentioned, about 1 in 300 women will develop gestational diabetes during their pregnancy. Circle one answer to each of the following questions to help you determine your risk for gestational diabetes.

| Question | Answer | |
|---|---|---|
| 1. From your previous lab experiences in chapter 4, did you determine that you have a healthy weight and body composition? | Yes | No |
| 2. Do you have a family history of any type of diabetes? | Yes | No |
| 3. Are you over 25 years of age? | Yes | No |
| 4. If you've already had a baby, was the baby's birth weight over 9 pounds? | Yes | No |
| 5. If you've already had a baby, did the baby suffer a birth defect or was it stillborn? | Yes | No |

Question 1: A "no" answer indicates that you have a body fat level that is not consistent with good health. Women who are obese ("overfat") have an increased risk for developing gestational diabetes.

Question 2: A "yes" answer indicates that you have a grandmother, mother, and/or sister who developed gestational diabetes. As with many diseases, a family history of that disease indicates a risk for other family members.

Question 3: A "yes" answer indicates a higher risk.

Question 4: A "yes" answer indicates a higher risk. A previous baby born with a high birth weight increases the risk for the mother to develop gestational diabetes in subsequent pregnancies.

Question 5: A "yes" answer indicates a higher risk. Health problems with previous babies indicate a higher risk for gestational diabetes in subsequent pregnancies.

## Exercise and Pregnancy

In addition to a regular aerobic training program at least three times weekly, pregnant women can benefit from the exercises that follow. The abdominal strengthening exercises help prevent diastasis recti and prepare you for labor and delivery; the postural exercises relieve or offset stress on your body from postural changes during pregnancy; and the pelvic floor exercises strengthen the pelvic floor muscles.

**10**

### Abdominal Exercises

Perform the test for diastasis recti (see page 258) each time before you perform these exercises. If there is more than 1 inch (2.5 centimeters) of separation, do not perform the exercises; consult your medical caregiver. When the separation becomes 1 inch or less, you can resume these exercises.

#### *Pelvic Tilting (Phase I)—Lying Down*

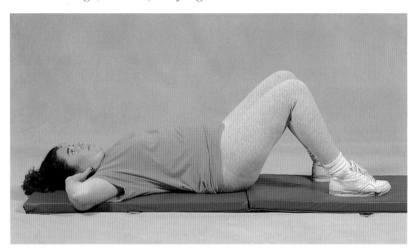

While lying on your back with your knees bent and feet flat on the floor, flatten your lower back against the floor by rolling the pelvis backward. Breathe out while performing this motion and contract the abdominal muscles as strongly as you can. Hold for 5 seconds, relax, and repeat. Once you can perform 10 pelvic tilts and understand the correct movements, you can progress to the next exercise.

#### *Pelvic Tilting (Phase II)—All Fours*

Performing a pelvic tilt on your hands and knees is more difficult because you're working against gravity. To begin, get down on your hands and knees and keep your back flat. The weight of the baby will make your back want to sag, *but don't let it!* Perform a pelvic tilt by contracting your abdominal

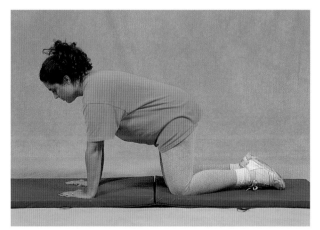
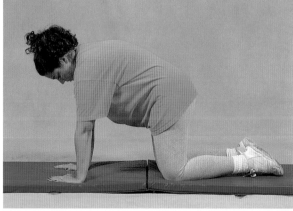

muscles and pressing up with your lower back. Hold for 3 to 5 seconds, then relax only enough to return to the neutral starting position. If you relax completely, your back will sag all the way down. When you first try this exercise, have a partner place a hand in the small of your back to let you know when your back is flat so you learn how much to relax. Repeat 5-10 times but stop before this if you're having difficulty keeping your back from sagging.

### Curl-Ups

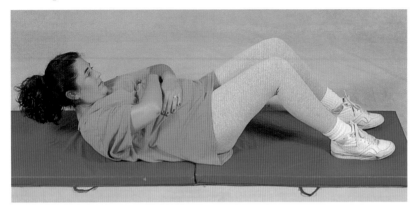

Don't start doing this exercise if you're already in your third trimester and haven't been performing it regularly throughout your pregnancy. Lie on your back with your knees bent, feet flat on the floor, and arms crossed over your abdomen for support. Pull each side of the abdomen toward the midline as you perform a pelvic tilt and raise your head and upper shoulders off the floor. Remember to breathe out as you slowly raise your head, then breathe in as you slowly lower back to the starting position. Repeat 10 times.

### Diagonal Curl-Ups

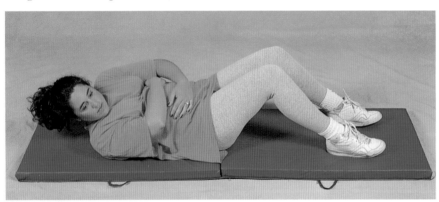

Again, don't start doing this exercise if you're already in your third trimester and haven't been performing it regularly throughout your pregnancy. Lie on your back with your knees bent, feet flat on the floor, and arms crossed over your abdomen for support. Tuck your chin to your chest, then breathe outward as you lift your right shoulder toward your left knee, then slowly lower yourself to the starting position. Repeat on the other side, performing five repetitions for each side. Remember to pull the sides of your abdomen toward the midline with your hands to prevent diastasis recti.

### Postural Exercises

Remember that women have increased lumbar lordosis during pregnancy. The pelvic tilting and abdominal exercises described earlier reverse the lordosis and provide a gentle stretch to the back extensors to help ease tension. In addition, the following two exercises are helpful for your upper back—by strengthening the muscles needed to help support the added weight of enlarged breasts and by gently stretching tight muscles.

### Shoulder Blade Squeeze

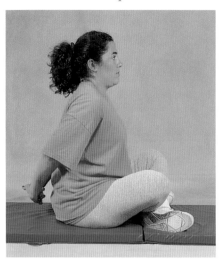

This exercise can be done in a standing or sitting position. Lightly clasp your hands behind your back and pull shoulders back while trying to squeeze your shoulder blades together. Hold for 30 seconds while breathing normally. Repeat three times.

### Wall Push-Ups

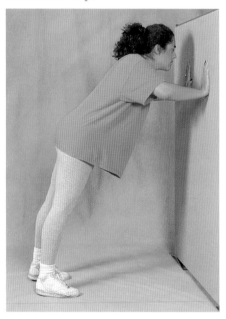

Stand facing a wall, about an arm's length away with your feet shoulder-width apart and toes pointing forward. Place your palms on the wall at shoulder height, then slowly bend your elbows, bringing your face toward the wall. Make sure not to tilt your pelvis forward or backward; keep your heels flat on the floor and your legs straight. Slowly push away from the wall to return to the starting position. Repeat 10-15 times.

### Pelvic Floor Exercises

To understand the sensation of "drawing up the pelvic floor" in the next three exercises, try this exercise. While in the bathroom, begin by purposely stopping and then restarting the flow of urine—this requires the contraction and relaxation of the pelvic floor muscles. Stop the flow of urine by drawing up the pelvic floor; contract the muscles, and hold for a few seconds. Then release the contraction to start the flow again. When you can do this, you're ready for the next three exercises from the YMCA's *Fit for Two* book.

### Contract and Release

Start in any comfortable position, either standing, sitting, or lying down. Draw up the pelvic floor by contracting the muscles and then releasing them. Hold for 3 to 5 seconds. Repeat 3 to 5 times frequently throughout the day, aiming for 50 total daily.

### Elevator

Start in any comfortable position. Imagine you're in an elevator, and draw up the pelvic floor a little more each time you go up one story. When you reach your limit, gradually "descend" floor by floor by relaxing the muscles a little each time. Repeat 3 to 5 times frequently throughout the day, aiming for 50 total daily.

### Super Kegels

Begin in any comfortable position. Contract the pelvic floor muscles and hold them for 20 seconds. Repeat 1 to 2 times frequently throughout the day, aiming for 50 total daily.

Chapter*11*

# Mental Health

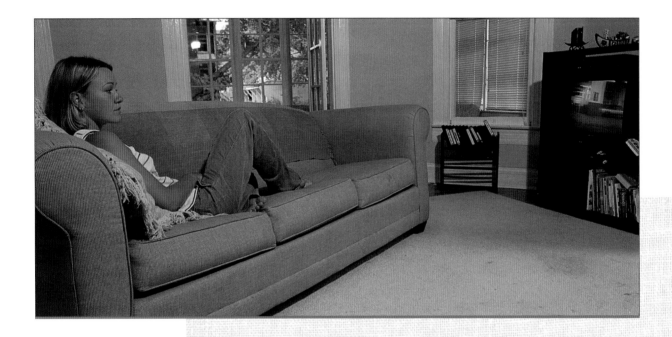

I've been really down lately. I don't know why I feel like this. I had fun in college last year. I look around me now and it seems like everyone else is having fun. I have no energy, I don't care about my classes, and I feel like crying most of the time. I do remember last year when I played tennis and took aerobics I'd feel pretty energized afterward, and feel pretty good about myself. Now I can't stand myself and don't even want to go outside of my room. I just want to sleep all day. I wonder if getting back into exercise can help me feel better?

—Maria, 19-year-old sophomore

*W*hat do you think?

Maria is certainly describing a depressed state, though it's hard to diagnose from her brief statement whether or not she's clinically depressed. However, if she is, she's not as alone as she thinks: about one in seven women in the United States between the ages of 15 and 54 has experienced an episode of depression within the past year. Maria's thoughts on exercise and depression are intriguing. *Can* physical activity alleviate the effects of depression? How might being physically active affect depression? Is depression just a "state of mind"—or does it have a physiological or neurological basis?

In this chapter we'll explore how physical activity affects depression, anxiety, and stress. We'll look at the symptoms of depression and anxiety and study their causes and treatments. We'll also explore differences in the ways stress affects people and examine the impact of physical activity on stress. Finally, we'll consider specific ways that physical activity improves mental health: by improving self-esteem and sleep and by causing biological adaptations that decrease depression and anxiety. The lab at the end of the chapter will give you ways to estimate your own levels of tension, perceived stress, and depression.

When most people think of physical activity's effects on a person, they think of the physiological benefits to physical health. In this chapter we'll learn how certain physiological adaptations can benefit *mental* health as well.

## DEPRESSION

About one in five people will experience an episode of *depression*—feelings of despair or hopelessness accompanied by a loss of pleasure—at some point in their lives; two of every three people who experience depression are women. Among different races, Hispanics tend to experience more depression than Caucasians, who in turn experience more depression than African-Americans. The annual rate of depression among teenagers and young adults is nearly twice that of adults 25 to 44 years old, and about four times the rate among people over age 65. Depression is more prevalent than coronary heart disease or heart attacks, and the occurrence of major depression in the United States has increased steadily during the past 50 years. (See figure 11.1 for the lifetime prevalence of depression, anxiety, and total psychiatric disorders.) Next to accidental deaths, suicide is the leading cause of death among college students—and depression is a major contributing factor to suicide. According to Greenberg et al. (1993), the annual direct and indirect costs of depression in 1990 were about $40 billion, nearly one-third of the United States' total mental health bill of $148 billion.

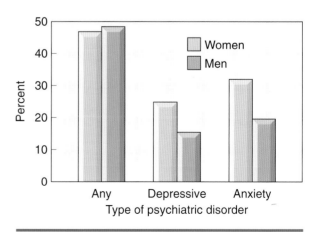

**FIGURE 11.1**  Lifetime prevalence of psychiatric disorders.
Data from Kessler et al. 1994.

In this section we'll look at the symptoms of major depression, its causes and treatments, and the ways in which physical activity affects it.

 Depression is more prevalent than coronary heart disease or heart attacks, and the occurrence of major depression in the United States has increased steadily during the past 50 years.

### HEALTHCHECK

**Why do women experience depression more often than men?**

Although it's not well understood, four hypotheses have been posed. First, men and women tend to think differently; women think more about their troubles while men often avoid thinking about them. Second, women may be in better tune with losses and feelings that can result in depression. They may be more likely to seek help for depression, thus skewing the numbers of those who are diagnosed as depressed. Third, women in many cultures have less control over their lives than men do, contributing to feelings of helplessness and despair. Fourth, fluctuations in estrogen and progesterone result in higher risk of depression for women during menstruation, during menopause, after childbirth, and while taking birth control pills. Women do benefit as much as men, or even more, from the protective effects of physical activity against depression.

### Symptoms of Major Depression

The most common form of clinically diagnosed depression is a *major depressive episode*. According to the American Psychiatric Association, people are going through a major depressive episode when they have experienced at least five of the following eight symptoms during the same two-week period and these symptoms represent a change from previous functioning. In addition, one of the symptoms must be depressed mood or marked loss of interest or pleasure (i.e., one of the first two symptoms from the following list).

- Depressed mood most of the day, nearly every day
- Marked loss of interest or pleasure in almost all activities most of the day, nearly every day
- Significant weight loss or weight gain when not dieting (e.g., more than 5% of body weight in a month); decrease or increase in appetite nearly every day
- Insomnia or hypersomnia nearly every day
- Psychomotor agitation or retardation nearly every day, observable by others
- Fatigue or loss of energy nearly every day
- Feelings of worthlessness or of excessive and inappropriate guilt nearly every day
- Recurrent thoughts of death (not just fear of dying); recurrent ideas of suicide with or without a specific plan; or a suicide attempt

When a person is experiencing a major depressive episode, these symptoms cause significant distress and impairment in social and occupational settings as well as in other areas of the person's life. Note that it's not considered a major depressive episode if the depression is caused by drug abuse or medication or a medical condition such as hyperthyroidism. Note also that many people have these symptoms within the first two months after a loved one has died, but it's not considered major depression unless the symptoms are associated with marked functional impairment, a preoccupation with worthlessness, ideas of suicide, psychotic symptoms, or psychomotor retardation.

### Causes and Treatments

Depression can be caused by diseases that have biological consequences for the brain—for instance, thyroid disease, diabetes, multiple sclerosis, hepatitis, and rheumatoid arthritis. It can result from psychological, catastrophic events such as the loss of a loved one through death or separation. Depression can stem from loss of self-esteem (for instance, students might feel unworthy when they don't meet academic goals). It can also be caused by overstimulation of the sympathetic nervous system and the hypothalamic-pituitary-adrenal cortical system resulting from persistent anxiety or other forms of emotional stress. (Later in the chapter we'll discuss how disruptions of these two systems contribute to depression.) And depression can occur for no apparent reason.

Regardless of the cause, depression is associated with imbalances in *neurotransmitters,* which are chemicals that influence the activity of the brain cells that regulate mood, pleasure, and rational thought. Research hasn't confirmed a direct genetic abnormality leading to depression, but some people are more vulnerable to depression when they are exposed to stress. Repeated exposure to uncontrolled stress appears to overtax the body's natural biological response to threatening circumstances. Two major neurotransmitters in the brain, *noradrenaline* and *serotonin,* modulate the nerve activity of other cells that stimulate behavioral (e.g., motivation) and physiological (e.g., heart rate, blood pressure, hormones) responses needed to cope with stress. After persistent stress, the nerves that manufacture and release noradrenaline and serotonin lose their ability to do so fast enough to keep pace with needs. As we'll discuss, drugs can help most people regain normal function of those cells within a few weeks. Importantly, growing evidence suggests that regular physical activity can both protect against loss of function and restore lost function in ways not too different from the actions of drugs.

 Depression is associated with imbalances in *neurotransmitters,* which are chemicals that influence the activity of the brain cells that regulate mood, pleasure, and rational thought.

Most depression is *unipolar,* characterized by depressed mood. A small percentage of people have *bipolar depression,* which is also known as *manic-depressive disorder.* People who have bipolar depression experience wild swings of emotions and feelings, ranging from depressed moods to elevated, expansive, or irritated moods; this type of depression can cause exaggerated self-confidence, risky or asocial behavior, and paranoia. People who have bipolar depression are often treated with a drug called lithium carbonate—a salt that influences how ions pass through brain cells and regulates nerve impulses that in turn regulate mood, pleasure, and rational thought.

Thankfully, about 9 of 10 people who seek treatment for depression can be effectively treated as outpatients through antidepressant medications, psychotherapy, or a combination of the two. People who don't respond to these treatments may be helped by electroconvulsive therapy, in which small amounts of electric current are passed through the brain.

Unfortunately, in studies among people who report having experienced symptoms or signs of depression, only about 3 in 10 actually seek the help of a mental health professional. About half the people who have an episode of clinical depression go undiagnosed or misdiagnosed. Of the people who are correctly diagnosed with depression and who would be helped by antidepressant drugs, half have never taken the drugs and less than one-third are prescribed the appropriate dose. Many antidepressants have negative side effects for many people; some side effects are serious (see table 11.1). These facts point to the importance of self-help behaviors that enhance mental hygiene. Many studies have shown that regular physical activity can prevent or reduce symptoms of depression.

## Physical Activity and Depression

Most studies that have evaluated exercise as treatment for depression were conducted with young to middle-aged adults; reductions in depression after exercise were similar for men and women. Fewer studies have been done with chil-

## Table 11.1 Common Antidepressant Drugs and Side Effects

| Antidepressant drug | Side effects of all |
|---|---|
| **_Tricyclics_** | |
| Anafranil (clomipramine)* | Low blood pressure, |
| Asendin (amoxapine) | blurred vision, |
| Aventyl (nortriptyline) | irregular heart beat, |
| Elavil (amitriptyline) | stomach and |
| Norpramin (desipramine) | intestinal upsets, |
| Sinequan (doxepin) | male sexual |
| Tofranil (imipramine) | dysfunction, toxicity |
| Vivactil (protriptyline) | with lithium |
| | |
| **_Monoamine oxidase inhibitors_** | |
| Marplan (isocarboxazid) | |
| Nardil (phenelzine sulfate) | |
| Parnate (tranylcypromine sulfate) | |
| | |
| **_Serotonin selective reuptake inhibitors_** | |
| Desyrel (trazodone) | |
| Ludiomil (maprotiline) | |
| Paxil (paroxetine) | |
| Prozac (fluoxetine) | |
| | |
| **_Serotonin and noradrenaline reuptake inhibitor_** | |
| Effexor (venlafaxine) | |

*The generic name of each drug appears in parentheses.

dren or people over age 65, though the mental health outcomes for these groups after exercise are nearly the same as for people of middle age. There's some evidence that the benefits of exercise for _reducing_ depression may diminish slightly as people age; however, older people have a lower prevalence of depression than young and middle-aged adults. In contrast, the benefits of physical activity for helping _prevent_ depression usually occur regardless of people's age, gender, race, or socioeconomic status.

The benefits of physical activity for helping prevent depression usually occur regardless of people's age, gender, race, or socioeconomic status.

## Preventing Depression

Numerous studies conducted around the world have shown that physical activity can play a role in preventing depression:

- The National Health and Nutrition Examination Survey I (NHANES I), a 1975 survey of nearly 7,000 Americans aged 25 to 74, found that people who said they got little or no exercise in their leisure time also reported more symptoms of depression (Stephens 1988).

- The Canada Fitness Survey of 22,000 Canadians aged 10 years and older yielded similar findings (Stephens 1988). In this 1981 survey, inactive people reported more symptoms related to negative moods in comparison to people who said they were moderately or very active in their leisure time.

- A study conducted in Germany between 1975 and 1984, of 1,500 people aged 15 and older, noted the prevalence of several types of depressive disorders for those who stated that they currently did not exercise for sports, as compared with those who stated that they did regularly exercise for sports (Weyerer 1992).

In all three studies, higher rates of depression occurred among inactive people regardless of physical illness, gender, age, and social class. It's important to note that the studies reported cross-sectional comparisons of active and inactive people. This means that the studies merely took a "snapshot" of physical activity and health measured at the same time. The studies didn't determine whether it was inactivity or depression that occurred first. It's possible that people became less active after becoming depressed, rather than becoming depressed due to inactivity.

However, about 1,500 of the people originally interviewed in NHANES I were interviewed again eight years later (Farmer et al. 1988). That follow-up survey first measured physical activity and then looked for the later occurrence of the symptoms of depression. Among the findings of the NHANES I follow-up were these:

- The rate of depression among sedentary Caucasian women who were *not* depressed in 1975 and who remained inactive was twice that of women who said they participated in a moderate amount of physical activity and who remained active over the eight years.

- Caucasian men who were depressed and inactive in 1975 and remained inactive were 12 times more likely to be depressed after eight years than those who were initially depressed but who had become physically active.

Again, these findings were observed regardless of age, education level, and socioeconomic status.

Finally, in a study of about 10,000 Harvard male alumni from the mid-1960s through 1977, physical activity was shown to reduce the likelihood of developing depression (Paffenbarger, Lee, and Leung 1994). Those who spent 3 or more hours per week playing sports during their leisure time reduced their risk of developing depression by 17% as compared with their less active peers.

### Treating Depression

About 2,500 years ago, Hippocrates prescribed exercise for his patients experiencing depression, which he called *melancholia*—a term still used today for deep depression. Modern studies show that Hippocrates knew quite well what he was doing. Physical activity can have a positive effect on depression, and the benefits of exercise have been found in patients whether or not they were medicated with antidepressant drugs.

In 1984, the U.S. National Institute of Mental Health concluded that regular exercise and physical fitness are associated with reduced depression; in 1992, a group of experts who convened at the Second International Consensus Symposium on Physical Activity, Fitness, and Health reached similar conclusions. These findings were corroborated in 1996 by the U.S. Surgeon General's report, *Physical Activity and Health.*

Most of the research showing that exercise improves self-ratings of mood has been done with people having normal mental health, but some experiments involving people diagnosed with mild unipolar depression have shown improvements in mood after several weeks of moderately intense exercise. When the exercise program lasted four to five months, the improvements in people's self-ratings of depression were as large as those usually seen after psychotherapy. The best results for fighting depression occurred when outpatients were in an exercise program and also received psychotherapy. A few studies of exercise programs lasting beyond five months showed improvements comparable to those typically seen after drug treatment. Although current evidence on the benefits of physical activity isn't strong enough to let us conclude that exercise is a substitute for drug treatment and psychotherapy, exercise *is* an important aid in reducing the likelihood of developing depression or anxiety.

### How Much Physical Activity Is Enough?

As we've seen, population studies indicate that being sedentary increases the odds that a person will become depressed. It's not clear how big the increased risk is, but it seems to be about twofold. This means the risk of depression among physically inactive people is nearly as great as their risk for developing coronary heart disease. However, unlike the investigations on exercise and heart disease, the population studies provided no clear evidence concerning how much physical activity will help prevent or treat depression. People who were very active did not report fewer symptoms of depression than people who were only moderately active; thus it appears that while being sedentary increases the risk for depression, high levels of physical activity may not be any more protective than moderate amounts of physical activity.

 Being sedentary increases the risk for depression, but high levels of physical activity may not be any more protective than moderate amounts of physical activity.

In the Canada Fitness Survey, people were seemingly protected from symptoms of depression if their daily leisure energy expenditure was at least 1 kilocalorie per kilogram of body weight per day, which is a low level of activity (e.g., about 20 minutes of walking). Risk of depression was not further reduced when the energy expenditure was raised to 2 to 5 kilocalories per kilogram of body weight per day. For example, the reduced rate of depression was similar for people who weighed 60 kilograms (132 pounds) whether they expended 120 calories (about 1.5 miles of walking) or 300 calories (about 3 miles of jogging).

Data from the Harvard alumni study did suggest a dose-dependent reduction in depression with increased exercise; this occurred after 2,500 kilocalories of expenditure per week. However, the significance of those findings is limited, because fewer than 1 in 10 adults in America expend this much energy in leisure-time physical activity.

Most people reported changes in self-ratings of depression after exercise whether or not their cardiorespiratory fitness had increased. Most of the studies used jogging as the mode of activity; a few used cycling or weight lifting. Training usually was prescribed based on the guidelines of the American College of Sports Medicine for the types and amounts of exercise recommended for cardiorespiratory fitness in otherwise healthy people (see table 2.1 on page 23). Because no adverse effects were reported in these studies, the following exercise guidelines should be appropriate for people with depression who are otherwise healthy:

• Three to five days a week
• 20 to 60 minutes each session
• 55% to 90% of maximal heart rate

Though beginners should always increase the intensity and length of their workouts gradually, gradual progress is especially important for someone who is depressed. Gradual progress helps to maximize feelings of success and control and minimize potential feelings of failure if the person can't stick with an exercise program because the program called for too quick a progression.

## HEALTHCHECK

### What type of exercise is best for improving mood?

Aerobic and resistance exercise each can reduce depression and mild anxiety; most studies have used running, swimming, and weight training. Some people may notice immediate benefits, but for most people the biggest changes occur after about four months of regular exercise.

## ANXIETY

*Anxiety disorders*—characterized by apprehension or worry accompanied by restlessness, tension, and elevated heart rate and breathing—are the most common mental illnesses in the United States, affecting about 23 million people (4% of women and 2% of men) each year. Anxiety disorders in the United States accounted for $46.6 billion in direct and indirect costs in 1990 (DuPont et al. 1996). While anxiety often occurs with depression, and chronic anxiety can contribute to the risk of depression, people most often experience anxiety apart from depression.

You've probably had feelings of anxiety before a big exam or a job interview. Anxiety disorders, however, are illnesses that cause people to feel frightened, distressed, and uneasy for extended periods of time for no apparent reason. Left untreated, these disorders can reduce productivity and diminish the quality of life. There are several types of anxiety disorders. The major ones include the following:

• Phobias—Intense fear of an object, place, or situation. People with a specific phobia experience extreme fear of something that poses little or no actual danger; the fear causes people to avoid these objects or situations and most likely limit their lives unnecessarily. People with social phobia have an overwhelming fear of scrutiny and embarrassment in social situations, which causes them to avoid many potentially enjoyable activities.

• **Panic disorder**—Repeated episodes of intense fear that strike without warning and without an obvious source. Physical symptoms include chest pain, heart palpitations, shortness of breath, dizziness, abdominal distress, and fear of dying.

• **Obsessive-compulsive disorder**—Repeated, unwanted thoughts or compulsive behaviors that seem impossible to stop, typified by repetitive acts or rituals to relieve anxiety.

• **Generalized anxiety disorder**—Recurrent or persistent excessive worry about everyday, routine life events and activities, lasting at least six months. This most prevalent type of anxiety disorder is accompanied by fatigue, trembling, muscle tension, headaches, or nausea. *State anxiety* can be used to describe this condition if the feelings of anxiety are temporary and fluctuate from moment to moment ("How do I feel right now?"); the term *trait anxiety* is used if these feelings and symptoms are constant and persistent ("How have I been feeling generally?").

As we've already mentioned, the signs and symptoms of anxiety disorders vary in number and severity. They include agitation, excessive alertness, confusion, muscle tension, tremors, high heart rates, palpitations, flushing, sweating, dry mouth, and urinary and gastrointestinal problems.

As with depression, young people tend to have more anxiety than do older people. People in the age group of 15 to 24 experience episodes of anxiety about 40% more often than people aged 25 to 54 years old. This is true regardless of race.

## Causes and Treatments

Just as people can have a depressive temperament, people can also, through genetics and early experiences, have an anxious temperament. And

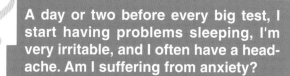

**HEALTHCHECK**

**A day or two before every big test, I start having problems sleeping, I'm very irritable, and I often have a headache. Am I suffering from anxiety?**

You probably are experiencing *state anxiety* if your symptoms only last for a few days and go away after you take the test. If you start to feel nervous before an exam, take a walk, try the relaxation response on page 280, and don't forget to allow yourself extra time to study!

fluctuations in anxiety are a major part of most people's emotional lives even for those who don't have an anxiety disorder. Anxiety, like depression and anger, is a stress emotion. Uncertainties about important events can lead to worry and apprehension, especially when a person feels a lack of control over how the event is going to turn out. Life events such as romance, divorce, paying bills, making good grades, making a good impression on others, and getting a good job contribute to anxieties that affect the quality of life. Smaller hassles of daily living, such as catching the bus on time, making it to class on time, and dealing with a noisy neighbor or a nagging friend or relative, can also add to stress emotions, including anxiety.

Anxiety can also be more subconscious, leading to tension, digestion problems, headaches, high blood pressure, and sleep problems, even when people don't report they are worried. Though feelings of helplessness can be common to the experience of both anxiety and depression, depression is distinguished by feelings of hopelessness and despair. A common view of scientists is that chronic anxiety can lead to depression for some people. Anxiety and depression share a common link in that the brain cells that help organize emotional and behavioral responses during real and imagined threat are either overactive (such as in anxiety) or become overtaxed during chronic stress (such as in depression). These cells lose their ability to maintain chemical balance in the brain and physiological balance of the cardiovascular, endocrine, and immune systems.

The two most effective forms of psychotherapy used to treat anxiety disorders are behavioral and cognitive-behavioral therapy. Behavioral therapy helps patients change their actions through breathing techniques or through gradual exposure to what is frightening them. Cognitive-behavioral therapy, in addition to these techniques, teaches patients to understand their thinking patterns so they can react differently to the situations that cause them anxiety.

The most effective short-term treatment of anxiety uses drugs called *benzodiazepines* (see table 11.2). Receptors in the parts of the brain that are important for emotions, particularly in the *hypothalamus* and the *limbic system*, bind benzodiazepine molecules to brain cells; this activates a bigger molecule that contains a receptor for gamma-aminobutyric acid, or GABA. The result is an inhibition of brain cells involved with anxiety. Cells that manufacture GABA are located throughout the brain, but are especially important in the hypothalamus, the limbic system, and the brain cortex. Some research suggests that exercise helps reduce anxiety by elevating GABA levels in the brain and altering the number of GABA receptors.

Excessive responses by nerves that manufacture and release noradrenaline contribute to signs and symptoms of anxiety, especially panic. Drugs that block receptors for noradrenaline, called beta-blockers, help reduce feelings of panic—especially those related to rapid heartbeat and palpitations. Inadequate responses by nerves that manufacture and release serotonin in the brain also contribute to anxiety, especially obsessive-compulsive disorder. Some drugs lengthen the time that serotonin stays in the synapse (the area between nerve cells that permits transmission of nerve signals) after it is released by serotonin nerves; these help manage anxiety.

## Physical Activity and Anxiety

There is no compelling evidence that increased physical activity or fitness changes a person's temperament from an anxious one to a calm, relaxed one. However, studies do show that a single session of physical activity can reduce state anxiety and that regular exercise can reduce trait anxiety. Because there is no evidence that physical activity causes the underlying sources of anxiety to disappear or causes people to perceive events as less threatening, how can these reductions in anxiety be explained?

A number of possible explanations have been put forth. One is that exercise distracts people from thoughts that cause anxiety or from symptoms of anxiety. This could explain reduced state anxiety. Another view is that physical activity, by improving body image and physical skills, increases self-esteem, which in turn reduces worry because it helps people feel more in control of the events that cause anxiety. Yet another view is that by becoming accustomed to the sensations of physical exertion, people are less threatened by the physical arousal that accompanies anxiety—a key element in panic attacks. Another explanation relates to the chance for social interaction that often occurs while people exercise. Because in any given year 9% of

### Table 11.2 Common Antianxiety Drugs and Side Effects

| Antianxiety drug | Side effects of all |
|---|---|
| **Benzodiazepines** | |
| Ativan (lorazepam)* | Sedation; low muscle tone; anticonvulsant effects; tolerance or dependence and withdrawal may develop |
| Centrax (prazepam) | |
| Paxipam (halazepam) | |
| Serax (oxazepam) | |
| Valium (diazepam) | |
| Xanax (alprazolam) | |
| **Barbiturates** | |
| Librium (chlordiazepoxide) | |
| Tranxene (clorazepate) | |
| **Serotonin antagonist** | |
| Buspar (buspirone) | |

*The generic name of each drug appears in parentheses.

## Learning to Relax: The Benson Relaxation Response

Regular physical activity helps many people manage tension and anxiety. However, some meditational practices, or even just resting or taking "time-out," can offer equally effective alternatives for anxiety reduction. Approaches such as these can be especially useful when an injury or illness prevents exercise, or if you find yourself overstressed or "stale" in your exercise routine.

Benson's Relaxation Response (Benson 1975) is based on the following ingredients:

▌ A quiet environment

▌ A mental symbol (mantra), such as a word or phrase, repeated in rhythmical cadence

▌ A passive attitude with no attention to any single thought

▌ A comfortable, stationary position

Find a quiet, isolated area and follow these instructions:

1. Sit quietly in a comfortable position.
2. Close your eyes.
3. Thoroughly relax all your muscles. Begin at your feet and continue up to your face. Keep the muscles relaxed throughout the entire session.
4. Breathe through your nose and become aware of your breathing. As you breathe out, silently say the word "One" (or substitute another word or phrase). For example, breathe IN . . . OUT ("One"), IN . . . OUT ("One"). Breathe easily and naturally.
5. Continue for 10 to 20 minutes. You may open your eyes to check the time, but do not use an alarm. When you finish, sit quietly for several minutes, at first with eyes closed and later with eyes open. Don't stand up for a few minutes.
6. Don't worry about whether you are achieving a deep level of relaxation. Maintain a passive attitude and permit relaxation to occur at its own pace. When distracting thoughts occur, don't dwell on them; return to repeating "One." With practice, the response should come with little effort. Practice the technique once or twice daily, but not within 2 hours after any meal; the digestive process interferes with the relaxation response.

women and 6% of men have social phobias (e.g., fear of groups), the potential benefits of the social environments of physical activity are not trivial. Case studies show that mild physical activity can help patients with panic disorders associated with a fear of being in public.

There are still other possible explanations for the effects of physical activity on anxiety and depression. These involve body warming during exercise; changes in brain blood flow, endorphins, and brain neurotransmitters; and biological adaptations to physical activity by the autonomic nervous system and the hypothalamic-pituitary-adrenal system that operate through mechanisms similar to those of antianxiety drugs. Several of these mechanisms, which we'll discuss later in more detail, appear similar to those involved with depression, because as we've noted earlier, chronic anxiety can lead to depression.

Physical activity may reduce anxiety and depression by temporarily distracting you from worries or symptoms; it may also produce more lasting changes in self-esteem, improved sleep, and several biological adaptations that help reduce anxiety and depression.

Aerobic exercise that lasts for about 30 minutes is associated with the largest reductions in self-rated symptoms of anxiety. This also is true for physiological signs of anxiety; exercise reduces resting muscle tension as measured by electromyography and changes electrical activity of the brain (especially by increasing the number of alpha waves, which are believed to indicate relaxed wakefulness). Anxiety is reduced the most about 20 to 30 minutes after exercise. In addition, studies show that the reduction in trait anxiety after four months of regular exercise training is about half the reduction that occurs after taking the most commonly prescribed antianxiety drugs (benzodiazepines).

Aerobic exercise that lasts for about 30 minutes is associated with the largest reductions in self-rated symptoms of anxiety, as long as the exercise intensity is between 55% and 90% of maximal heart rate.

As with depression, people in the Canada Fitness Survey reported fewer symptoms of anxiety if their daily leisure-time energy expenditure was at least 1 kilocalorie per kilogram of body weight per day. Risk for developing symptoms of anxiety was not further reduced by increasing the energy expenditure to 2 to 5 kilocalories per kilogram of body weight per day. Most people can reduce their risk of anxiety by expending about 50 to 80 extra calories per day—which usually occurs in about a 1-mile walk.

Although the relationship of exercise to anxiety hasn't been studied as much as that between exercise and depression, Breus and O'Connor

## HEALTHCHECK

### Should I be concerned about "exercise addiction?"

It's true that some people are so committed to exercise that they abuse it—they let it take priority over school, job, family, and social responsibilities and work out even if they are injured or sick. But this addiction is not caused by exercising. It occurs in people who are vulnerable to abusive behavior—and it's not very common. Only 10% of Americans are active enough to become fit; surely few of them are "addicted" in a bad way. When regular exercisers are forced to be inactive, they usually report a worsened mood after a few days, but they don't have the physiological signs of withdrawal, which are the hallmark of addiction. The health risks—both physical and mental—of being sedentary are clearly a greater concern for the public than the potential risk of abusive exercise.

(1998) found that college women with higher-than-average trait anxiety experienced a greater-than-usual reduction in state anxiety after 20 minutes of cycling at a mild intensity (40% of aerobic capacity).

## STRESS

As we've seen, depression and anxiety are stress emotions. They differ in their subjective aspects (e.g., despair or fear), but they have some common roots in how people respond physiologically during stressful events. Stress occurs when the harmony or balance of bodily functions (i.e., homeostasis) is disrupted by real or imagined threat. Stress produces feelings of strain that are often accompanied by abnormal physiological changes in the skin, digestion, muscle tension, heart rate and rhythm, brain activity, and hormone levels. Catastrophic events cause stress, but so do daily hassles. Even positive life events or daily uplifts in spirit can be stressful—but in good ways. It's when you feel overwhelmed by responsibilities, have too much to do in too little time, or are uncertain about important consequences that seem out of your control that you are a candidate for chronic stress, which strains cells, organs, and body systems. This chronic wear and tear can contribute to a poor quality of life and to increased risk for diseases such as coronary heart disease and hypertension and for suppression of the immune system. Depression, anxiety, and anger are stress emotions that can threaten homeostasis when they occur too often or are not controlled.

 **KEY POINT** The chronic wear and tear of stress can contribute to a poor quality of life and increased risk for diseases such as coronary heart disease and hypertension and for suppression of the immune system.

Though it is true that some people simply are exposed to more events that cause stress or strain (e.g., family conflicts, money problems, relationship problems, loss of a loved one, too many hard exams), it is also true that personality and

### Good and Bad Stress

If chronic stress can increase your risk of conditions such as heart disease, high blood pressure, a suppressed immune system, eating disorders, headaches, sleep disorders, and ulcers, you might be wondering if you should attempt to remove *all* stress from your life. The answer is no. A certain amount of stress is needed for optimum health and performance—life without stress would be very boring! Stress researcher Hans Selye made a clear distinction between *distress* ("bad stress") and *eustress* ("good stress"). Some level of stress (eustress) is desirable for optimal performance and well-being; however, each person can reach a point where stress can become too much (distress) and it starts to inhibit our mental, emotional, and physiological abilities to function effectively (see the figure below).

Excessive stress can blunt positive emotions such as love, joy, and surprise and exaggerate negative emotions such as anger, sadness, and fear. Exercise can contribute to your levels of good stress when it is enjoyable and isn't so intense that it causes strain or so frequent that you don't recuperate. Moderate exercise performed regularly can offset negative stress emotions and possibly enhance positive stress emotions.

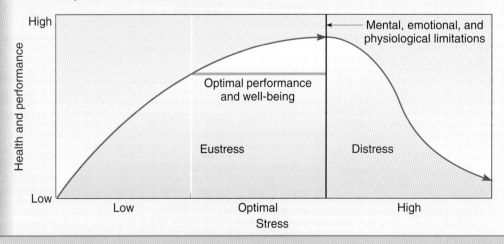

coping skills can lessen one's vulnerability to stress. About 50% of your temperament—whether it's usually calm or usually nervous or fiery—is explained by heredity and early childhood learning. Nonetheless, you can improve your ability to deal with stress by learning skills to reduce your exposure to stressful events or to change your outlook on life. People who view change as a challenge or an opportunity for success, who feel in control, and who have a strong commitment to a purpose in their lives (e.g., career, other people, spirituality) seem to deal better with misfortune than people whose outlook interprets change as a threat, who feel out of control, and who lack a guiding purpose in their lives. Avoiding fatalistic, all-or-none thinking (e.g., "I must," "I can't") or catastrophic thinking (i.e., making mountains out of molehills) can help control emotions by helping you become more rational in your thinking. Doing nothing but worrying about the stressful situation exacerbates stress. Taking positive steps to deal with the situation can alleviate the stress. In other words, if you're stressed out about exams coming up, the best solution is to study!

Nonetheless, exercise is another good way to cope with stress once it occurs. Though exercise usually won't eliminate the source of stress, it can provide a temporary distraction from the problem. An exercise program might increase feelings of control or commitment; it can provide a sense of success in doing something important for yourself, which buffers the impact of stressful events.

## HOW PHYSICAL ACTIVITY IMPROVES MENTAL HEALTH

We've already stated that, in addition to preventing physical disease and developing fitness, physical activity can help improve your mental health by preventing or reducing depression, anxiety, and perceived stress. In the following sections, we'll discuss in more detail how physical activity may produce lasting changes in self-esteem, improved sleep, and several biological adaptations that help reduce anxiety and depression.

## Improved Self-Esteem

*Self-esteem* is the value people place on their conception or view of themselves. It is a composite of specific personal features—including physical attributes such as appearance, endurance, strength, and sport skills—and social, academic or professional, emotional, and spiritual attributes. Self-esteem is the cornerstone of mental health and behavior.

Depression and anxiety are often associated with low self-esteem. Because body image is related to general self-concept, an improvement in body image or physical skills can contribute to general self-esteem in people who place high value on physical attributes relative to the other aspects of self-concept. Positive comments from others about fitness or physique, or merely expectations of increased fitness, can improve self-esteem even when actual fitness hasn't been improved. A sense of achievement is the key.

The U.S. Preventive Services Task Force of the U.S. Office of Disease Prevention and Health Promotion concluded in 1989 that regular exercise can improve self-esteem. Students tend to improve self-esteem more after fitness training than after participating in competitive sports (where success and feelings of accomplishment are less predictable). The biggest gains in self-esteem usually occur for people who value physical fitness or appearance and aren't satisfied with their current status in these areas. Believing you are doing something positive for yourself may be enough to improve self-esteem. Supporting this idea is a study by Desharnais et al. (1993) in which college students improved their self-esteem after participating in an exercise program whose stated goal was to improve psychological well-being. Students in the same study who were *not* told of the goal did *not* report improvements in self-esteem—even though they showed similar fitness improvements.

People who improve their fitness can gain an increased sense of mastery over physical tasks. Some evidence suggests that this confidence can extend beyond physical activity settings to enhance overall self-concept and life adjustment, therefore helping to reduce anxiety and depression and enhance positive moods.

## Improved Sleep

About one-third of all adults will experience insomnia sometime in their lives. Chronic insomnia increases mortality and psychiatric problems and decreases work productivity. People experiencing depression or anxiety commonly have disturbed sleep. Most people who have sleep disturbances don't seek medical treatment, but of those who do, about half will receive a prescription drug to aid sleep. This is often a drug from the benzodiazepine family (refer back to table 11.2), similar to the drugs used to treat anxiety. Many who don't seek treatment from a physician buy over-the-counter sleep aids. Because drugs often don't address the source of the sleep problem, are expensive, and can have negative side effects (see table 11.3), exercise is frequently included as a component of good sleep hygiene.

The small number of studies of the effects of regular physical activity on normal sleepers indicate small-to-moderate effects of increased slow-wave (deep) sleep and total sleep time, with decreases in the time needed to fall asleep, in wakefulness during sleep, and in REM (rapid eye movement) sleep. How exercise facilitates sleep is unknown; possible but unconfirmed explanations include body restitution, energy conservation, anxiety reduction, body warming, and increased production of melatonin and adenosine, body chemicals that help regulate sleep.

In 1997, several studies were published that examined whether regular exercise promotes sleep for people with sleep problems. Stanford University researchers found that elderly patients with insomnia reported improvements in self-rated sleep after a 16-week exercise program of moderate intensity consisting of 30 to 40 minutes of aerobic exercise four times a week (King et al. 1997). Tufts University researchers reported that a 10-week, three-days-a-week, resistance-training program improved self-ratings of sleep in depressed adults with sleep problems (Singh, Clements, and Fiatarone 1997).

## Biological Adaptations

Physical activity is unique among behavioral treatments for mental health. The increased metabolism of physical exertion produces several responses during exercise, as well as more long-lasting adaptations to an exercise program, which appear to improve mental health. Possible explanations for reduced depression or anxiety after exercise include increases in body warming, brain blood flow, and endorphins; regulation of pituitary-adrenal stress hormones; and changes in the autonomic nervous system, brain noradrenaline, and brain serotonin.

### Body Warming

Increases in body temperature in the range that occurs with moderate to intense exercise under normal environmental temperatures have been associated with reduced muscle tension. The speculation that reduced anxiety after exercise is dependent on increased body temperature is

| Table 11.3 Common Sleep-Aiding Drugs and Side Effects | |
|---|---|
| Sleep aid | Side effects |
| **Benzodiazepines** | |
| Ativan (lorazepam)* | Toxicity with |
| Dalmane (flurazepam) | barbiturates; |
| Dormalin (quazepam) | dependency may |
| Halcion (triazolam) | develop |
| Restoril (temazepam) | |
| **Barbiturates** | |
| Amytal (amobarbital) | Toxicity; |
| Nembutal (pentobarbital) | dependency may |
| Seconal (secobarbital) | develop |

*The generic name of each drug appears in parentheses.

biologically plausible, but the handful of studies testing the idea have not supported it. Changes in anxiety after acute exercise have not corresponded with manipulations of body temperature before or during exercise. However, the studies that simulated natural exercise did a poor job controlling temperature or used inadequate nonexercise control conditions. A study that effectively controlled temperature during exercise did so in an unnatural exercise setting: subjects cycled in shoulder-deep water. It remains plausible that increased temperature during typical exercise contributes to reduced anxiety, but body warming probably isn't the sole or direct cause of the reduced anxiety or improved mood.

### Brain Blood Flow

The speculation that increased brain blood flow during an exercise session can cause changes in mood also is plausible but unverified. Studies using estimates of blood flow in both humans and animals show that blood flow to the brain is increased during acute exercise, but researchers haven't examined whether the increased flow occurs in the areas of the brain that are important in generating emotional responses and moods.

### Endorphins

Endorphins and enkephalins are proteins with analgesic properties that occur naturally in the brain, spinal cord, adrenal gland, gut, and sympathetic nerves. They help modulate body temperature and the cardiovascular system during stress; they can elevate mood and reduce pain, with effects similar to those of the powerful drug morphine. The speculation that endorphins influence mood or anxiety following exercise may be true, but it has been perpetuated as fact by the popular media without a scientific basis. One type of endorphin, β-endorphin, has opiate-like effects; but its appearance in the blood during vigorous exercise comes from the pituitary gland, not the parts of the brain involved with the experience of emotions or moods. The influence of β-endorphins on mood is not established. In

nearly all studies, drugs that block the binding of endorphins or opiates within brain cells did not prevent mood changes after exercise. Further, β-endorphin is naturally blocked from entering the brain from the bloodstream. Though studies with rats and mice show increased levels of endorphins after acute exercise, the importance of this for behavior, emotion, and physiology is unknown.

So, while runners (and others exercising aerobically and performing resistance exercises) may indeed experience positive moods after exercise, it's not just because of endorphins. Other explanations range from mental states such as feelings of accomplishment to other brain chemicals, such as noradrenaline, serotonin, dopamine, and GABA, that affect mood.

### HEALTHCHECK

#### Is "runner's high" fact or fiction?

The release by exercise of endorphins—proteins that occur naturally in the brain—is commonly understood to produce "runner's high," a euphoric feeling that results for some people after moderate to intense exercise. However, there's no good research that supports this theory. Though endorphins play a role in feelings of euphoria and analgesia (i.e., pain reduction), the endorphins that have been measured in humans after exercise come from the pituitary gland, not the parts of the brain involved with mood—so it is unlikely that they are important for mood after exercise. Also, the biochemical basis of mood after exercise is more complex than can be explained by a single chemical system.

### Autonomic Nervous System

Many people experiencing depression or anxiety have an imbalance between the sympathetic and parasympathetic branches of the autonomic nervous system. The sympathetic nervous system (SNS) stimulates energy expenditure, while the parasympathetic nervous system (PNS) helps store and conserve energy. The two systems work together to maintain a balance of the body's energy resources both at rest and during stress. Normally, for example, heart rate and blood pressure are restrained by the vagus nerve of the PNS. Under mild emotional or exercise stress, the vagal restraint is withdrawn and heart rate and blood pressure increase. As stress becomes greater, the sympathetic nerves increase their activity to elevate heart rate and blood pressure even more. Sympathetic nerves stem from the portions of the spinal cord in the areas of the trunk and stimulate organs such as the heart, adrenal glands, and arteries (see figure 11.2). Under physical or emotional stress the sympathetic nerves stimulate the heart to beat faster and more forcefully, the adrenal glands to secrete adrenaline and noradrenaline, and the arteries supplying the heart and skeletal muscles to dilate so that blood flow increases. During physical or emotional stress, systolic blood pressure rises to help drive blood to the muscles; the nervous, cardiovascular, and endocrine systems are preparing for a threatening situation—the "fight-or-flight" response to danger. When people are constantly under emotional stress but not responding physically by "fighting or fleeing," brain, heart, and vessel tissues are damaged. This can contribute to diseases such as coronary heart disease and to suppression of the body's immune system.

*Noradrenaline* is the main nerve chemical of the SNS. It modulates behavior during threat, as well as hormonal release, cardiovascular function, sleep, and responses to pain. About half of the cells that manufacture noradrenaline in the brain are located in a small area of the upper brain stem called the *locus coeruleus*. These cells send nerve fibers to other parts of the brain involved with stress and emotion—the limbic system—and to the spinal cord. Noradrenaline is also manufactured in bundles of nerves, or *ganglia,* located next to the spinal cord, and in the center of the adrenal glands located above the kidneys. As happens during many other types of stress, during exercise noradrenaline is secreted into the blood from the sympathetic nerves that

go to the heart and skeletal muscles. During heavy exercise the adrenal glands can also secrete noradrenaline and its related hormone, adrenaline. The increased heart rate during exercise results from stimulation of the heart muscle by SNS nerves and by the action of blood levels of noradrenaline and adrenaline.

These responses by the SNS adapt to regular exercise. Vigorous exercise training increases the capacity of the SNS to respond to maximal exercise but lowers the SNS response to a constant submaximal exercise. For example, people who through training improve their best mile time from 8 minutes to 7 minutes have lower levels of noradrenaline in the blood than they had before training. Exercise training increases the capacity of the sympathetic nerves to respond to maximal exercise while lessening the SNS response to submaximal exercise.

Though this is yet another example of how increasing one's level of fitness decreases the strain of typical physical activity, the more intriguing question for this chapter is whether this adaptation to exercise also extends to mental stress. Indeed, studies show that people with high fitness maintain lower heart rates during mental stress. Levels of noradrenaline or adrenaline in the blood do not explain the lower heart rate. People with high fitness have the same levels of these chemicals during mental stress as do people with low fitness. This is important for health because people with lower heart rates tend to have lower risk for developing cardiovascular disease.

Rather, heart rate during most types of mental stress depends more on excitement of the heart by SNS nerves than by adrenal hormones. This is illustrated by responses to stress by heart-transplant patients who have no SNS nerves to the heart muscle and must rely on adrenal hormones to increase heart rate during stress. During exercise, heart-transplant patients can increase heart rate to nearly the same level as people with a complete nerve supply to the heart by the action of adrenal hormones on the heart. However, they do not have increased heart rate during most

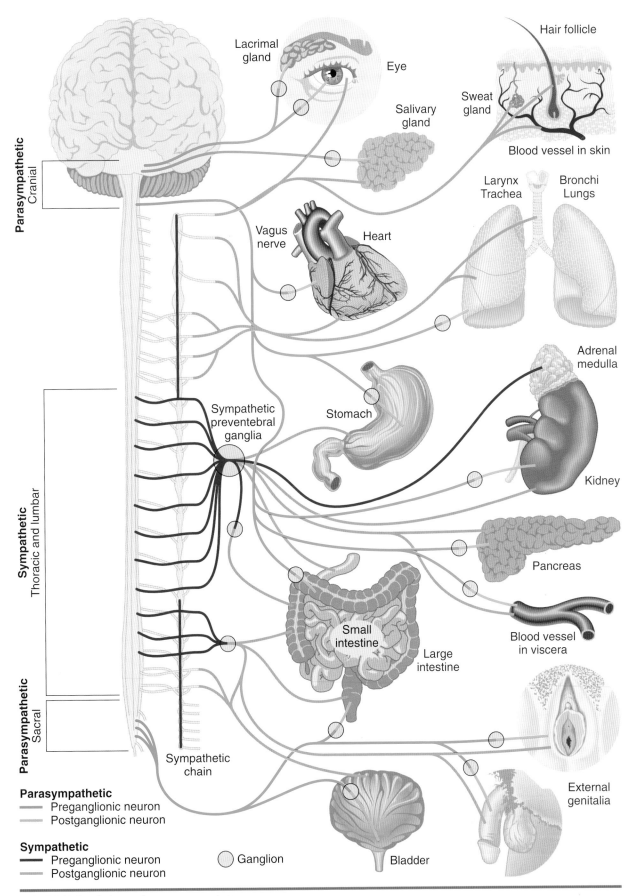

**FIGURE 11.2** Autonomic nervous system.

From Neil R. Carlson, *Physiology of Behavior*, 6th edition, Copyright ©1998 by Allyn & Bacon. Adapted by permission.

kinds of mental stress, which elevates heart rate by 10 to 30 beats per minute in people with normal hearts.

There is no evidence that people with higher levels of fitness perceive stressful events differently than people with lower levels of fitness. People with high fitness probably have lower heart rates during stress because they have less sympathetic nerve activity on the heart or because they have what is known as increased *cardiac vagal tone*. The vagus nerve slows the heart's frequency and force of beating and relaxes or dilates arteries that supply blood to skeletal muscle. So, a person who has increased vagal tone after exercise training can better offset the effects of the sympathetic nerves on heart and blood vessels, and thus have lower heart rate and blood pressure at rest and during stress. Increased cardiac vagal tone helps reduce some of the prominent features of anxiety and depression and also decreases the risk for coronary heart disease and sudden death.

### Hypothalamic-Pituitary-Adrenal Cortex System

During stress, the brain stimulates energy production through the hypothalamic-pituitary-adrenal cortex system (see figure 11.3). The front half of the pituitary gland co-releases β-endorphin and a hormone called *adrenocorticotropin (ACTH),* which stimulates the outer part of the adrenal gland to secrete *cortisol.* Cortisol repairs tissues and maintains blood glucose levels during stress.

When the hypothalamic-pituitary-adrenal system is functioning properly, cortisol levels return to normal as the hypothalamus and part of the limbic system sense that enough cortisol has been released. In major depression and panic anxiety disorder, this feedback is abnormal—resulting in abnormally high ACTH and cortisol levels. When cortisol levels are elevated too frequently or remain high, tissues become damaged and the immune system is suppressed.

Highly fit people can secrete more ACTH and cortisol during maximal exercise than people who have low fitness levels, but ACTH and cortisol during submaximal exercise are lowered by exercise training. Thus, similar to the adaptation by the SNS, fit people have an increased capacity to respond to severe stress and possibly a dampened response to mild stress.

### Brain Noradrenaline and Serotonin

Noradrenaline and serotonin influence attention and vigilance, hormone release, cardiovascular function during stress, fatigue, and sleep. They play important roles in depression and anxiety by modulating the nerve activity of other brain cells in the cortex, limbic system, and hypothalamus. During an episode of depression, people have reduced blood flow and nerve activity in the left frontal lobe of the brain; people with an anxiety disorder often have exaggerated brain activity in the right frontal lobe.

A quick lesson in the structure and function of nerve cells will help you understand the roles of noradrenaline and serotonin in these responses. People with depression and anxiety often have impaired function of the nerve cells that manufacture noradrenaline and serotonin. Cells that manufacture noradrenaline (found in the locus coeruleus) and serotonin (found in a region of the brain stem called the *raphe nuclei*) send nerve fibers to other parts of the brain involved in stress and emotion—the limbic system—and to the spinal cord.

Like all cells, nerves have a body where the cell nucleus is located, containing DNA (deoxyribonucleic acid). The cell body also contains the machinery to translate the DNA into the chemicals that allow the nerve to transmit an impulse to another cell through an extension of the cell body called an *axon.* The region of near-contact between two nerve cells is called the synapse. When a nerve is excited electrically, the axon releases chemicals such as noradrenaline and serotonin that then bind with special receptors, much like a lock and key. Then, through a series of other chemical events, the second cell is either excited or inhibited depending on the type of chemical and the type of receptor.

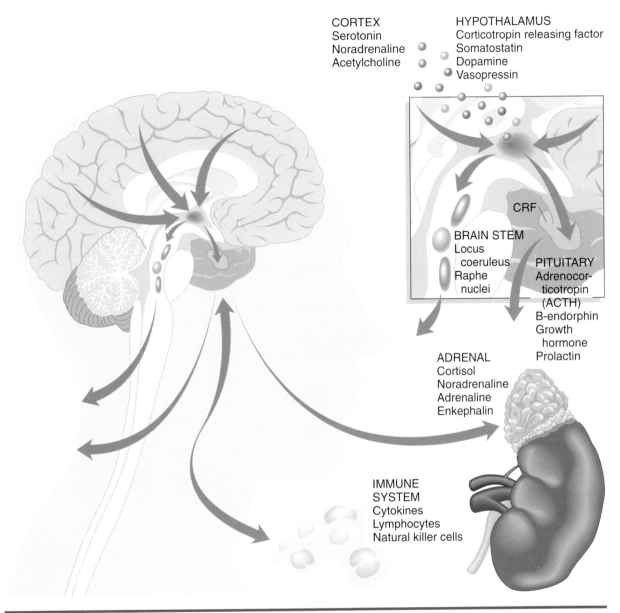

CORTEX
Serotonin
Noradrenaline
Acetylcholine

HYPOTHALAMUS
Corticotropin releasing factor
Somatostatin
Dopamine
Vasopressin

CRF

BRAIN STEM
Locus
coeruleus
Raphe
nuclei

PITUITARY
Adrenocor-
ticotropin
(ACTH)
B-endorphin
Growth
hormone
Prolactin

ADRENAL
Cortisol
Noradrenaline
Adrenaline
Enkephalin

IMMUNE
SYSTEM
Cytokines
Lymphocytes
Natural killer cells

**FIGURE 11.3** Responses of the hypothalamic-pituitary-adrenal cortex system and the sympatho-adrenal medullary system during stress.

Adapted from Black 1995.

Several popular antidepressant drugs such as Prozac block serotonin release or reuptake by the nerve after release. Other antidepressants and antianxiety drugs block the release or reuptake of noradrenaline. Two main effects of the drugs are to keep noradrenaline or serotonin in the synapse longer and to decrease the number or sensitivity of their receptors. As a consequence, drug therapy returns to normal the rate of synthesis and release of brain chemicals. Drugs also help to stabilize the electrical discharge of the nerve cells that receive and use noradrenaline and serotonin.

Though studies with humans have shown that exercise can be as effective as drug therapy in treating mild depression if people stay active for at least five months, researchers haven't tested whether noradrenaline or serotonin explains the benefits of exercise. This is so because a strong case hasn't yet been made that exercise reduces depression in ways similar to drugs and psychotherapy. However, studies with rats show that regular exercise has some effects on noradrenaline and serotonin cells that are similar to those seen after drug therapy. First, exercise training leads to higher levels of noradrenaline in the pons, limbic system, and cortex. Second, the release of noradrenaline during stress is reduced by chronic exercise. Third, the metabolism of serotonin during stress is lower after chronic physical activity. Fourth, the number of β-receptors for noradrenaline in the cortex is reduced by chronic exercise, just as it is by antidepressant drugs. As a mild stress, exercise stimulates the brain—apparently enhancing its ability to manufacture and conserve noradrenaline and serotonin during more severe stress.

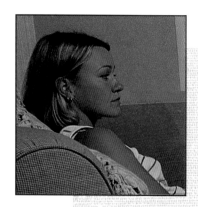

# Health Concepts

As you'll recall from the beginning of the chapter, Maria wondered if physical activity could help her recover from her depressed state. She noted that her moods were elevated when she had been regularly physically active. The good news is that regular exercise can both help prevent and treat depression. Numerous studies have shown that those who are more physically active have fewer symptoms of depression than those who are less active. And this isn't simply because those who are depressed are less likely to be active; recall the NHANES I follow-up study of the 1,500 men and women after eight years. Of the men who had been depressed at the outset of the study and who had been inactive, those who *became* active over the years showed a marked decrease in the symptoms of depression when compared with those who had remained inactive. So physical activity can have a significant positive effect on mental health.

## SUMMARY

▌ About one in five people will experience an episode of depression at some point in their lives; two of every three people who have depression are women. The annual rate of depression among teenagers and young adults is nearly twice that of adults 25 to 44 years old, and about four times the rate among people over age 65. Depression is more prevalent than coronary heart disease or heart attacks, and the occurrence of major depression in the United States has increased steadily during the past 50 years.

▌ Major symptoms of depression (that can be felt or noted nearly every day) include depressed mood; marked loss of interest in activities; significant weight loss or gain when not dieting; fatigue or loss of energy; feelings of worthlessness or inappropriate guilt; and recurrent thoughts of death or suicide.

■ Depression can be caused by physical illnesses such as thyroid disease, by catastrophic events, by loss of self-esteem, and by chronic anxiety and stress. Depression is associated with imbalances in *neurotransmitters,* which are chemicals that influence the activity of the brain cells that regulate mood, pleasure, and rational thought.

■ Physically inactive people report more symptoms of depression than physically active people. Physical activity can be used both to prevent depression and to treat it.

■ Anxiety disorders are a major mental health problem affecting about 23 million Americans (4% of women and 2% of men) each year.

■ There are several types of anxiety disorders. Symptoms include agitation, excessive alertness, confusion, muscle tension, tremors, high heart rates, palpitations, flushing, sweating, dry mouth, and urinary and gastrointestinal problems. As with depression, young people tend to have more anxiety than do older people.

■ Most people can reduce their risk of anxiety by expending about 50 to 80 extra calories per day—which usually occurs in about a 1-mile walk.

■ Stress results from real or imagined threats to a person's sense of control and from a disturbed physiological balance. It produces feelings of strain that are often accompanied by abnormal physiological changes in the skin, digestion, muscle tension, heart rate and rhythm, brain activity, and hormone levels. Chronic stress strains cells, organs, and body systems, and can increase the risk for diseases such as coronary heart disease and hypertension, as well as for suppression of the immune system.

■ Though exercise usually won't eliminate the source of stress, it can provide a temporary distraction from the problem. An exercise program might increase feelings of control or commitment; it can provide a sense of success in doing something important for yourself—which buffers the impact of stressful events.

■ Physical activity may reduce anxiety and depression through cognitive mechanisms such as temporary distraction from worries or symptoms. It may also produce more lasting changes in self-esteem, improved sleep, and several biological adaptations in the brain, the autonomic nervous system, and the endocrine system that help reduce anxiety and depression and improve the ability to cope with stress. The social interaction often gained through physical activity can also have a positive effect on mental health.

*As you've just learned, physical activity can have a positive effect on mental health. Next we're going to switch gears and consider physical activity's impact on aging. In the next chapter we'll look at how physical activity can enhance your quality of life as you age.*

## KEY TERMS

anxiety disorders

adrenocorticotropin (ACTH)

benzodiazepines

cortisol

depression

hypothalamus

limbic system

locus coeruleus

neurotransmitters

noradrenaline

raphe nuclei

self-esteem

serotonin

state anxiety

trait anxiety

# 11

# Gauging Your Levels of Stress and Depression

## THE PURPOSES OF THIS LAB EXPERIENCE ARE TO

▮ gauge your tension level,

▮ assess your level of perceived stress, and

▮ assess your level of depression.

## Gauge Your Tension Level

**Indicate whether each statement below describes you by marking "yes" or "no."**

Are you often troubled by feelings of tenseness, tightness, restlessness, or inability to relax?                                                                Yes _____ No _____

Are you often bothered by nervousness or shaking?                               Yes _____ No _____

Do you often have trouble sleeping or falling asleep?                           Yes _____ No _____

Do you feel under a great deal of tension?                                      Yes _____ No _____

Do you have trouble relaxing?                                                   Yes _____ No _____

Do you often have periods of restlessness so that you cannot sit for long?    Yes _____ No _____

Have you often felt that difficulties were becoming too much for you to handle?                                                                           Yes _____ No _____

Tally the number of "yes" answers. A score of 2 is common among men; 3 is common among women. A score of 5 or more for men indicates that risk for developing high blood pressure is increased twofold. Tension measured by this scale is not related to developing high blood pressure in women. (Adapted from Haynes et al. 1978.)

Name_____Section_____Date_____

## Assess Your Level of Perceived Stress

The questions in the following scale (adapted from Cohen et al. 1983) ask you about your feelings and thoughts during the last week. In each case you'll be asked to circle the number that corresponds best to *how often* you felt or thought a certain way. Although some of the questions are similar, there are differences between them and you should treat each one as a separate question. The best approach is to answer each question fairly quickly. That is, don't try to count the number of times you felt a particular way. Rather, indicate the answer that seems a reasonable estimate.

| In the last week: | Never | Almost never | Sometimes | Fairly often | Very often |
|---|---|---|---|---|---|
| 1. How often have you been upset because of something that happened unexpectedly? | 0 | 1 | 2 | 3 | 4 |
| 2. How often have you felt that you were unable to control the important things in your life? | 0 | 1 | 2 | 3 | 4 |
| 3. How often have you felt nervous and "stressed?" | 0 | 1 | 2 | 3 | 4 |
| 4. How often have you dealt successfully with irritating life hassles? | 4 | 3 | 2 | 1 | 0 |
| 5. How often have you felt that you were effectively coping with important changes occurring in your life? | 4 | 3 | 2 | 1 | 0 |
| 6. How often have you felt confident about your ability to handle your personal problems? | 4 | 3 | 2 | 1 | 0 |
| 7. How often have you felt that things were going your way? | 4 | 3 | 2 | 1 | 0 |
| 8. How often have you found that you could not cope with all the things you had to do? | 0 | 1 | 2 | 3 | 4 |
| 9. How often have you been able to control irritations in your life? | 4 | 3 | 2 | 1 | 0 |
| 10. How often have you felt that you were on top of things? | 4 | 3 | 2 | 1 | 0 |
| 11. How often have you been angered because of things that happened that were outside of your control? | 0 | 1 | 2 | 3 | 4 |
| 12. How often have you found yourself thinking about things you have to accomplish? | 0 | 1 | 2 | 3 | 4 |
| 13. How often have you been able to control the way you spend your time? | 4 | 3 | 2 | 1 | 0 |
| 14. How often have you felt that difficulties were piling up so high you could not overcome them? | 0 | 1 | 2 | 3 | 4 |

Tally the total sum of the numbers you circled in the survey. The lowest possible score is 0, and the highest is 56. A score of 30 or less is common for college students; if your score is higher, you may be experiencing an excessive amount of stress.

Name_____Section_____Date_____

## Assess Your Level of Depression

Indicate how often you have felt this way *during the past week.* Circle the number that best corresponds with your choice for each response.

| | Most of the time (5-7 days) | Occasionally (3-4 days) | Some of the time (1-2 days) | Rarely or never (less than 1 day) |
|---|---|---|---|---|
| 1. I was bothered by things that don't usually bother me. | 3 | 2 | 1 | 0 |
| 2. I didn't feel like eating; my appetite was poor. | 3 | 2 | 1 | 0 |
| 3. I felt that I could not shake off the blues even with help from my family or friends. | 3 | 2 | 1 | 0 |
| 4. I felt that I was just as good as other people. | 0 | 1 | 2 | 3 |
| 5. I had trouble keeping my mind on what I was doing. | 3 | 2 | 1 | 0 |
| 6. I felt depressed. | 3 | 2 | 1 | 0 |
| 7. I felt that everything I did was an effort. | 3 | 2 | 1 | 0 |
| 8. I felt hopeful about the future. | 0 | 1 | 2 | 3 |
| 9. I thought my life had been a failure. | 3 | 2 | 1 | 0 |
| 10. I felt fearful. | 3 | 2 | 1 | 0 |
| 11. My sleep was restless. | 3 | 2 | 1 | 0 |
| 12. I was happy. | 0 | 1 | 2 | 3 |
| 13. I talked less than usual. | 3 | 2 | 1 | 0 |
| 14. I felt lonely. | 3 | 2 | 1 | 0 |
| 15. People were unfriendly. | 3 | 2 | 1 | 0 |
| 16. I enjoyed life. | 0 | 1 | 2 | 3 |
| 17. I had crying spells. | 3 | 2 | 1 | 0 |
| 18. I felt sad. | 3 | 2 | 1 | 0 |
| 19. I felt that people disliked me. | 3 | 2 | 1 | 0 |
| 20. I could not get going. | 3 | 2 | 1 | 0 |

Tally the total sum of the numbers you circled in the survey. The lowest possible score is 0, and the highest is 60. A score of less than 16 is common for college students. A score higher than 16 suggests a risk for depression; see a psychologist or physician for a clinical interview that will determine if you are suffering from depression. (Only the questions in this lab experience were taken from the CES-D scale, National Institute for Mental Health [NIMH]. The scoring system that NIMH developed for use with the full CES-D scale does not apply to this scale in this publication.)

# Lifetime Physical Activity, Health, and Fitness

Part IV addresses perhaps the most important question for you: What do you do once you finish this course, in terms of your health and lifestyle? It's been said that the two certainties of life are death and taxes. Add two more certainties to that list: as long as you're alive, you'll grow older and your life circumstances will change. Part IV helps you adjust to those changing circumstances and maintain a healthy lifestyle. In chapter 12, you'll learn about the effects of aging on your physical and mental health, as well as about the effects of exercise on aging. Chapter 13, our final chapter, explores the barriers that keep many people from being physically active over a lifetime, and it details how people can change their behavior to become more active. Part IV offers a good understanding of future health and fitness challenges that you'll face, along with sound plans for meeting those challenges and living a healthy, active life.

# Chapter 12

# Healthy Aging

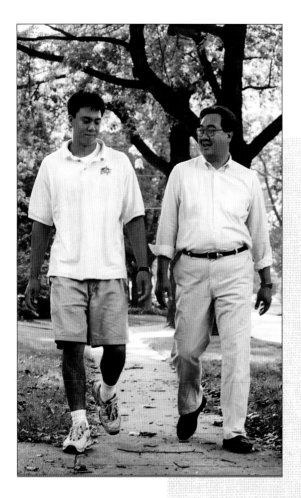

Today is my dad's 60th birthday. He joked around a lot about being old. He said when he was young he couldn't wait until he got old so he wouldn't have to take a nap—and now he'd love to be able to take an afternoon nap again. When he was a teenager he couldn't wait to drive; now he wishes someone would drive *him* through all the traffic. And when he got to college he couldn't wait to get out. Now he's going back, taking a course "just for the fun of it." (What a novel idea!)

But he also moaned and groaned about aches and pains that he didn't used to have. I know he's been more concerned about his health and quality of life. He's always been active, but he's not sure if he should slow down as he gets older. He's not sure if his body can take it any more. He wants to stay active, but he's not sure how much—or what—to do.

—Sean, 22-year-old senior

# What do you think?

It *is* common to get more aches and pains as you age. Does this mean you should gradually cut back on your physical activity as you grow older? Can exercise continue to improve your quality of life in your later years? Just what are the effects of exercise on aging?

In this chapter we'll examine the physical effects of aging and explore how older people respond to physical activity—how their cardiorespiratory endurance and muscular strength are affected. And we'll consider the implications of regular, lifelong physical activity for younger people—how such activity will affect their health and vitality as they grow older. In the lab at the end of the chapter you'll assess your knowledge of aging and analyze some of the health risks associated with the aging process.

## PHYSICAL ACTIVITY AND AGING

If you reach 65 years of age, you can expect to live between 15 and 20 years longer. An increasing number of people are living beyond the average life expectancy in America of 76 years (73 for males and 79 for females). This means that most people will live a significant number of years in old age. (We define *old* as 65 to 84, and *very old* as 85 and beyond.) The health or lack of health of older people has a direct impact on you right now as Americans debate the political, financial, and budgetary issues related to health care expenses for older adults. And it will certainly have a direct impact on you when you reach old age! The lifestyle behaviors you follow now and throughout your life will greatly affect your health and need for medical services during your later years. Physical activity and good nutrition bring you physical, mental, and financial rewards not only now but also in your future.

Americans are joining these older age groups in increasing numbers and at increasing rates.

**KEY POINT** The lifestyle behaviors you follow now and throughout your life will greatly affect your health and need for medical services during your later years.

The 3.1 million Americans who were 65 or over in 1900 represented 4.1% of the U.S. population (see figure 12.1). The 33.9 million Americans age 65 or over in 1996 represented 13% of the population. The statistics are even more dramatic for those 85 or older: their numbers are 31 times greater than they were in 1900. This growth in the older population won't stop. By the year 2030, it's projected that 69.4 million Americans will be 65 or older, representing 20% of our population.

Why are the numbers of older people increasing? As discussed in chapter 1, modern medi-

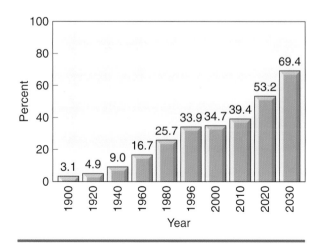

**FIGURE 12.1** Actual and projected numbers of Americans 65 years of age and older, in millions.

Data from U.S. Bureau of the Census 1997.

cine has prevented many early deaths due to infectious disease and has lowered the rate of infant mortality. But the life span after reaching 65 years is also increasing. The average length of life after 65 is 17.5 years (18.9 for females and 15.7 for males). Girls born in 1997 have an average life expectancy of 79 years; boys born the same year have an average life expectancy of 73 years.

This growing part of our population has created dramatic changes in our society from social, moral, economic, political, and health perspectives. As you'll learn in the next section, aging is an ongoing process that results in numerous psychological and physiological changes. The better you understand those changes, the better you can live and age so that you can still be vibrant and healthy in your later years.

## EFFECTS OF AGING

Aging is a process that begins from the moment you are conceived until the moment you die. While it is a natural process, you do have some control over it through the lifestyle you choose. In figure 12.2 you can see how *functional capacity*—the mental and physical ability to perform—changes over the typical lifetime. Note the peaks for both physically active people and

sedentary people from age 20 to 30. From there, a gradual decline begins; but note too that the peak of the physically active person is much higher than that of the sedentary person, and also that functional capacity for physically active people remains higher throughout their lifetime.

The changes that occur through aging include

- **Decreased sensations:** taste, smell, vision, hearing
- **Decreased mental ability:** memory, judgment, speech
- **Decreased organ function:** digestive system, urinary, liver, kidney
- **Decreased bone and muscle mass:** lean body weight, bone mineral content (osteoporosis)
- **Decreased physical fitness:** cardiorespiratory fitness, strength, flexibility, muscular endurance, reaction and movement times, balance

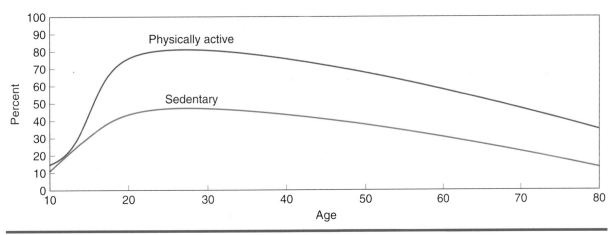

**FIGURE 12.2** Changes in the functional capacity of physically active and sedentary persons.

These mental, physical, and physiological declines lead to health problems for older people. Older adults have the highest rates of any age group of coronary heart disease, stroke, cancer, diabetes, osteoporosis, and arthritis.

According to the Administration on Aging, this loss of functional capacity and the high rates of chronic disease cause 28% of older persons (compared to 10% for all persons) to rate their health as fair or poor. In 1994, those 65 and older reported an average of 35 days of restricted activity with 14 of those days in bed due to illness or injury. One of the ways functional capacity is measured is through the assessment of *activities of daily living (ADL)*. Examples of ADLs are bathing, dressing, eating, transferring from bed or chair, walking, getting outside, and using the toilet. Over 50% of people between ages 65 and 84 report having difficulty with the necessary tasks of daily life. That percentage increases for those 85 or over.

These high rates of serious chronic diseases and inability to perform ADLs have led to a tremendous growth in the cost of the care of older persons. In 1995, older people were responsible for 38% of all hospital admissions and 48% of all days spent in hospitals, although they represented only about 13% of the population. *Medi-*

*care*, the federal health care program for older adults, cost $203.1 billion in 1996 and will cost an estimated $450 billion in 2005. The huge and increasing cost for health care services for older people is one of the main reasons for the health care crisis in the United States.

**KEY POINT**
Over 50% of people between ages 65 and 84 report having difficulty with the necessary tasks of daily life. That percentage increases for those 85 or over. While aging is a natural process, you do have some control over it through the lifestyle you choose.

---

### HEALTHCHECK

**Older people have the highest rates of hip fractures of any population group. Why?**

Their physiological and fitness declines provide the answer. Many older people suffer from osteoporosis; they also lose strength, flexibility, reaction time, movement time, and balance. These factors result in more falls—and more serious consequences because of the falls.

---

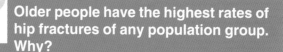

### Ten Tips for *Healthy Aging*

The Administration on Aging offers these 10 tips for improving your chances of living a long and healthy life:

- Eat a balanced diet.
- Exercise regularly.
- Get regular health checkups.
- Don't smoke; if you do, stop.
- Practice safety habits to prevent falls; wear a seat belt when in a car.
- Stay in contact with family and friends; stay active.
- Avoid overexposure to the sun and to cold temperatures.
- Use alcohol in moderation; never drink and drive.
- Begin and maintain a sound long-term financial plan.
- Keep a positive attitude and do things that make you happy.

## PHYSICAL RESPONSES TO REGULAR EXERCISE

Just as with younger people, older people need to be physically active to improve their health, functional capacity, and quality of life. But how do older people's bodies respond to physical activity? Do older people improve their cardiorespiratory endurance, body composition, muscular strength and endurance, and flexibility at the same rates that younger people do? Let's take a look at two of those components: cardiorespiratory endurance and muscular strength.

Hagberg et al. (1989) conducted a cardiorespiratory endurance training study with men and women ages 70 to 79. The participants trained for six months to improve their cardiorespiratory endurance. As you can see from figure 12.3, they improved their maximal oxygen consumption ($VO_2$max) by 22%—an improvement not often seen even in younger adults. This study demonstrates that older people respond positively to cardiorespiratory endurance training. Further research in this area has shown that the improved cardiorespiratory endurance is due to the same physiological changes observed in younger adults. Other studies have demonstrated that meaningful improvements in the cardiorespiratory endurance of older people can occur with lower exercise intensities than are recom-

mended for younger adults. This is significant, because the lower intensity also lowers the risk of musculoskeletal injuries in older people.

Fiatarone, O'Neill, and Ryan (1994) studied high-intensity strength training in more than 100 men and women whose average age was 87 years and who were described as frail nursing home residents. As figure 12.4 shows, the men and women made dramatic improvements in strength, gait (walking) speed, and stair-climbing power. (Walking speed and stair-climbing power are typically used as relevant measures of functional capacity in older people.) Strength training can produce dramatic increases in strength in frail older people. The improvements were much greater than those seen in younger adults who had not already lost much of their strength, and the training produced improvements in functional capacity as well. These men and women also gained 3% muscle mass in their thighs, which indicates that older people can improve their lean body mass through strength training. Several other studies have shown that older people can improve their strength and functional capacity through strength training. It's safe to say that fitness training in older people improves cardiorespiratory endurance, lean body mass, muscular endurance, strength, flexibility, balance, reaction time, and coordination—thus improving their quality of life.

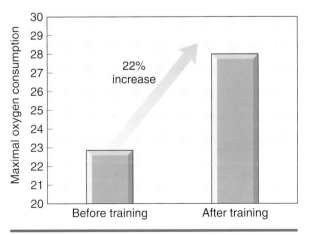

FIGURE 12.3 Improvements in cardiorespiratory endurance in older persons.

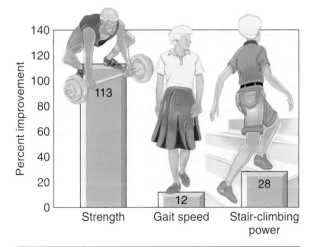

FIGURE 12.4 Effects of strength training in older frail persons.

## Ducking Quacks

Quacks—people who provide unproven products, remedies, or services—have bilked money out of people throughout history. Schemes and scams are as varied as the people who operate them. A small sampling of such scams includes investment and insurance "opportunities," balms and ointments to cure baldness and all sorts of medical diseases, "miracle" weight loss programs, and on and on.

Older people are prime targets for quacks, many of whom read the obituaries and then approach the surviving spouse at a most vulnerable time with a scheme that is truly too good to be true. But younger adults also fall prey to a variety of scams. And the health area is a prime one for quacks to operate in, for the simple reason that people value their appearance and their health and may be desperate enough or gullible enough to try "quick fixes." Typically all they end up with is less money in the bank and egg on their faces.

You can usually recognize quackery through the following:

▮ You're pressured to buy quickly.
▮ You're promised a quick or painless cure.
▮ You can obtain the necessary "special" or "secret" formulas only through the mail.
▮ The only evidence of value comes from "testimonials" or "case histories."
▮ The product claims to cure a wide variety of health problems.
▮ The product is a "new discovery" that is not backed by scientific knowledge.

Remember, if it's too good to be true—it probably *isn't* true. If you have questions about a product or service, contact the Better Business Bureau, the Federal Trade Commission, the U.S. Postal Service, or the Food and Drug Administration, depending on the type of product or service.

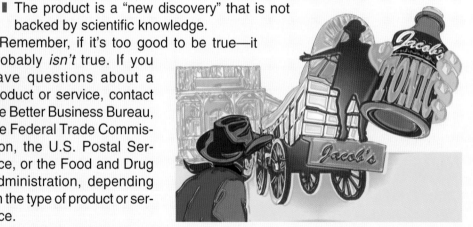

## IMPLICATIONS OF LIFELONG PHYSICAL ACTIVITY

The research on physical activity and older people is conclusive: exercise training that establishes an appropriate overload with suitable frequency, intensity, and duration will produce positive physiological and physical adaptations similar to those observed in younger people. These fitness changes lead to improvements in the quality of life of older people. But an appropriate question for most readers of this book is "What will a lifetime of physical activity do for *my* quality of life?"

Figure 12.5, which summarizes the relationship between cardiorespiratory endurance and the aging process for three groups of men, provides a partial glimpse into the future. Observe that age had its negative effects no matter the level of physical activity (highly trained runners, joggers, or sedentary, untrained men). All three groups declined in cardiorespiratory endurance as they aged. But the active groups achieved and maintained a higher level of cardiorespiratory endurance across the entire age range. Note that active men at age 60 had higher cardiorespiratory endurance than sedentary men 20 to 30 years old!

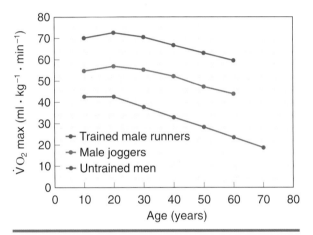

**FIGURE 12.5** Decline in $\dot{V}O_2$max in trained and untrained subjects.

Adapted from Wilmore and Costill 1994.

 Exercise training that establishes an appropriate overload with suitable frequency, intensity, and duration for older people will produce positive physiological and physical adaptations similar to ones observed in younger people.

People who are physically active throughout their lives have a better quality of life than those who are sedentary. Research by Breslow and Breslow (1993) has shown that you can increase your life span by nine years and lower your risk of disability by 50% by living a healthy lifestyle—one that includes

- no smoking,
- moderate alcohol use,
- daily breakfast,
- limited snacking,

- 7 to 8 hours of sleep per night,
- regular physical activity, and
- maintaining a healthy weight.

In addition, *Physical Activity and Health: A Report of the Surgeon General* (U.S. Department of Health and Human Services 1996) provides several key messages for older adults:

- Older adults, both men and women, can benefit from regular physical activity.
- Physical activity doesn't need to be strenuous in order for older adults to achieve health benefits.
- Older adults can obtain significant health benefits with a moderate amount of physical activity, preferably daily. A moderate amount of activity can be obtained in longer sessions of moderately intense activities (such as walking) or in shorter sessions of more vigorous activities (such as fast walking or stair walking).
- Older adults can gain additional health benefits through greater amounts of physical activity by increasing either the duration, intensity, or frequency. Because risk of injury increases at high levels of activity, people need to take care not to engage in excessive amounts of activity.
- Previously sedentary older adults who begin physical activity programs should start with short intervals of moderate physical activity (5 to 10 minutes) and gradually build up.
- Older adults should consult with their medical caregiver before beginning a new physical activity program.
- In addition to aerobic activity, older adults can benefit from muscle-strengthening activities. Stronger muscles help reduce the risk of falling and improve the ability to perform the routine tasks of daily life.

Finally, the American College of Sports Medicine (ACSM) released a position statement regarding exercise and physical activity for older adults in 1998. This position stand recommends that older adults perform regular exercise to improve their cardiorespiratory endurance, strength, postural stability, and flexibility. The ACSM also indicated that older adults generally respond to increased activity levels and receive important health and fitness benefits similarly to younger adults. In addition, older adults gain improved mental and psychological functioning with increased physical activity, and regular supervised physical activity can enhance the function and quality of life for the very old and frail. Physical activity programs might need to be adjusted for the age and fitness level of older persons, but the bottom line is that consistent levels of moderate activity can be valuable to older adults. Convinced yet?

It's very clear that we are growing older as a population, and our life span is increasing. But what about the *quality* of life and freedom from disease while we are enjoying these longer lives? As you can see in the health continuum shown in figure 12.6, we progress from birth as a healthy (usually!) baby toward physical death—no one can escape this fact. A healthy lifestyle will decrease your risk for an early death and increase your chances for a longer life. We also move through temporary periods of health and illness throughout our lives—a healthy lifestyle will allow you to spend a much longer portion of your life on the healthy end of the continuum. On the other hand, an unhealthy lifestyle increases your risk of spending much of your lifetime, especially in older age, on the illness side of the continuum. Remember the old saying, "If you don't have health, you don't have anything!"

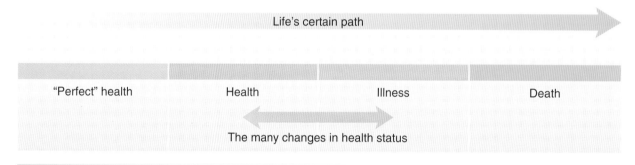

**FIGURE 12.6**  Health continuum.

## OF INTEREST

### POINT

### The Health Care Crisis: The Financial Problems of Medicare

Medicare has been very successful in aiding older persons with their medical expenses. For instance, Medicare might cover 85% of the costs of a coronary bypass surgery that costs about $100,000. But medical costs of the program have grown faster than funds to cover the costs. In 1995, the trust fund created to pay hospital costs showed a yearly deficit for the first time, and it will be completely without funds early in the twenty-first century. The problem is growing in part because of the increase in the number of older persons and their increasing life spans. The Board of Trustees of the Social Security System has declared Medicare's hospital funding system financially unsound and in need of major changes; as this book was being written, the federal government was locked in a political struggle to save the future of Medicare—and of those people who depend on it.

The best individual response to this crisis is to keep in good health as you age and keep your demand for health care services to a minimum. Indeed, if the *majority* of Americans—instead of the minority—would follow healthy lifestyles, the health care crisis might be averted.

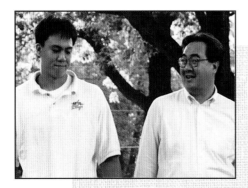

# Health Concepts

As you'll remember, Sean's father, who had just turned 60, was concerned about his health and quality of life—and wondered if he should decrease his physical activity as he got older. All the evidence points to what's also true for younger adults: physical activity can improve cardio-respiratory endurance, lean body mass, muscular endurance, strength, flexibility, balance, reaction time, and coordination—thus improving health and quality of life—regardless of age.

## SUMMARY

▌ The lifestyle behaviors you follow now and throughout your life will greatly affect your health and need for medical services during your later years.

▌ Functional capacity—the mental and physical ability to perform—changes over the typical lifetime. Peaks for both physically active people and sedentary people occur from ages 20 to 30. From there a gradual decline begins.

▌ The changes that occur through aging include decreased sensations, decreased mental ability, decreased organ function, decreased bone and muscle mass, and decreased physical fitness (cardiorespiratory fitness, strength, flexibility, muscular endurance, reaction and movement times, and balance).

▌ Over 50% of people between ages 65 and 84 report having difficulty with the necessary tasks of daily life. That percentage increases for those 85 or over.

▌ Older people respond positively to cardiorespiratory endurance training. They experience the same physiological changes observed in younger adults.

▌ Strength training can produce dramatic increases in strength in frail older people.

*Physical activity can have positive effects on older people who want to maintain a good quality of life. It obviously can also have a good impact on you—no matter what your circumstances are! In the next chapter we'll look at how you can put a physical activity plan together—so you can make sure you experience all these benefits we've been talking about.*

## KEY TERMS

activities of daily living (ADL)    Medicare

functional capacity    old

healthy aging    very old

# 12

# Assessing Your Knowledge of Aging and Analyzing Health Risks

## THE PURPOSES OF THIS LAB EXPERIENCE ARE TO

▮ assess your knowledge of issues related to aging and

▮ analyze various health risks.

## Assess Your IQ on Aging

The following assessment is from the National Institute on Aging.

| | True | False |
|---|---|---|
| 1. Baby boomers are the fastest growing segment of the population. | ❑ | ❑ |
| 2. Families don't bother with their older relatives. | ❑ | ❑ |
| 3. Everyone becomes confused or forgetful if they live long enough. | ❑ | ❑ |
| 4. You can be too old to exercise. | ❑ | ❑ |
| 5. Heart disease is a much bigger problem for older men than for older women. | ❑ | ❑ |
| 6. The older you get, the less you sleep. | ❑ | ❑ |
| 7. People should watch their weight as they age. | ❑ | ❑ |
| 8. Most older people are depressed. Why shouldn't they be? | ❑ | ❑ |
| 9. There's no point in screening older people for cancer because they can't be treated. | ❑ | ❑ |
| 10. Older people take more medications than younger people. | ❑ | ❑ |
| 11. People begin to lose interest in sex around age 55. | ❑ | ❑ |
| 12. If your parents had Alzheimer's disease, you will inevitably get it. | ❑ | ❑ |
| 13. Diet and exercise reduce the risk for osteoporosis. | ❑ | ❑ |
| 14. As your body changes with age, so does your personality. | ❑ | ❑ |
| 15. Older people might as well accept urinary accidents as a fact of life. | ❑ | ❑ |
| 16. Suicide is a problem mainly for teenagers. | ❑ | ❑ |
| 17. Falls and injuries "just happen" to older people. | ❑ | ❑ |
| 18. Everybody gets cataracts. | ❑ | ❑ |
| 19. Extremes of heat and cold can be especially dangerous for older people. | ❑ | ❑ |
| 20. "You can't teach an old dog new tricks." | ❑ | ❑ |

## Answers:

1. **False.** The population age 85 and older is the fastest growing age group in the United States.

2. **False.** About 4 in 5 older men and 3 in 5 older women live in family settings. Only 1 in 20 live in nursing homes.

3. **False.** Alzheimer's disease and a myriad of other diseases can cause confusion and serious forgetfulness, but these diseases and conditions are limited to older people.

4. **False.** Exercise at any age can help strengthen the heart, lungs, and muscles and lower blood pressure.

5. **False.** By age 65, both men and women have a one in three chance of showing symptoms of heart disease.

6. **False.** *Quality* of sleep declines, but total sleep time doesn't.

7. **True.** Most people gain weight as they age.

8. **False.** Most older people are not depressed.

9. **False.** Many older people can beat cancer, especially if it's detected early.

10. **True.** Older people often have a combination of conditions that require drugs. They consume 25% of all medications.

11. **False.** Most older people can lead an active, satisfying sex life.

12. **False.** The overwhelming number of people with Alzheimer's disease have not inherited the disorder.

13. **True.** Women are at a particular risk for osteoporosis. People can prevent bone loss by eating calcium-rich foods and exercising regularly.

14. **False.** Except for change that results from disease such as Alzheimer's, personality is one of the few constants of life.

15. **False.** Urinary incontinence is a symptom, not a disease. A variety of treatment options are available.

16. **False.** Suicide is most prevalent among those 65 and older.

17. **False.** Many such injuries can be avoided through practicing good safety habits and having regular vision and hearing tests.

18. **False.** Cataracts are more common among older people, but not everyone gets them. About 18% of people between the ages of 65 and 74 have cataracts; about 40% between the ages of 75 and 85 have them.

19. **True.** The body's thermostat tends to function less efficiently with age; older people are less able to adapt to heat or cold.

20. **False.** People at any age can learn new information and skills.

## Health Risk Analysis

The following survey (reprinted from Sharkey 1997) will help you analyze health risks in these areas: coronary heart disease, health habits, medical factors, safety factors, personal factors, psychological factors, and a category for women only. Tabulate your scores to discover what your risks are in each area—and then consider how you may be able to add years to your life by changing behaviors and lifestyle.

**12**

| I  Coronary Heart Disease (CHD) Risk Factors | | | | | |
|---|---|---|---|---|---|
| **Cholesterol, total cholesterol/high density lipoprotein ratio** | | | | | |
| Under 160 | 160-200 | 200-220 | 220-240 | Over 240 | |
| < 3 | 3-4 | 4-5 | 5-6 | > 6 | |
| +2 | +1 | −1 | −2 | −4 | _____ |
| **Blood pressure (systolic/diastolic)** | | | | | |
| 110 | 110-130 | 130-150 | 150-170 | 170 | |
| 60-80 | 60-80 | 80-90 | 90-100 | > 100 | |
| +1 | 0 | −1 | −2 | −4 | _____ |
| **Smoking** | | | | | |
| never | quit | smoke cigar or pipe or close family member smokes | 1 pack cigarettes daily | 2 or more packs daily | |
| +1 | 0 | −1 | −3 | −5 | _____ |
| **Heredity** | | | | | |
| no family history of CHD | 1 close relative over 60 with CHD | 2 close relatives over 60 with CHD | 1 close relative under 60 with CHD | 2 or more close relatives under 60 with CHD | |
| +2 | 0 | −1 | −2 | −4 | _____ |
| **Body weight (or fat)** | | | | | |
| 5 lb below desirable weight (< 10% fat—M; < 16% fat—F) | 5 lb below to 4 lb above desirable weight (10-15% fat—M; 16-22% fat—F) | 5-20 lb overweight (15-20% fat—M; 22-30% fat—F) | 20-35 lb overweight (20-25% fat—M; 30-35% fat—F) | 35 lb overweight (> 25% fat—M; > 35% fat—F) | |
| +2 | +1 | 0 | −2 | −3 | _____ |
| **Sex** | | | | | |
| female under 45 years | female over 45 years | male | stocky male | bald, stocky male | |
| 0 | −1 | −1 | −2 | −4 | _____ |
| **Stress** | | | | | |
| phlegmatic, unhurried, generally happy | ambitious but generally relaxed | sometimes hard-driving, time-competitive | hard-driving, time-conscious, competitive (Type A) | Type A with repressed hostility | |
| +1 | 0 | 0 | −1 | −3 | _____ |

Physical activity

| high-intensity, over 30 minutes daily | intermittent, 20-30 minutes 3-5 times/week | moderate, 10-20 minutes 3-5 times/week | light, 10-20 minutes 1-2 times/week | little or none | |
|---|---|---|---|---|---|
| +2 | +2 | +1 | 0 | −2 | _____ |

**Total:   I CHD Risk Factors** _____

## II   Health Habits (associated with good health and longevity)

Breakfast

| daily | sometimes | none | coffee | coffee and doughnut | |
|---|---|---|---|---|---|
| +1 | 0 | −1 | −2 | −3 | _____ |

Regular meals

| 3 or more | 2 daily | not regular | fad diets | starve and stuff | |
|---|---|---|---|---|---|
| +1 | 0 | −1 | −2 | −3 | _____ |

Sleep

| 7-8 hours | 8-9 hours | 6-7 hours | 9 hours | 6 hours | |
|---|---|---|---|---|---|
| +1 | 0 | 0 | −1 | −2 | _____ |

Alcohol

| none | women 3/week | men 1-2 daily | 2-6 daily | 6 daily | |
|---|---|---|---|---|---|
| +1 | +1 | +1 | −2 | −4 | _____ |

**Total:   II Health Habits** _____

## III   Medical Factors

Medical exam and screening tests (blood pressure, diabetes, glaucoma)

| regular tests, see doctor when necessary | periodic medical exam and selected tests | periodic medical exam | sometimes get tests | no tests or medical exams | |
|---|---|---|---|---|---|
| +1 | +1 | 0 | 0 | −1 | _____ |

Heart

| no history of problems self or family | some history | rheumatic fever as child, no murmur now | rheumatic fever as child, have murmur | have ECG abnormality and/or angina pectoris | |
|---|---|---|---|---|---|
| +1 | 0 | −1 | −2 | −3 | _____ |

## III Medical Factors *(continued)*

Lung (including pneumonia and tuberculosis)

| no problem | some past problem | mild asthma or bronchitis | emphysema, severe asthma, or bronchitis | severe lung problems | |
|---|---|---|---|---|---|
| +1 | 0 | −1 | −2 | −3 | _____ |

Digestive tract

| no problem | occasional diarrhea, loss of appetite | frequent diarrhea or stomach upset | ulcers, colitis, gall bladder, or liver problems | severe gastrointestinal disorders | |
|---|---|---|---|---|---|
| +1 | 0 | −1 | −2 | −3 | _____ |

Diabetes

| no problem or family history | controlled hypoglycemia (low blood sugar) | hypoglycemia and family history | mild diabetes (diet and exercise) | diabetes (insulin) | |
|---|---|---|---|---|---|
| +1 | 0 | −1 | −2 | −3 | _____ |

Drugs

| seldom take | minimal but regular use of aspirin or other drugs | heavy use of aspirin or other drugs | regular use of amphetamines, barbiturates, or psychogenic drugs | heavy use of amphetamines, barbiturates, or psychogenic drugs | |
|---|---|---|---|---|---|
| +1 | 0 | −1 | −2 | −3 | _____ |

**Total: III Medical Factors** _____

## IV Safety Factors

Driving in car

| 4,000 miles/ year, mostly local | 4,000-6,000 miles/ year, local and some highway | 6,000-8,000 miles/ year, local and highway | 8,000-10,000 miles/ year, highway and some local | 10,000 miles/ year, mostly highway | |
|---|---|---|---|---|---|
| +1 | 0 | 0 | −1 | −2 | _____ |

Using seat belts

| always | most of time (75%) | on highway only | seldom (25%) | never | |
|---|---|---|---|---|---|
| +1 | 0 | −1 | −2 | −3 | _____ |

Risk-taking behavior
*(motorcycle, skydive, mountain climb, fly small plane, etc.)*

| some with careful preparation | never | occasional | often | try anything for thrills | |
|---|---|---|---|---|---|
| +1 | 0 | −1 | −1 | −2 | _____ |

**Total: IV Safety Factors** _____

## V   Personal Factors

### Diet

| low-fat, high complex carbohydrates | balanced, moderate fat | balanced, typical fat | fad diets | starve and stuff | |
|---|---|---|---|---|---|
| +2 | +1 | 0 | −1 | −2 | _____ |

### Longevity

| grandparents lived past 90, parents past 80 | grandparents lived past 80, parents past 70 | grandparents lived past 70, parents past 60 | few relatives lived past 60 | few relatives lived past 50 | |
|---|---|---|---|---|---|
| +2 | +1 | 0 | −1 | −3 | _____ |

### Love and marriage

| happily married | married | unmarried | divorced | extramarital relationship | |
|---|---|---|---|---|---|
| +2 | +1 | 0 | −1 | −3 | _____ |

### Education

| postgraduate or master craftsman | college graduate or skilled craftsman | some college or trade school | high school graduate | grade school graduate | |
|---|---|---|---|---|---|
| +1 | +1 | 0 | −1 | −2 | _____ |

### Job satisfaction

| enjoy job, see results, room for advancement | enjoy job, see some results, able to advance | job OK, no results, nowhere to go | dislike job | hate job | |
|---|---|---|---|---|---|
| +1 | +1 | 0 | −1 | −2 | _____ |

### Social

| have some close friends | have some friends | have no good friends | stuck with people I don't enjoy | have no friends at all | |
|---|---|---|---|---|---|
| +1 | 0 | −1 | −2 | −3 | _____ |

### Race

| white or Asian | black or Hispanic | American Indian | | | |
|---|---|---|---|---|---|
| 0 | −1 | −2 | | | _____ |

**Total:   V Personal Factors** _____

## VI   Psychological Factors

### Outlook

| feel good about present and future | satisfied | unsure about present or future | unhappy in present, don't look forward to future | miserable, rather not get out of bed | |
|---|---|---|---|---|---|
| +1 | 0 | −1 | −2 | −3 | _____ |

## VI   Psychological Factors *(continued)*

**Depression**

| no family history of depression | some family history—I feel OK | family history and I am mildly depressed | sometimes feel life isn't worth living | thoughts of suicide | |
|---|---|---|---|---|---|
| +1 | 0 | −1 | −2 | −3 | _____ |

**Anxiety**

| seldom anxious | occasionally anxious | often anxious | always anxious | panic attacks | |
|---|---|---|---|---|---|
| +1 | 0 | −1 | −2 | −3 | _____ |

**Relaxation**

| relax or meditate daily | relax often | seldom relax | usually tense | always tense | |
|---|---|---|---|---|---|
| +1 | 0 | −1 | −2 | −3 | _____ |

**Total:   VI Psychological Factors** _____

## VII   For Women Only

**Health care**

| regular breast and Pap exam | occasional breast and Pap exam | never have exam | treated disorder | untreated cancer | |
|---|---|---|---|---|---|
| +1 | 0 | −1 | −2 | −4 | _____ |

**Birth control pill**

| never used | quit 5 years ago | still use, under 30 years of age | use pill and smoke | use pill, smoke, over 35 | |
|---|---|---|---|---|---|
| +1 | 0 | 0 | −2 | −3 | _____ |

**Total:   VII For Women Only** _____

| Category | Score (+/− years) | | Life expectancy | |
|---|---|---|---|---|
| | | | *Nearest age* | *Expectancy* |
| I.   CHD risk factors | _____ | | | |
| II.   Health habits | _____ | | 30 | 74 |
| III.   Medical factors | _____ | | 35 | 74 |
| IV.   Safety factors | _____ | | 40 | 75 |
| V.   Personal factors | _____ | | 45 | 76 |
| VI.   Psychological factors | _____ | | 50 | 76 |
| VII.   For women only | _____ | | 55 | 77 |
| | | | 60 | 78 |
| _____ + _____ = _____ | | | 65 | 80 |
| Total   Life   Longevity expectancy   estimate | | | 70 | 82 |

Now go back and see how you can add years to your life by improving behaviors and lifestyle. Check each category for possible changes you would like to make in your current lifestyle.

# Chapter 13

# Leading a Physically Active Life

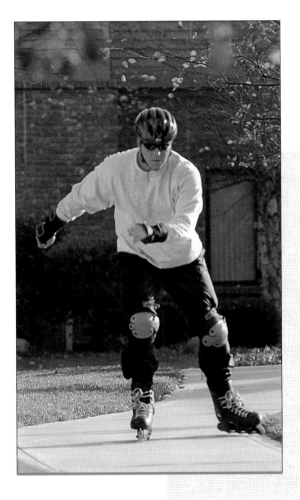

I don't know how I got this out of shape—except that I'm not getting much regular exercise. Getting more exercise is always one of my New Year's resolutions, and I usually work out hard before spring break—but I never keep it going. If I feel this out of shape when I'm only 20, I hate to think what it will be like when I'm 40 or 60. I wish I could find a way to stick with some type of regular exercise. My dad always told me good habits are as easy to keep as bad habits—but I'm beginning to wonder if I can change my habits at all!

—Aaron, 20-year-old junior

*What do you think?*

Despite the medical and scientific evidence that physical activity promotes health, about 6 in 10 Americans are not regularly active, and another 1 in 4 are not active at all. Why is it so hard to adopt and maintain a physically active lifestyle? What are the barriers that keep so many people from being physically active? How can people change their behaviors to become more active?

The most dramatic decrease in physical activity occurs during late adolescence—the last years of high school and first years of college. It becomes even more difficult for young adults to stay physically active when they enter the workforce. Whereas 70% of 12-year-old children report that they engage in vigorous physical activity, by age 21 these rates drop off to 40% for men and 30% for women.

All you've learned in the previous chapters will be of little use if you don't maintain a physically active lifestyle. Yet most adults have difficulty doing so. In this chapter, then, we'll look at the common roadblocks people face in trying to become more active and examine the psychological factors influencing physical activity. We'll consider ways to overcome those barriers by changing behavior, and we'll help you understand how to *stick with* a more physically active lifestyle. In Lab 13 you'll look at your own motivation and decision-making regarding regular physical activity and set activity goals for yourself.

## GOOD INTENTIONS, POOR RESULTS

The dropout rate in the first three to six months of exercise programs has averaged 50% for the past 20 years (see figure 13.1). While there has been a slight decrease in recent years in the percentage of Americans leading inactive lifestyles (see figure 13.2), it's still true that the majority of Americans aren't regularly physically active. Many inactive people have at least tried to be-

come more active, but they haven't stayed with it. The vast majority of Americans believe that being active is healthy for them, yet most remain sedentary. Why?

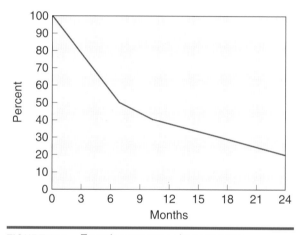

**FIGURE 13.1**  Exercise program dropout rates.

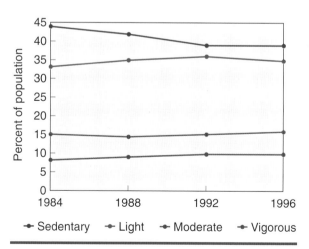

**FIGURE 13.2**  Physical activity trends among Americans.

Data from Centers for Disease Control (Atlanta), U.S. Department of Health and Human Services 1996.

First, it's important to realize that exercise does not spring from a single behavior. It derives from a set of distinct acts, including planning for participation, initial adoption of physical activity, continued participation or maintenance, and periodicity (stops and starts and seasonal variation). Second, the idea that a better attitude or greater motivation alone will solve the problem appears to be false. Studies have identified about 50 reasons why people are, or become, inactive (see "Common Barriers to Physical Activity"). Although it isn't yet clear which factors are most critical, it appears that for many people certain beliefs held about exercise—often misconceptions about what works and how quickly—combine with poor *self-regulation* to make being physically active another unfulfilled New Year's resolution.

 The vast majority of Americans believe that being active is healthy for them, yet most remain sedentary.

Attitudes toward being physically active, and to a lesser extent *social norms* about exercise, influence a person's intent to exercise, but intentions are often fleeting. Intentions themselves are influenced by changing priorities and by personality factors such as *willpower* or *self-motivation*. The intent to exercise can also be influenced by actual and perceived personal control over one's ability to exercise—that is, available time and facilities for exercising.

People who adopt challenging exercise goals that they believe they can meet have a good chance for success. However, confidence to meet exercise goals is best increased by past success in exercise, thus creating a "catch-22" situation. Confidence increases *exercise adherence*, but adherence is needed in order for confidence to grow. Nothing breeds success like success; most people need more than encouragement and role models.

In this chapter we're particularly concerned with the barriers that limit physical activity. We'll look at the barriers as well as at common views of motivation. Motivation is synonymous with needs, drives, incentives, and an impetus to action. Many approaches toward understanding and increasing physical activity have focused on motivation; less attention has been directed at understanding how barriers add to and interact with motivation to determine the direction, intensity, and persistence of physical activity.

## HEALTHCHECK

### Are physical activity habits inherited?

Research suggests that only about 20% of the variation in a person's physical activity is explainable by genetic inheritance, although families can also transmit a home culture that promotes or hinders physical activity. Social cultures outside the home can create barriers to physical activity. That's why it's important to understand the social and environmental influences that might be changed to increase physical activity.

## COMMON BARRIERS TO PHYSICAL ACTIVITY

Costs and barriers associated with a behavior have been recognized as important influences on behavior since theories about how people make decisions began to proliferate in the 1950s. While not enough is known about the roles of barriers in determining physical activity, most of what *is* known relates to four categories of barriers: personal, environmental, social, and exercise history and exertion barriers.

 Barriers to physical activity can be categorized as personal, environmental, social, and exercise history and exertion barriers. Lack of time and poor accessibility to facilities or equipment are the two main barriers people report for not adopting or maintaining an exercise program.

## Personal Barriers

The personal barriers to physical activity can be divided into demographic and cognitive variables. Demographics are attributes that put people at risk for being inactive, but aren't necessarily direct causes of inactivity; they can be difficult to change. Cognitive variables are more likely to be direct causes of physical inactivity and are usually changeable.

### Demographic Variables

Occupation, ethnicity, education, income, and obesity are examples of personal demographics that can present barriers to being physically active (see table 13.1). They may also be sentinel markers of habits or circumstances that reinforce sedentary living. For example, blue-collar workers in low-exertion occupations are among the least active Americans in their leisure time. Many of these workers feel their jobs require enough physical activity for health and fitness; but as a result of advances in technology, most workers—even in blue-collar and hourly positions—lift and carry less and expend less energy than workers in similar positions 50 years ago. Smoking and being overweight are also direct barriers for high-intensity activities and can indicate lifestyles of unhealthy behaviors.

Obesity makes weight-bearing activities physically harder than for normal-weight people. An obese person who has had bad experiences with physical activity, such as being embarrassed, can become negative toward physical activity and especially toward exercise classes with normal-weight people. The typical obese person loses about 22 pounds in a weight loss program but then regains about one-third of it within a year and all of it within three to five years. This high rate of failure to maintain weight loss may lead to even lower confidence about staying with an exercise program.

Some barriers differ according to age and gender. For example, pregnancy and early child-rearing can present unique barriers to physical activity among women. Aging is associated with activity limitations due to deteriorating health. Also, older people may not know the benefits of being physically active. Perceived control over exercise and health is slightly lower in older persons. Older men perceive a lack of support for being in a physical activity program. Many older people may not view exercise as appropriate for their age. This is unfortunate, because age doesn't necessarily predispose people to lowered activity (see chapter 12). Indeed, barriers associated with a person's job or with disposable income may diminish during retirement years.

### Cognitive Variables

People of similar age, education, income, and social circumstances vary greatly in how physically active they are. Cognitive variables such as *beliefs*, *values*, and *attitudes* help explain why some people are active despite circumstances that would predict an inactive lifestyle, and why others are sedentary even though they have the opportunities and resources to be physically active. After all, many older people are active despite their age, many high school dropouts are active despite their lack of education, and many smokers exercise despite their unhealthy habit.

 Beliefs, attitudes, and values help explain why some people are active despite circumstances that would predict an inactive lifestyle, and why others are sedentary even though they have the opportunities and resources to be physically active.

Beliefs and values, expected outcomes, intentions, and the confidence people have in their ability to maintain an exercise program are especially important in motivating people to take the first steps toward being physically active. Other factors such as self-motivation influence how successfully people can adopt and maintain a new behavior once they've decided to do so. People set goals, monitor their progress, and reward and punish themselves as they attempt to maintain new behavior.

While people who are motivated to exercise are one step ahead of those who lack motivation, motivation isn't the only key. People who receive strong *social support* may stick with a program even if they lack self-motivation. Nonetheless, self-motivation can help offset intentions that waver or wane.

People can also be hindered in their physical activity if they lack knowledge about what's appropriate or have negative or indifferent beliefs and attitudes about the benefits. However, knowing that physical activity is healthy doesn't guarantee that someone will start or stay with an exercise program. Many people are motivated to *begin* exercising by the benefits they expect to receive, but they are more likely to *maintain* exercise when they achieve personal goals and enjoy exercise. Willpower can help you overcome personal barriers. But people don't need excessive amounts of willpower to be active. If you lack willpower, plan so that you'll enjoy your physical activity and it will fit in with your other interests. All the willpower in the world, though, won't help you overcome a bad plan.

Many people are motivated to *begin* exercising by the benefits they expect to receive, but they are more likely to *maintain* exercise when they attain personal goals and enjoy the exercise.

## Table 13.1 Personal Factors Influencing Physical Activity

| Factor | Influence |
|---|---|
| ***Demographics*** | |
| Increasing age | Negative |
| Blue-collar occupation | Negative |
| Higher level of education | Positive |
| Gender (male) | Positive |
| High risk for heart disease | Negative |
| Higher socioeconomic status | Positive |
| Injury history | Unclear |
| Overweight/obesity | Negative |
| Race (nonwhite) | Negative |
| Pregnancy and early child-rearing | Negative |
| ***Cognitive variables*** | |
| Positive attitude | Positive |
| Perceived barriers to exercise | Negative |
| Control over exercise | Unclear |
| Enjoyment of exercise | Positive |
| Expected benefits | Positive |
| Value of expected outcomes | Positive |
| Health locus of control | Positive |
| Intention to exercise | Positive |
| Knowledge of health and exercise | Neutral |

## Environmental Barriers

In early studies of supervised exercise programs, dropouts reported that their failure to attain goals and program inconvenience (e.g., facilities weren't easily accessible, or the exercise schedule conflicted with other commitments such as work) were environmental barriers that kept them from maintaining an exercise program (see table 13.2 for environmental factors influencing physical activity). For example, Oldridge (1979) found that about 20% to 30% of heart patients in exercise programs dropped out for medical reasons but that up to 40% dropped out because of nonmedical barriers such as work conflicts, relocation, and inaccessibility of exercise facilities.

Perceived lack of time and poor accessibility to facilities or equipment are the two main barriers people report for not adopting or maintaining an exercise program. In a study of a community in southern California (Sallis et al. 1990),

**Table 13.2 Environmental Factors Influencing Physical Activity**

| Factor | Influence |
| --- | --- |
| Climate/season | Negative |
| Perceived lack of time | Negative |
| Easy access to facilities | Positive |
| Home equipment | Unknown |

adults who had more commercial exercise facilities located within 1 kilometer of their home were more likely to report that they exercised at least three times a week, regardless of age, education, and income. In contrast, other studies have shown that dropouts from exercise programs actually had more leisure time and lived closer to exercise facilities than did their peers who remained active. This suggests that removing barriers related to time and place (e.g., providing flexible scheduling or home programs) does not translate into an increase in physical activity. Changing people's perceptions about barriers or teaching time-management skills may help. However, those who report time and inconvenience as problems may simply place low priority on being physically active, and it may be that no amount of time or convenience will sway them to become more active.

Lack of time can represent a true barrier, a perceived barrier, a lack of time-management skills, or an excuse for not wanting to be active. A good way to tell the difference is to ask someone which current leisure activity the person is willing to give up to exercise. While adding exercise to an already busy schedule merely invites a schedule conflict or makes lack of time an easy excuse, being unwilling to replace a current activity with exercise probably signals that exercise isn't a high priority.

Lack of access to activity programs is a barrier that often results in attempts to exercise alone at home (or not exercise at all). Access to facilities is even more of a problem for people who depend on others for transportation or who have health conditions that limit their mobility (e.g., those who are disabled or institutionalized).

*Where* people do the activity may also matter. In another study by Sallis et al. (1986) in southern California, half the adults reported exercising at home. In fact, in one of the first clinical studies of the use of exercise to rehabilitate a group of heart patients, the investigators found that allowing the men to exercise at home increased their amount of exercise—a finding replicated among healthy men and women by researchers at Stanford University (King et al. 1991).

Though home exercise adds convenience, it isn't the only answer to America's inactivity. According to the National Sporting Goods Manufacturing Association, money spent in the United States on exercise machines increased from $1.2 billion in 1986 to about $3 billion in 1996. Television shoppers spent $100 million on exercise equipment in 1994. During the abdominal-machine craze in late 1996 and early 1997, peak sales reached about $1 million *a day*. From 1986 to 1996, however, Americans increased actual participation in moderate and vigorous physical activity by only 2%. A lot of that exercise equipment ended up in closets collecting dust.

## Social Barriers

Social factors can create or break down barriers to physical activity (see table 13.3). Through word and deed, family and friends can help or hinder your efforts to be physically active. Encouragement, praise, sharing chores in order to free up time for exercise, or being an "exercise buddy" can help. Excessive nagging or distraction from exercise goals (e.g., going to movies, parties, or just "hanging out") can hurt. You also learn attitudes and habits from watching and listening to family and friends.

Andrew et al. (1981) found that a lack of spousal support for involvement was associated with a threefold increase in the dropout rate in a large Canadian study of exercise in men who were recovering from a heart attack. In another study (Heinzelmann and Bagley 1970), the attitudes

## Benefits of—and Barriers to—Physical Activity

Though specific benefits and barriers to exercise can vary according to age, gender, or other personal circumstances (e.g., pregnancy, illness, change in work schedule), according to Steinhardt and Dishman (1989) the general categories of perceived benefits and perceived barriers to physical activity are remarkably similar for men and women from college age through middle age.

**Perceived benefits**
1. Stay in shape
2. Make me feel better in general
3. Good health
4. Maintain proper body weight
5. Improve appearance
6. Enhance self-image and confidence
7. Positive psychological effect
8. Reduce stress and relax
9. Fun and enjoyment
10. Help cope with life's pressures
11. Lose weight
12. Companionship

**Perceived barriers**
1. Lack of motivation
2. Too lazy
3. Too busy
4. Not enough time
5. Interferes with school
6. Too tired
7. Interferes with work
8. Too inconvenient
9. Bad weather
10. Lack of facilities
11. Exercise is boring
12. Fatigued by exercise
13. Family obligations
14. Limiting health reason

### Table 13.3 Social Factors Influencing Physical Activity

| Factor | Influence |
|---|---|
| Class size | Unknown* |
| Exercise role models | Unknown* |
| Good group cohesion | Positive* |
| Physician influence | Positive |
| Past family influences | Positive |
| Social support (friends/peers) | Positive |
| Social support (spouse/family) | Positive |
| Social support (staff/instructor) | Positive |

*Experts predict the influence of these factors, but not enough research has been done to draw firm conclusions.

toward exercise held by wives of heart patients were better predictors of participation than were the attitudes held by the men who had been advised by physicians to exercise.

## Exercise History and Exertion Barriers

Past habits can also be a barrier to adopting a physical activity program. The habits that make up a sedentary lifestyle can be hard to break. People develop an "inactive inertia" when they spend too much of their leisure time engaged in sedentary activities. Too much time spent looking at the television, surfing the Internet, watching movies, or reading (perhaps while eating extra calories!) creates huge barriers to starting an exercise program that takes time and effort and may not initially feel as good as your sedentary options (see table 13.4). On the positive side, the best predictor of someone's future physical activity is that person's past leisure physical activity. So you can develop a new "active inertia," but you must take the first step. And you don't have to have been an athlete to be a successful

**Table 13.4  Exercise History and Exertion Factors Influencing Physical Activity**

| Factor | Influence |
| --- | --- |
| Past adult activity | Positive |
| Diet | Unclear |
| Television watching | Negative |
| Past childhood activity | Unknown |
| School sports | Neutral |
| School sports | Unrelated (men) |
| | Positive (women) |
| Smoking | Unclear |
| Exercise intensity | Negative |
| Exercise frequency | Negative |
| Exercise duration | Negative |
| Perceived effort of exercise | Negative |

exerciser now. Playing school sports doesn't necessarily have influence on leisure-time physical activity after the school years. Dishman (1988) found that men who had been athletes in high school or college were not more physically active during the middle-age years than former nonathletes. However, one study of alumnae from colleges in Boston found that women who had participated in college athletics or intramural sports reported that they were more active after college compared with nonparticipants (Frisch et al. 1987). The people surveyed in those studies were in school in the 1920s to 1950s; cultural changes in relation to the role of sports in society, as well as changing opportunities for widespread sport participation by males and females, may paint a different picture in today's world.

The habits that make up a sedentary lifestyle can be hard to break. The best predictor of how physically active people will be in the future is how active they have been in the past.

The types of activity people choose also impact their success at maintaining the activity. Choosing an activity you enjoy and exercising at an intensity that is challenging but not uncomfort-

able are important for planning an exercise program you'll stick with.

Choosing an activity you enjoy and exercising at an intensity that is challenging but not uncomfortable are important for planning an exercise program you'll stick with.

As we mentioned in chapter 2, the Borg scale uses the exerciser's *rating of perceived exertion (RPE)* as a subjective rating of how hard physical activity feels. It is a perception that sums up all of the sensations you experience during exertion, including muscular force or pain, achy joints, heavy breathing, body and skin temperature, and sweat. Rating of perceived exertion should be used along with your target heart rate (see chapter 2, page 37) to help you pick the intensity of exercise that is challenging without being too uncomfortable (see table 13.5). For example, following the American College of Sports Medicine guidelines from table 2.1 on page 23, you would want to exercise at a target rate of 55% to 90% of your maximal heart rate, which translates into an RPE somewhere between 12 and 16, reflecting intensities from moderate to heavy.

Using RPE to help you monitor your exercise intensity is also important because it is possible to make errors when using your heart rate alone. The target heart rate approach to selecting exer-

## Table 13.5 Classifying Exercise Intensity

| Maximum heart rate (% of maximal heart rate) | RPE | Intensity classification |
|---|---|---|
| < 35% | < 10 | Very light |
| 35% to 54% | 10 to 11 | Light |
| 55% to 69% | 12 to 13 | Moderate (somewhat hard) |
| 70% to 89% | 14 to 16 | Hard |
| ≥ 90% | > 16 | Very hard |

The intensity of exercise is based on 20 to 60 minutes of endurance training.

cise intensity that was introduced in chapter 2 is the most widely used and practical approach to determine a target intensity, but this approach isn't perfect. Even when variability in age and training level is accounted for, the standard deviation of your maximal heart rate can be about 11 beats per minute (so if you're 22 and figure your maximal heart rate to be 198 by subtracting your age from 220, your actual maximal heart rate could be anywhere from 187 to 209). This error can occur in about 30% of the adult population. Thus, using heart rate alone to determine your exercise intensity can lead to large over- or underestimates. Because RPE during exercise is influenced less by heart rate than it is by the amount of oxygen consumed (expressed as a percent of aerobic capacity, or $\dot{V}O_2$max), it isn't surprising that some exercisers who are using only age-predicted target heart rate ranges feel that the exercise intensity is either too easy or too hard. For the most part, studies show that when people exercise at a pace not exceeding what feels "somewhat hard," their breathing is not too labored and their pulse rate will likely be in the range of 120-150 beats per minute. At this level, most healthy people can safely and comfortably increase their fitness and health.

If previously sedentary people choose an intensity that they perceive as too hard, they're less likely to stick with exercising. Typically, people who are just beginning to exercise prefer a more comfortable level of exertion. If you're just beginning an exercise program, you may find it easier to make the permanent change from a sedentary to an active lifestyle if you choose an intensity toward the lower end of the ACSM recommendations (i.e., exercise for 20 minutes 3 days per week) and build up gradually. Studies have shown that the dropout rates from exercise programs increase when the duration exceeds 45 minutes and/or the frequency exceeds 5 days per week.

However, in a recent one-year study of middle-aged sedentary people (King et al. 1991), those who worked out at high intensities (74% to 88% maximal heart rate) were as successful at sticking with the exercise as the group who exercised at lower intensities (60% to 73%). The authors did note that each group gradually moved toward a common RPE level between about 12 and 13, which is moderately hard. During cycling or treadmill walking, young and middle-aged men preferred intensities about 60% of $\dot{V}O_2$max with an RPE of 11 to 14, again moderately hard. After endurance-exercise training, your preferred level of exercise intensity should increase while your RPE decreases. For example, in a study of running for 30 minutes (Farrell 1982), trained runners preferred intensities of about 75% of $\dot{V}O_2$max, which they rated between 9 and 12 on Borg's scale.

## SUCCESSFUL BEHAVIOR CHANGE

People can create their own environments for prompting and rewarding physical activity. Many psychologists believe that people can learn to overcome barriers to behavior change through goal setting, *self-monitoring*, and *self-reinforcement*. These aspects of self-regulation are particularly important in explaining whether or not people maintain physical activity.

Successful behavior change requires that a person be ready to change. This readiness can vary depending on past experiences and current circumstances. You should view successful behavior change as an ongoing endeavor, not as a

# Ten Tips for Success

**#1** **Set specific long-term and short-term exercise goals.**
The long-term goals don't even have to be realistic—an ideal goal you can never reach can be a good incentive. But you must plan shorter-term step-by-step goals that you *can* attain and that will bring you closer to your ultimate objective. Don't change distant goals, but be flexible with your daily goals. Avoid all-or-none thinking; if you miss a workout, all is not lost.

**#2** **Enter in for the long haul.**
Don't expect a quick fix; for instance, if you're becoming more physically active to lose weight, stay off the scales for the first month. And realize that most promises from commercial fitness companies are distortions or half-truths. It typically takes 10 to 20 weeks of consistent physical effort to show a noticeable fitness gain. Expecting too much too soon will only frustrate you—and increase the chances of your dropping out.

**#3** **Make physical activity fun.**
It doesn't have to be a *work*out. If exercise is "too hard" or "no fun," then make it fun (or at least make it easy). Walk and talk with a friend. Plant a garden. Do something active that you enjoy. You don't have to sweat or ache to improve your health.

**#4** **Motivate yourself through rewards.**
If you aren't motivated to carry out good intentions to exercise just by knowing the fitness and health benefits, pick rewards that are more important to you and make a personal commitment to not indulge yourself until you meet your daily exercise goal—for example, no newspaper until you've exercised. Following through on this will reduce your guilt and make both activities more enjoyable. Keep a chart of your promises so you can't conveniently forget them or lie to yourself when you don't keep them.

**#5** **Schedule your physical activity.**
Schedule your workout. Pick a time and place. Things that aren't scheduled often aren't accomplished. Many people find exercise at lunchtime or at the end of the day invigorating. Others feel too tired by the end of the day; these people should schedule exercise for earlier. Good intentions often weaken by day's end. Make exercise a top priority by actions, not just words.

# Ten Tips for Success

**#6** **Try something new.**

Seek pleasure. Try different activities and pick those you enjoy, and do them in places you enjoy. The type of exercise you do and when you do it are much less important than the time you spend doing it. Once you start moving, you can try other less enjoyable but healthful activities. They can become rewarding later. Having options reduces the chance that you will relapse if vacations, illness, or other interruptions break into your favorite routine.

**#7** **Make it difficult to *not* exercise.**

Engineer your environment so it is difficult to talk yourself out of exercising. Put exercise equipment beside your bed at night so it's the first thing you see in the morning. Keep workout clothing in your car, dorm, or house so you can't say "I don't have it with me" when a workout opportunity arises. Put exercise signs or cartoons on your door or on the refrigerator. When you have second thoughts, take the first step; this usually leads to another. You can always decide to stop after you start moving—but usually you won't.

**#8** **Exercise to feel better.**

Don't judge the benefits of your exercise by fitness gains alone. Exercise can also enhance your health and make you feel better. Exercise doesn't just add years to your life—it adds life to your years. This enhanced quality of life may be the key to sustaining an active lifestyle. Exercise should make you feel better. If it doesn't, change it until it does.

**#9** **Work out with a friend.**

Find a buddy. Make a commitment with a friend who shares your interests. Substitute an active leisure choice for a passive one; meet a friend for a bike ride instead of lunch. People often keep commitments they make to others when individually, they would let themselves down.

**#10** **Finish workouts feeling good.**

Choose an intensity that allows you to feel at least as good when you finish as when you started. Remember, you'll still receive most of the health benefits from exercise when you exercise in shorter, repeated bouts (e.g., three 10-minute walks) rather than a single, longer bout. So pick a type of exercise you enjoy, a time that best fits your schedule, and an intensity that allows you to enjoy the exercise and feel good when you finish.

329

final product. Reaching a new physical activity goal doesn't necessarily mean you have permanently changed. To retain the goal, you need to maintain the behaviors that helped you to reach the goal in the first place. This usually requires ongoing effort.

 Successful behavior change requires that a person be ready to change. This readiness can vary depending on past experiences and current circumstances. You should view successful behavior change as an ongoing endeavor, not as a final product.

## Why Some Behavior-Change Plans Fail

Those who plan to change their behavior often fail because they have unrealistic expectations about exercise outcomes or because they haven't developed an effective exercise plan that will help them sustain the new behavior. The first key to planning a program you can stick with is to set realistic yet challenging goals about increasing your physical activity and fitness.

Often we expect quick fixes but are quickly disappointed. While some health outcomes may not require much time or effort, other outcomes of exercise that are valued by many people, such as weight loss or improved body image, may require more time and effort. Many measurable or noticeable fitness gains require 10 to 20 weeks of sustained effort. Thus, there may be a time-effort paradox in sustaining an exercise program. Many sedentary people may be more likely to adopt an exercise program of low time and effort. However, the sedentary people who are also expecting a great increase in fitness or dramatic change in physique will likely be frustrated by small or no gains of this kind if they invest only the minimal time or effort in the exercise program.

It's reasonable, for example, to try to lose 1 or 2 pounds per week through exercise and diet. But don't gauge progress in the first few weeks by scale weight. Trained muscles grow; they store sugar for energy and retain water. Because lean tissue is dense, you can lose fat but gain muscle weight early on. Also, don't expect to "spot reduce." People have patterns of fat loss, and trying to reduce in certain spots just doesn't work. Finally, later improvements in fitness occur more slowly than initial ones, so you should expect plateaus. As you maintain your physical activity throughout the months, you can decide whether further advances are worth the increased effort they'll require.

Results from the health risk appraisals and fitness tests you completed in the previous lab experiences provide a starting point—and in many cases, motivation—for goal setting. However, don't expect any boost in motivation to be enough to keep you going. Researchers commonly find that people initially increase their intentions to be active after fitness testing and health risk appraisals but within a few weeks or months lose motivation and become as inactive as before. This happens because health risk appraisals and fitness testing don't teach the behavioral skills people need to convert their intentions into actions. We'll cover this important concept next.

## How to Modify Behavior Successfully

Many people plan to exercise consistently, but not as many possess the necessary behavioral skills to bring that plan to fruition. People may highly value goals such as better health, weight loss, or improved appearance; but such goals are remote and require long-term diligence before rewarding changes are seen. Also, as we've noted in earlier chapters, later gains occur more slowly than initial ones. This frustrates people who expect constant improvements. The only reward that many health gains offer is the knowledge that gains are being made. This is good enough for some people, but those who are least active often need more tangible rewards in order to keep going.

*Behavior modification* applies principles of associational learning (i.e., stimulus-response) to modify behavior. Changes in behavior result from associations between external stimuli and the consequences of a specific behavior. The role of people's thoughts, motives, and perceptions is minimized. What precedes and what follows a behavior will influence the frequency of that behavior; that is, behavior is cued and reinforced. The key to behavior change lies in identifying a target behavior (e.g., walking at lunchtime, or stationary cycling while studying) and using effective *cues* and *reinforcers*. Many people have also successfully changed their behaviors through the use of written agreements and contracts, and stimulus and reinforcement control.

*Cognitive behavior modification* is based on the idea that people's beliefs and behavioral skills are the key links between the environment and behavior. Unhealthy behaviors result from irrational or unproductive thoughts. Learning or insight can serve to restructure or replace faulty thoughts with behaviorally effective beliefs and skills. Simply put, thoughts and feelings moderate behavior, and they can be changed. People can be educated about the relationship between knowledge, feelings, and behaviors and can be taught skills to identify and control antecedents and consequences that prompt and reinforce behavior. Cognitive-behavioral approaches (e.g., self-monitoring, goal setting, feedback, and the *decision-balance* technique) have been effective in increasing exercise adherence when used alone or when combined in intervention packages.

In short, exercise is maintained when it is cued and reinforced by aspects of your environment. The key tactic to successfully attaining an exercise habit is to make environmental changes that will support physical activity while weakening the impact of other behaviors that compete for your leisure time. Three ways to make these changes are

1. developing prompts or cues using stimulus-control techniques,

2. adapting the physical activity itself (e.g., incorporating skill training or modifying the exercise intensity or duration to fit your needs), and

3. ensuring the outcome of physical activity, using contingency management, goal setting, contracts, and so forth.

### Behavioral Antecedents

Habits are cued by aspects of your physical environment. *Stimulus control* involves manipulating these cues to prompt a behavior. For example, the sight and smell of food are powerful cues to eat. Seeing a television after work is a cue to sit down and relax for the rest of the night. In the same way, the clock striking noon can become your cue to head to your workout. Cues can be verbal, physical, or symbolic.

The aim is to increase cues for the desired behavior and decrease cues for competing behaviors. Examples of cues you can use to increase exercise behavior are posters, slogans, and self-adhesive notes; keeping exercise equipment in visible places, recruiting social support, and exercising at the same time and place every day will also provide cues. Maintaining records of your personal exercise progress (one self-monitoring technique) can also be especially helpful in providing a cue to exercise, especially if you keep the records in a place where you'll see them regularly. Exercising the first thing in the morning is an example of lessening the risk of encountering distracting cues and being tempted by other options. If you travel to a fitness center, choose a route that doesn't take you past your favorite bar or restaurant. If you exercise at home, don't let yourself be distracted by the television, your roommate or family, or a comfortable sofa until you get your workout in. The more often you exercise at a particular time and in a particular place, the more powerful a cue those circumstances become. The downside, of course, is that those cues can disappear if you're part of a formal exercise program (e.g., a fitness class) that ends or is interrupted by illness or vacation.

Once your exercise habit becomes routine, try to diversify the type of exercise you do and the location in which you do it so that these, rather than just the time and place, can become cues.

### Behavioral Consequences

As we've already noted, behavior is determined, especially when you're working to form a habit, by its immediate consequences rather than by long-term outcomes such as living longer or being more healthy. Consequences that occur during or right after exercise will be more powerful influences on your future exercise habits than those that do not occur until some time in the distant future (whether it be weeks, months, or years from now)—which is another reason to make exercise as fun as possible!

*Reinforcement control* involves using reinforcement during or after a behavior (in this case exercise) to increase or decrease the occurrence of a behavior. There are two kinds of reinforcers: positive and negative. Positive reinforcers (also called rewards) involve the presentation of a stimulus during or following a behavior. For example, an exercise class instructor who praises a person for finishing a hard routine is positively reinforcing the behavior (the workout). Reinforcement can also be negative: negative reinforcers are ongoing stimuli or events that are withdrawn during or following a behavior. If something is taken away to shape the desired behavior, the reinforcement is negative. For example, if someone who has been nagging you to exercise stops nagging when you start to exercise, you may be more likely to exercise. On the other hand, this tactic may backfire: you might just avoid the nagging person!

It should be clear that positive reinforcement is key. Positive reinforcement comes in many forms. Social reinforcement through verbal praise and encouragement from an instructor, friend, or family member—or simply through the chance to interact with others—can be a powerful reward. Watching the miles mount on an odometer or pedometer while you're biking or walking can encourage you to want to add more.

*Goal setting* can be used to attain something by a certain time or date. Goals can be as simple and focused as getting to your next class on time, or as arduous and distant as the aim of competing in a triathlon. Goals regulate behavior by providing direction, mobilizing effort, and instigating the search for ways to attain them. Through goal setting, people can devise a plan that directs activity and emphasizes the link between behavior and outcome. Specific, measurable goals are easier to monitor and make adjustments for; also, when goals are specific, it's easier to know when they have been reached. Keeping a cumulative chart of your exercise and creating a goal that you can compare your progress to can provide a particularly positive reinforcer.

 Through goal setting, people can devise a plan that directs activity and emphasizes the link between behavior and outcome. Specific, measurable goals are easier to monitor and make adjustments for; it's also easier, when goals are specific, to know when they have been reached.

Short-term goals should be reasonable and realistic. For example, losing 2 pounds a week through diet and exercise is reasonable, but it may be almost impossible for the mother of three who works outside the home unless she can change her meal planning and get extra help to allow a little more time for exercise (or involve her spouse or children in her exercise!) Unrealistic short-term goals ultimately doom a person to failure, which can damage self-confidence and undermine other reasons for being physically active. To be the most helpful, goals should be specific and should take the form of a statement about what you actually need to do to achieve them. For example, "I'm going to be more active" and "I'm going to reduce my resting heart rate to 60 beats per minute" aren't helpful. The first goal is not specific, and the second isn't formulated to explain what you'll do to achieve it. "I'm going to take three 30-minute walks this week" and "I'm going to ride my bike 20 miles this week" are more helpful, assuming that they are also realistic for you.

### Stage-Specific Interventions

The success of any behavior-change tactic depends on whether the tactic fits the readiness of the person. One popular view, applied to exercise by Prochaska and Marcus (1994), proposes that when people try to change behavior they move through five stages. The stages are

- precontemplation,
- contemplation,
- preparation,
- action, and
- maintenance.

One popular view proposes that when people try to change behavior they move through five stages: precontemplation, contemplation, preparation, action, and maintenance.

The goal in the *precontemplation stage,* in the case of physical activity, is to make people more aware of their lack of physical activity and of the positive consequences of being active. People in this stage need to have the benefits of exercise emphasized and the costs minimized. Health risk appraisals and fitness testing can prompt contemplation and enhance motivation to become more active.

The objective with people in the *contemplation stage* is to bolster their intentions to become more active and help them take action. Marketing and media campaigns that promote physical activity and provide accurate, easy-to-understand information about how to start an exercise program can help move people into the *preparation stage,* during which they begin to form their intentions. Intentions to start exercising are affected by role models, perceived barriers and benefits, and self-confidence. People move through the stages of change more efficiently

when they evaluate how past habits, environments, and social influences create barriers for physical activity. Goal setting is an important tactic for people in the preparation stage. People should also evaluate environmental and social supports and barriers, and plan to maintain or enhance the supports and overcome the barriers in order to adopt a more active lifestyle.

Self-regulation skills such as goal setting and self-monitoring come into play in moving from preparation to the *action stage,* during which intentions become reality. Fitness assessments and self-monitoring can be useful strategies at this point to help in goal setting. For example, a fitness assessment can help establish the type and intensity of exercise necessary to accomplish certain goals, and self-monitoring can help identify scheduling changes needed to fit in an exercise routine.

People in the action phase are at a high risk of dropping out of an exercise program; social support is critical at this stage. In the *maintenance stage,* the use of self-regulatory skills such as stimulus control, reinforcement management, and self-monitoring of progress, along with tactics to prevent relapse into inactivity, is necessary to maintain the more active lifestyle.

---

### HEALTHCHECK

#### What type or amount of exercise will help keep me active?

Most aspects of health that are improved by physical activity rely more on moving your body than on precisely what the activity is and how intensely it's performed. So choose an activity that you enjoy and pick an intensity that's comfortable (between 55% and 90% of your maximal heart rate) and do the activity for 20 to 30 minutes each session, several times a week. Even sessions that are shorter than 20 minutes may temporarily help with anxiety, although they probably won't have as many fitness benefits. You may notice benefits immediately, but for most people the biggest changes occur after about four months of regular exercise.

## A Little Is Better Than None

By now you know the minimal recommendations for exercise: moderate intensity for at least 30 minutes a day on most if not all days of the week. But only about 4 in 10 Americans exercise at *any* intensity for this frequency and duration. Would lowering the standards help people stick with regular physical activity and reduce the rate of sedentary living?

Some evidence suggests that this may be the case. In a study of California adults (Sallis et al. 1986), more men (11%) than women (5%) adopted vigorous exercise such as running during a year's time, but more women (33%) than men (26%) took up moderate activities such as walking, stair climbing, and gardening. Both sexes were more likely to adopt regular activities of a moderate intensity than high-intensity fitness activities. Moderate activities showed a dropout rate (25% to 35%) roughly one-half of that seen for vigorous exercise (50%). Regardless of exercise intensity, injuries from weight-bearing exercise (e.g., running) can directly lead to dropout. However, this often doesn't occur unless previously untrained people exercise for 45 minutes or longer five days or more per week. When older people walk as their physical activity, they are less likely to sustain injuries that cause them to stop walking.

The bottom line? A little is better than none. And moderate or even low intensity is better than high intensity—especially if high intensity leads to relapsing to inactivity again.

## STICKING WITH PHYSICAL ACTIVITY

Being ready to change doesn't mean it will be easy to maintain regular physical activity. Even seasoned exercisers may have their exercise programs interrupted or ended by unexpected changes in their routines. Relocation, travel, and illnesses and injuries are just a few of the types of events that can disrupt a routine and create activity barriers.

*Relapse prevention,* designed to help smokers and drug abusers, has also helped people maintain new exercise programs. Following are the main components of relapse prevention:

1. Identify situations that put you at high risk for relapse.

2. Plan to avoid or cope with these situations (e.g., reducing activity barriers and using

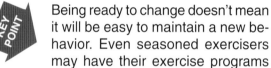

**KEY POINT** Being ready to change doesn't mean it will be easy to maintain a new behavior. Even seasoned exercisers may have their exercise programs interrupted or ended by unexpected changes in their routines.

time-management, relaxation, and confidence-building skills).

3. Put the consequences of not exercising in proper perspective. For example, if you're tired at the end of your day, you may expect to feel refreshed if you rest rather than exercise. But the actuality may be that you feel guilty resting, whereas the activity would likely have been invigorating.

4. Expect and plan for lapses. For example, schedule alternative activities while on vacation or after injury.

5. Don't have an "all-or-nothing" attitude. A temporary lapse is not the end of the world, but feeling that it is can lead to loss of confidence and complete cessation.

6. Enjoy exercise rather than viewing it as an obligation.

7. Block self-talk and images that focus on the benefits of not exercising.

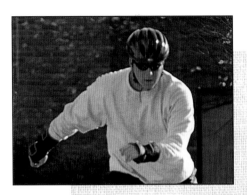

## Health Concepts

As you'll remember, Aaron wanted to figure out ways to stick with a regular exercise program. He was concerned that he'd never be able to change his inactive lifestyle. The good news is that people *can* change and become regularly active. By choosing exercises that they enjoy and intensities that are challenging but not overly difficult, people can make physical activity a regular part of their lives—and improve their health, fitness, and energy levels through the process.

## SUMMARY

▊ Barriers to physical activity can be categorized as personal, environmental, social, and personal exercise history and exertion barriers. People report lack of time and poor accessibility to facilities or equipment as the two main barriers for not adopting or maintaining an exercise program.

▊ The habits that make up a sedentary lifestyle can be hard to break. The best predictor of how physically active people will be in the future is how active they have been in the past.

▊ Psychological factors such as beliefs, attitudes, and values help explain why some people are active despite circumstances that would predict an inactive lifestyle, and why others are sedentary even though they have the opportunities and resources to be physically active.

▊ Many people are motivated to begin exercising by the benefits they expect to receive, but they are more likely to *maintain* exercise when they attain personal goals and enjoy the exercise.

▊ Successful behavior change requires that a person be ready to change. Readiness varies depending on past experiences and current circumstances. View successful behavior change as an ongoing endeavor, not as a final product.

▌ People often fail to change their behaviors because they have unrealistic expectations about exercise outcomes, or they haven't developed an effective plan that will help them sustain the new behavior. The first key to planning a program you can stick with is to set realistic yet challenging goals about increasing your physical activity and fitness.

▌ Goal setting provides a plan of action that focuses and directs activity and emphasizes a clear link between behavior and outcome. Specific, measurable goals make it easier to monitor progress and make adjustments; when goals are specific, it's also easier to know when they have been reached.

▌ One popular view proposes that when people try to change behavior they move through five stages: precontemplation, contemplation, preparation, action, and maintenance.

▌ Being ready to change doesn't mean that adopting and maintaining a new behavior will be easy. Even people who are regularly active may have their exercise programs interrupted or even terminated by unexpected changes in their routines.

## KEY TERMS

| | |
|---|---|
| attitude | relapse prevention |
| behavior modification | self-monitoring |
| beliefs | self-motivation |
| cognitive behavior modification | self-regulation |
| cues | self-reinforcement |
| decision-balance | social support |
| exercise adherence | stimulus control |
| rating of perceived exertion (RPE) | values |
| reinforcement control | willpower |
| reinforcers | |

**13**

# Determining Current Physical Activity Status and Motivation, Making Decisions to be Physically Active, Setting Goals, and Determining Perceived Exertion

**THE PURPOSES OF THIS LAB EXPERIENCE ARE TO**

▌ determine your current physical activity status,

▌ assess your motivation to be regularly physically active,

▌ consider gains and losses in deciding to become more regularly active,

▌ set goals regarding physical activity, and

▌ determine your rating of perceived exertion.

## Determine Your Current Physical Activity Status

Choose the *one* number below that best describes your current level of physical activity or your interest in physical activity. Don't include activities that you do as part of a job.

*Vigorous* exercise includes activities such as jogging, running, fast cycling, aerobics classes, swimming laps, singles tennis, and racquetball. Count as vigorous any activity that makes you work as hard as jogging and lasts at least 20 minutes at a time. These activities increase your heart rate and usually make you sweat (don't count weight lifting).

*Moderate* exercise includes activities such as brisk walking, gardening, slow cycling, dancing, and doubles tennis. Count as moderate any activity that makes you work as hard as brisk walking and that lasts at least 30 minutes at a time.

---

**Current Physical Activity Status**

1. I don't exercise or walk regularly now, and I don't intend to start in the near future.
2. I don't exercise or walk regularly, but I have been thinking of starting.
3. I'm trying to begin exercising or walking, or I do exercise or walk infrequently.
4. I'm doing vigorous exercise less than three times per week, or I'm doing moderate exercise less than five times per week.
5. I've been doing moderate exercise more than five times per week (or more than 2.5 hours per week) for the last one to six months.

*(continued)*

---

6. I've been doing moderate exercise more than five times per week (or more than 2.5 hours per week) for the last seven months or more.

7. I've been doing vigorous exercise three to five times per week for the last one to six months.

8. I've been doing vigorous exercise three to five times per week for the last seven months or more.

If you rated your activity status as 1, go to the "Getting Out of Your Chair" section.

If you rated your status from 2 to 4, go to the "Planning the First Step" section.

If you rated your status from 5 to 8, go to the "Keeping the Pace" section.

## Getting Out of Your Chair

Physical Activity Status Score: 1

In assessing your current physical activity status, you indicated that you're not very interested in physical activity. Remember that physical activity can help you

- feel better,
- look better, and
- be healthier.

What would be the two most important benefits of physical activity *for you*? Be specific.

1. _____

2. _____

Do you know that you can get most of the benefits of physical activity by just *walking* regularly?

Many things can interfere with physical activity. Here are some of the reasons people give for not being physically active. Check the ones that apply most to you.

| | |
|---|---|
| _____ Exercise is hard work. | _____ I don't enjoy exercise. |
| _____ I am usually too tired to exercise. | _____ I hate to fail, so I won't start. |
| _____ I don't have anyone to exercise with. | _____ I don't have a safe place to exercise. |
| _____ The weather is too bad. | _____ Exercise is boring. |
| _____ I don't have a convenient place to exercise. | _____ I don't have the time. |
| _____ I am too overweight. | _____ I'm too old. |

What are the two main things that keep you from being physically active?

1. _____

2. _____

Consider these reasons as roadblocks that you can get around. You can change the roadblock itself (e.g., "I will get up earlier to make time to exercise"), or you can change your attitude about the roadblock (e.g., "I really can make time to exercise").

| Roadblock | How to get past it |
|---|---|
| _____ Exercise is hard work. | Pick an activity that you enjoy and that is easy for you. "No pain, no gain" is a myth. |
| _____ I don't have time. | Thirty minutes a day can be gained from most schedules. Give up a TV show. Work out three times for 10 minutes each. |
| _____ I don't enjoy exercise. | Don't "exercise." Begin a hobby or a way of playing that gets you moving. |
| _____ I'm usually too tired to exercise. | Tell yourself "This exercise will give me more energy." Then try it and see if it doesn't happen. |
| _____ I don't have a safe place to exercise. | If your neighborhood isn't safe, walk at work or with a group. |
| _____ I don't have anyone to exercise with. | Ask a friend, a neighbor, a family member. Join an exercise group. Or choose an activity you like doing by yourself. |
| _____ I don't have a convenient place to exercise. | Choose an activity you can do near your home, school, or workplace. Walk around your neighborhood or do aerobics to a TV show at home. |
| _____ I'm afraid of being injured. | Walking is safe and is an excellent activity to improve your health. |
| _____ The weather is too bad. | There are many activities you can do in your home. |
| _____ Exercise is boring. | Listen to music while you exercise. Walking, biking, or running can take you past interesting scenery. |
| _____ I'm too overweight. | You can benefit from physical activity regardless of your weight. Choose an activity that you're comfortable with, such as walking. |
| _____ I'm too old. | It's never too late to start. Older people benefit greatly from exercise. If you're ill, talk to your doctor before beginning any exercise program. |

How can you get around the two main roadblocks that you listed earlier?

1. _____

2. _____

## Planning the First Step

Physical Activity Status Score: 2 to 4

Congratulations. In assessing your physical activity status, you indicated that you're ready to make physical activity a regular part of your life. It's recommended that you perform moderate activity at least five days a week, or vigorous activity three to five days a week. The form provided should help you begin an activity program that you can stick with.

What are the two main benefits you hope to derive from being active? Write them here and think of them often.

1. _____

2. _____

Following are examples of moderate and vigorous activities. Consider which activities you will do, based on your responses to these questions:

- Do you enjoy it?

- Do you have a convenient place to perform the activity?

- Can you realistically fit the activity into your schedule? (Consider rearranging your schedule if possible.)

- How long do you plan to do the activity? (Build gradually; start with a 5- to 10-minute workout and build to 30 to 60 minutes of moderate activity or 20 to 40 minutes of vigorous activity.)

- Who will support you in the activity? (It's ideal to have a friend be active with you.)

Moderate Activities

- Walking
- Regular gardening
- Hiking
- Slow cycling

- Folk, square, or popular dancing
- Ice or roller skating
- Doubles tennis
- Taking the stairs

Vigorous Activities

- Jogging
- Aerobic dance
- Basketball
- Fast cycling
- Cross-country skiing

- Swimming laps
- Singles tennis
- Other racket sports
- Soccer

Following are roadblocks to physical activities. Mark the ones that apply to you and consider ways to get past them.

| Roadblock | How to get past it |
|---|---|
| \_\_\_\_\_ I don't have time. | Thirty minutes a day can be gained from most schedules. Give up a TV show. Work out three times for 10 minutes each. |
| \_\_\_\_\_ I don't enjoy exercise. | Don't "exercise." Begin a hobby or a way of playing that gets you moving. |
| \_\_\_\_\_ I'm usually too tired to exercise. | Tell yourself "This exercise will give me more energy." Then try it and see if it doesn't happen. |
| \_\_\_\_\_ The weather is too bad. | There are many activities you can do in your home. |
| \_\_\_\_\_ Exercise is boring. | Listen to music while you exercise. Walking, biking, or running can take you past interesting scenery. |
| \_\_\_\_\_ I get sore when I exercise. | Build up gradually, and stretch after the activity. |

## Activity Log

Use this log to track your physical activity. Note any roadblocks that discourage you, and note how you can get around them. When this log is full, make one of your own.

| Date | Activity | Minutes | Feelings/Comments |
|---|---|---|---|
| \_\_\_\_\_ | \_\_\_\_\_ | \_\_\_\_\_ | \_\_\_\_\_ |
| \_\_\_\_\_ | \_\_\_\_\_ | \_\_\_\_\_ | \_\_\_\_\_ |
| \_\_\_\_\_ | \_\_\_\_\_ | \_\_\_\_\_ | \_\_\_\_\_ |
| \_\_\_\_\_ | \_\_\_\_\_ | \_\_\_\_\_ | \_\_\_\_\_ |
| \_\_\_\_\_ | \_\_\_\_\_ | \_\_\_\_\_ | \_\_\_\_\_ |
| \_\_\_\_\_ | \_\_\_\_\_ | \_\_\_\_\_ | \_\_\_\_\_ |
| \_\_\_\_\_ | \_\_\_\_\_ | \_\_\_\_\_ | \_\_\_\_\_ |
| \_\_\_\_\_ | \_\_\_\_\_ | \_\_\_\_\_ | \_\_\_\_\_ |
| \_\_\_\_\_ | \_\_\_\_\_ | \_\_\_\_\_ | \_\_\_\_\_ |

**Keeping the Pace**

Physical Activity Status Score: 5 to 8

Congratulations. You are regularly physically active. Sometimes you may even lose sight of the physical and mental health benefits you get from being active. What motivates you to stay active?

1. _____

2. _____

3. _____

Review Your Program

Review your activities to see if you need to make any changes. The goal is to improve your chances of *remaining* active.

What types of activities do you usually do? _____

How many times a week? _____

How long each time? _____

Who helps you or does the activity with you? _____

Have you had any injuries? _____

What parts of your activity plan are you most satisfied with?

_____

What parts of your activity plan are you least satisfied with?

_____

What changes might you make in your activity plan to make it more enjoyable, convenient, or safe?

_____

Looking Ahead for Roadblocks

Even people who are normally regularly active have stopped their activity—sometimes for a few weeks, sometimes for a year or more. Answering these questions now can help you get past roadblocks later.

If you've stopped regular activity before, what caused you to stop?

_____

What could you have done differently that would have helped you stay active or what helped you to get back on track quickly?

_____

What situation or thing is most likely to make you stop being active?

_____

What can you do to prevent or prepare for this roadblock?

_____

What is the best way for you to get back on track if you stop?

_____

## Keeping the Pace

How confident are you that you can continue to be regularly physically active for the next three months?

No confidence _____

Low confidence _____

Medium confidence _____

High confidence _____

What reduces your confidence, and what can you do to improve your confidence?

_____


## How to Get Back on Track

- Remind yourself it's okay to have a pause in your activity once in a while. Don't be hard on yourself. Feeling guilty will make it more difficult to get back on track.

- You may need some extra help to get going again. Ask family and friends to help and encourage you.

- Ask someone to exercise with you.

- It may help to tell important people in your life that you are restarting your activity plan.

- Use an activity log to track your activity.

- Reward yourself. Use things that give you enjoyment, and don't make the rewards either too easy or too hard to attain.

- Try new activities.

- Go back to what worked for you in the past.

## Assess Your Self-Motivation to Be Regularly Physically Active

Read each statement below and circle the number that best describes how you feel about the statement.

|  | Very unlike me | Somewhat unlike me | Neither like me nor unlike me | Somewhat like me | Very much like me |
|---|---|---|---|---|---|
| I get discouraged easily. | 5 | 4 | 3 | 2 | 1 |
| I'm good at making decisions and standing by them. | 1 | 2 | 3 | 4 | 5 |
| I seldom if ever let myself down. | 1 | 2 | 3 | 4 | 5 |
| I'm good at keeping promises, especially ones I make to myself. | 1 | 2 | 3 | 4 | 5 |
| If something gets to be too much of an effort, I'm likely to just forget it. | 5 | 4 | 3 | 2 | 1 |
| I'm just not the goal-setting type. | 5 | 4 | 3 | 2 | 1 |

Add the numbers you circled in the assessment above, adapted from Dishman and Ickes (1978). If you scored less than 18, you're probably prone to dropping out. The lower your score, the more likely it is that you may discontinue a regular exercise program.

Also, if your body fat estimate is equal to or greater than 20% (men) or 25% (women), you're probably prone to dropping out. The higher percentage of body fat, the more likely you will eventually stop exercising.

If your self-motivation score or body fat percent indicates that you're a dropout candidate, view this as a challenge to remain active. And remember, these are general indicators that apply to groups of people, not to each individual within a group. Some highly motivated people who are lean do drop out, and some with lower motivation and more body fat do adhere to regular exercise.

## Consider Gains and Losses From Being Physically Active

A decision-balance sheet like the one below (adapted from Wankel 1984a), can help you consider the potential gains and losses of an action, such as participating in a fitness program. Through this process, people often think of benefits and difficulties they weren't initially aware of. This helps in planning to obtain benefits and reduce undesired outcomes. By considering the potential costs and benefits you can make a better-informed decision and be more likely to stick with the decision. Fill in the categories on the balance sheet as completely as you can. "Tactics" refers to maximizing gains and minimizing losses.

| Gains to self | Losses to self | Tactics |
| --- | --- | --- |
| Gains to others | Losses to others | Tactics |
| Approval from others | Disapproval from others | Tactics |
| Self-approval | Self-disapproval | Tactics |

Once you make a decision to be active, follow up with a written commitment. This may help you stick with your decision. The contract might be as simple as this:

"I will spend at least 30 minutes in some type of physical activity in my spare time four or five days each week for the next two months."

My signature _____      Witness _____

Both you and the witness should keep a copy of the contract. You can build rewards or punishments into the contract to strengthen its effect.

## Setting Goals

All people have basic needs to achieve and gain recognition for accomplishments, to feel worthy and accepted by others and by themselves, and to feel good and derive pleasure from activities. In terms of physical activity, the need to achieve leads to task-oriented goals focusing on an outcome: to lose weight, improve aerobic fitness, increase strength, learn new activities, and so on. The need to belong, on the other hand, is based more on acceptance than on obtaining an outcome. That is, people have a basic desire to feel worthy and be accepted by others or to accept themselves. People also are active for the immediate pleasure of the activity.

Examples of these types of goals are:

Achievement goals—to lose 10 pounds; to run a mile in under 10 minutes

Person (worthiness/acceptance) goals—to feel good about my body and myself; to feel I am an accepted member of a group

Pleasure goals—to reduce anxiety or tension; to feel energized and exhilarated

Understanding how your reasons for being physically active fit into these categories of motivation can help you set goals and devise tactics to reach them. Overemphasizing one goal increases the likelihood that you will stop being active if you don't reach that goal.

This lab experience (adapted from Wankel 1984b) will give you a chance to consider the goals that you have for your physical activity program. After you identify these goals we'll ask you to identify how you, your instructor, or your friends or family can act to help you meet your goals.

What specific task outcomes do you want to achieve through physical activity? Indicate the importance of each outcome by circling the appropriate number (1 = not at all important, 5 = very important).

1. _____ 1  2  3  4  5

2. _____ 1  2  3  4  5

3. _____ 1  2  3  4  5

What specific behaviors (actions, words) of the following people will help you reach these goals?

Yourself                    Instructor                    Friends or family

1. _____    _____    _____

2. _____    _____    _____

3. _____    _____    _____

What person goals (e.g., feelings and relationships) do you want to satisfy through physical activity? Indicate the importance by circling the appropriate number (1 = not at all important, 5 = very important).

1. _____ 1  2  3  4  5

2. _____ 1  2  3  4  5

3. _____ 1  2  3  4  5

What specific behaviors (actions, words) of the following people will help you reach these goals?

Yourself                Instructor                    Friends or family

1. _____    _____             _____

2. _____    _____             _____

3. _____    _____             _____


What pleasure goals (e.g., feelings during physical activity) do you want to satisfy through physical activity? Indicate the importance by circling the appropriate number (1 = not at all important, 5 = very important).

1. _____  1   2   3   4   5

2. _____  1   2   3   4   5

3. _____  1   2   3   4   5


What specific behaviors (actions, words) of the following people will help you reach these goals?

Yourself                Instructor                    Friends or family

1. _____    _____             _____

2. _____    _____             _____

3. _____    _____             _____

## Ratings of Perceived Exertion

Borg's RPE scale is one way to assess exercise intensity. One formula used to test the similarity between perceived exercise intensity as determined by RPE and actual exercise intensity as determined by heart rate is RPE × 10 = HR at any given exercise intensity. The following laboratory experience, adapted from Falls, Baylor, and Dishman (1988), will help you determine how closely this formula depicts your RPE.

A class can do this lab as a group, with an instructor timing and recording, or students can pair up. Use the work sheet provided on page 352 to record your RPE and heart rate at each of the exercise intensities outlined at the bottom of the page, and follow the instructions for carrying out the walks and runs to be used for obtaining the RPE.

As you are exercising at each intensity, you should estimate how hard you *feel* the activity is: rate the degree of perceived exertion you feel. This perceived exertion includes the total amount of exertion and physical fatigue you experience and should be a combination of all the sensations of physical stress, effort, and fatigue you feel. Don't concern yourself with only one factor, such as leg discomfort or shortness of breath, but try to concentrate on your *total, inner* feeling of overall exertion. Try to estimate honestly and as objectively as possible. Use Borg's RPE scale to rate your exercise intensity (note that it is necessary to read *Borg's Perceived Exertion and Pain Scales* to fully understand the scale and its administration).

For this lab you'll need a 400-meter (436-yard) running track or other suitable running area with 50-meter (55-yard) intervals marked off; a stopwatch or wristwatch with a second hand; and a whistle (please note that this lab can also be modified for use with a cycle ergometer, or even swimming). Before beginning the lab, you'll need to determine your resting heart rate. To do this, count your pulse for one minute first thing in the morning, before getting out of bed.

After a brief warm-up period, the goal is for each person to complete one lap of the track at each of the six speeds (in miles per hour) listed in the table on page 352. Make sure to take a break between each lap so that your heart rate recovers to within 10 beats of your resting heart rate. If at the end of any stage your heart rate is equal to or exceeds 90% of your age-predicted heart rate, or, your RPE is equal to or exceeds 17, stop the exercise portion of the lab at that speed.

As an aid in exact pacing, your instructor or partner will give a whistle blast at each of the elapsed times called for in the table. Remember, you need to keep with the pacing to complete this exercise successfully. During the last few seconds of each 400-meter (436-yard) walk or run, choose an RPE value from the Borg scale. The number you choose should be your best estimate of how intense the exercise actually is. Report this number to your partner. *Immediately* after you rate your perceived exertion and have stopped walking or running, locate your pulse (see figure 2.4); count the number of beats in 15 seconds and multiply by 4 to calculate the beats per minute. Always rate and record your RPE *before* your heart rate. Record both of these values in the appropriate spaces on the work sheet.

| 6 | No exertion at all |
|---|---|
| 7 | |
| 8 | Extremely light |
| 9 | Very light |
| 10 | |
| 11 | Light |
| 12 | |
| 13 | Somewhat hard |
| 14 | |
| 15 | Hard   (heavy) |
| 16 | |
| 17 | Very hard |
| 18 | |
| 19 | Extremely hard |
| 20 | Maximal exertion |

Borg RPE scale
© Gunnar Borg, 1970, 1985, 1994, 1998

## Elapsed Times for Different Walks and Runs*

| | Walks | | Runs | | | |
|---|---|---|---|---|---|---|
| | (1) | (2) | (1) | (2) | (3) | (4) |
| | 3 mph | 4 mph** | 5 mph | 6 mph | 6.67 mph | 7.5 mph |
| 1st 50 m | 0:37.5 | 0:28.0 | 0:22.5 | 0:19.0 | 0:17.0 | 0:15.0 |
| 2nd 50 m | 1:15.0 | 0:56.0 | 0:45.0 | 0:37.5 | 0:34.0 | 0:30.0 |
| 3rd 50 m | 1:52.5 | 1:24.0 | 1:07.5 | 0:56.5 | 0:51.0 | 0:45.0 |
| 4th 50 m | 2:30.0 | 1:52.0 | 1:30.0 | 1:15.0 | 1:07.5 | 1:00.0 |
| 5th 50 m | 3:07.5 | 2:20.0 | 1:52.5 | 1:34.0 | 1:24.0 | 1:15.0 |
| 6th 50 m | 3:45.0 | 2:48.0 | 2:15.0 | 1:52.5 | 1:41.0 | 1:30.0 |
| 7th 50 m | 4:22.5 | 3:16.0 | 2:37.5 | 2:11.5 | 1:58.0 | 1:45.0 |
| 8th 50 m | 5:00.0 | 3:44.0 | 3:00.0 | 2:30.0 | 2:15.0 | 2:00.0 |

*Times are in minutes and seconds.
**Some individuals may have difficulty walking 400 meters at this speed.

After you've completed all of the exercise intensity levels and recorded all RPE and heart rate values, connect each RPE point with a solid line and each heart rate point with a dashed line. Compare the slopes of the two lines. How similar are they? They should be reasonably close. As another way to view your personal results with Borg's model, multiply your RPE by 10 at each activity level. Compare this new plot with your measured heart rate at each intensity and determine how close they are.

This model has been found to be about 80% accurate, so it isn't unusual to have some discrepancy between your RPE × 10 and your actual heart rate at each exercise intensity level. Is there a consistent difference in the values? For example, do you need to add or subtract 20 beats per minute to make your heart rate and RPE agree? The important idea to take with you is that careful monitoring of your RPE can help you avoid working at an intensity that is too high (or too low) for your individual fitness level in the beginning stages of your fitness program. This will help prevent excessive stress and discomfort resulting from too much exercise or from exercising in high heat or humidity, which can inhibit even a highly conditioned exerciser.

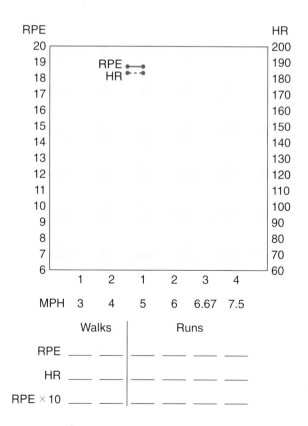

# Glossary

**activities of daily living (ADL)**—Basic necessary tasks of life that are measured in older persons to determine their functional status.

**adenosine triphosphate (ATP)**—The chemical compound that is the immediate source of energy for physical activity.

**adrenocorticotropin (ACTH)**—A hormone released from the hypothalamus that stimulates the secretion of cortisol from the adrenal gland during stress.

**aerobic**—Producing energy for physical activity with oxygen.

**anaerobic**—Producing energy for physical activity without oxygen.

**android obesity**—The distribution of more body fat above the waist (apple-shaped). This distribution of body fat is associated with an increased risk for cardiovascular disease.

**angina**—Chest pain due to insufficient blood flow to part of the heart.

**anorexia nervosa**—A medical condition in which people starve themselves by restricting caloric intake.

**anxiety disorders**—The most common mental illnesses in the United States, characterized by apprehension or worry accompanied by restlessness, tension, and elevated heart rate and breathing. Anxiety disorders include phobias, panic disorder, obsessive-compulsive disorder, and generalized anxiety disorder.

**arrhythmia**—An abnormal heartbeat caused by a breakdown of the heart's electronic impulses.

**arthritis**—General term used to describe more than 100 diseases that cause joint inflammation and loss of movement. The most common forms are osteoarthritis and rheumatoid arthritis.

**atherosclerosis**—The process of the buildup of plaque on the inner walls of the arteries, which restricts blood flow.

**atrophy**—A decrease in muscle size that occurs in response to inactivity or immobilization.

**attitude**—A belief that carries an emotional component and predisposes someone to act.

**ballistic stretching**—A stretching exercise that includes dynamic action (for example, bouncing).

**basal metabolic rate (BMR)**—The metabolic rate necessary to sustain life.

**behavior modification**—The use of stimulus-response learning to change behavior by manipulating cues and reinforcers in the environment.

**beliefs**—Expectations about the outcomes that result from participating in physical activity.

**benign tumor**—Noncancerous tumor that remains localized and usually is treated with little risk of death.

**benzodiazepines**—A family of antianxiety and sleep drugs that promote relaxation without sedation.

**bioelectric impedance**—A method of estimating percent body fat by measuring the speed with which an electric current passes through the body. Since electrical current passes more easily through lean tissue than through fat tissue, the time the current takes to travel through the body reflects the amount of fat.

**body composition**—The parts or components of body tissues. For health purposes, body composition consists of lean and fat tissue.

**body density**—The body's weight divided by its volume (the compactness of the body). A leaner person of a given weight has a higher density than a fatter person of the same weight.

**body mass index (BMI)**—A measure of body composition in which a person's weight in kilograms is divided by the square of the height in meters.

**bone mineral density**—Mineralized bone mass. The measure of bone mineral density is the best predictor of bone strength.

**bulimia**—A medical condition in which people go through a cycle of bingeing (massive calorie consumption) and purging (reducing the effects of calorie consumption through vomiting, taking laxatives, and exercising).

**bursitis**—Inflammation of a bursa.

**caloric balance**—A state in which calorie consumption equals caloric expenditure so that there is no change in body weight.

**cancer**—A complex group of diseases characterized by the uncontrolled growth and spread of abnormal cells.

**carbohydrates**—Compounds consisting of carbon, hydrogen, and oxygen. Some carbohydrates (sugars and starches) are digestible and provide the body with energy. Others (insoluble fiber) are not digestible but still have important functions.

**cardiorespiratory**—Pertaining to the cardiac (heart) and respiratory (lung) systems.

**cellulite**—Term used to represent fatty deposits on the thighs and arms. Cellulite is not supported by science as a specific type of fat.

**cerebral hemorrhage**—Bleeding into the brain that occurs when an artery within the brain bursts because of a weak spot (an aneurysm) in the arterial wall or because of a head injury.

**cerebral thrombosis**—Clotting of blood that occurs when atherosclerosis creates blockage in an artery in the brain or an artery bringing blood to the brain.

**cholesterol**—A fatlike substance found in the body's cells and bloodstream.

**cognitive behavior modification**—The use of *behavior modification* to alter psychological skills that people can use to self-regulate behavior changes.

**complementing proteins**—Combining protein-rich foods in such a way that the limiting amino acid in one food is "completed" by the abundance of that specific amino acid in another food.

**complex carbohydrates**—A form of carbohydrate commonly referred to as starch that consists of hundreds of simple carbohydrates (sugars) linked together.

**concentric muscle action**—Movement in which a muscle produces force by shortening (contracting).

**contusion**—A deep muscle bruise.

**coronary thrombosis**—A heart attack caused by blockage of a coronary artery.

**cortisol**—A steroid hormone released by the cortex of the adrenal gland that repairs tissues and regulates blood glucose levels during stress.

**creeping obesity**—The gradual and consistent increase in body fat weight over the years.

**cross training**—Participation in one sport to improve performance in another, or use of several different types of training to achieve a goal.

**cues**—Environmental events or objects that prompt behavior.

**cumulative trauma disorder**—See *overuse injury.*

**decision-balance**—A judgment that contrasts the positive and negative consequences of a change in behavior; used in *cognitive behavior modification* to persuade a person to change behavior.

**delayed onset muscle soreness (DOMS)**—Muscle soreness that occurs 24 to 48 hours after muscular activity performed at higher-than-accustomed intensity.

**depression**—Feelings of despair or hopelessness accompanied by a loss of pleasure; signs include significant weight loss or gain, insomnia or hypersomnia, psychomotor agitation or retardation, fatigue, feelings of worthlessness or guilt, and suicidal thoughts or attempts.

**desirable body weight**—The body weight that should produce a desirable body composition. This weight is often used as a simple goal in a weight loss program.

**diabetes mellitus**—A metabolic disorder resulting in the inability to properly metabolize carbohydrates and control blood sugar levels because the normal insulin mechanism is ineffective.

**diastasis recti**—Condition seen during the third trimester of pregnancy in which the rectus abdominis muscles separate into two parts down the center of the abdomen.

**diastolic blood pressure**—Blood pressure as measured when the heart is not contracting.

**eccentric muscle action**—Movement in which a muscle produces force by lengthening.

**epidemiology**—The study of the incidence and distribution of diseases, injuries, and accidents in human populations.

**essential amino acids**—Amino acids that the body cannot produce itself and must take in through the diet.

**estrogen**—Hormone whose level rises during pregnancy and stimulates growth of the breasts and uterus.

**exercise adherence**—Maintaining an exercise program; generally used to describe the problem of starting and maintaining a physical activity habit.

**fat-soluble vitamins**—Vitamins (A, D, E, and K) that need to dissolve in fat to be transported into and around the body.

**fats**—Compounds consisting of carbon, hydrogen, and oxygen that do not dissolve in water.

**flexibility**—The range of motion a person can achieve at any joint through any particular movement.

**functional capacity**—The basic mental and physical ability to accomplish necessary and desired tasks of daily living.

**genes**—The microscopic structures in every cell that contain the genetic codes determining to a large degree our appearance, personality, body composition, intelligence, natural resistance to disease, and fitness level.

**gestational diabetes**—A form of diabetes that develops during pregnancy and typically disappears after the baby is delivered.

**gynoid obesity**—The distribution of more body fat below the waist (pear-shaped).

**health**—Freedom from disease with sufficient energy and vitality to accomplish daily tasks and active recreational pursuits without undue fatigue.

**health-related fitness**—One aspect of fitness that is focused on areas affecting overall health and energy and our ability to perform daily tasks and activities. Its components include cardiorespiratory fitness, body composition, and musculoskeletal fitness.

**healthy aging**—The use of lifestyle choices to maximize longevity and increase quality of life.

**high density lipoproteins (HDL)**—Lipoproteins that combine with cholesterol to form HDL-cholesterol, the "good" cholesterol that is transported through the bloodstream to the liver for further metabolism or excretion.

**hydrostatic weighing**—Method used to determine the difference between a person's scale weight and weight underwater. A leaner person of a given weight will weigh more under water than a fatter person of the same weight.

**hypertension**—A condition that occurs when a person's blood pressure is continuously abnormally high.

**hyperthermia**—The condition in which the body's internal temperature rises to a life-threatening level.

**hypertrophy**—An increase in muscle size that occurs in response to strength training and is associated with increased strength.

**hypoglycemia**—Abnormally low blood sugar.

**hypotension**—A condition that occurs when a person's blood pressure is continuously abnormally low.

**hypothalamus**—A part of the brain that regulates cardiovascular, endocrine, and behavioral responses during stress.

**hypothermia**—The condition in which the body's internal temperature declines to a life-threatening level.

**hypoxia**—A condition in which insufficient oxygen is going to the fetus during pregnancy.

**inflammation**—A tissue's initial response to injury; signs of inflammation are heat, redness, pain, and swelling.

**insoluble fiber**—A type of complete carbohydrate that is not digested by the human body. Aids in absorption and elimination in the lower intestines.

**insulin**—Hormone that regulates carbohydrate, fat, and protein metabolism.

**isokinetic muscle action**—Movement in which a muscle produces force by moving the joint at a constant rate and through the same range of motion.

**isometric muscle action**—Force production by a muscle that involves no change in muscle length.

**isotonic muscle action**—Movement in which a muscle produces force against a constant resistance, such as a barbell, by shortening or lengthening.

**kilocalories**—Units of heat that measure the energy in food. A kilocalorie is actually 1,000 calories, but most people simplify the term to just calories and the two terms are used interchangeably.

**kyphotic curves**—Areas of the spine that are convex (curving outward) when viewed from the side.

**limbic system**—Network of brain regions, including the amygdala, hippocampus, and hypothalamus, that are important for generating emotional and behavioral responses during stress.

**lipoprotein**—A fat/protein compound that carries fat in the blood.

**locus coeruleus**—A small area of the upper brainstem; this group of cells manufactures noradrenaline, modulates other brain areas during stress, and helps initiate responses.

**lordotic curves**—Areas of the spine that are concave (curving inward) when viewed from the side.

**low density lipoproteins (LDL)**—Lipoproteins that combine with cholesterol to form LDL-cholesterol, which is the "bad" cholesterol because not all of it is transported and metabolized or excreted; high levels of LDL-cholesterol hasten the process of atherosclerosis.

**lumbar lordosis**—Normal curvature in the lumbar region of the spine.

**maximal oxygen consumption ($\dot{V}O_2$max)**—The maximum amount of oxygen the body can extract and utilize during extreme exercise. It is measured in milliliters of oxygen per minute per kilogram of body weight.

**Medicare**—A program of the Social Security system that is designed to help older persons cover their medical expenses.

**melanoma**—A deadly type of skin cancer. The principal sign of melanoma is any noticeable change in a mole or dark-pigmented area of the skin.

**metastasize**—The spread of cancerous cells to other areas of the body.

**minerals**—Chemical elements such as calcium, iron, and sodium that are essential for numerous body processes and structures.

**moderate physical activity**—Physical activity that uses approximately 150 kilocalories of energy per day, or 1,000 kilocalories per week.

**muscular endurance**—A muscle's ability to produce force over and over again.

**myocardial infarction**—A heart attack.

**negative energy balance**—State in which more calories are expended than are consumed. A negative energy balance will lead to weight loss.

**neurotransmitters**—Biochemicals that influence the activity of the brain cells regulating mood, pleasure, and rational thought; necessary to transduce an electrical impulse from a nerve cell to another cell.

**noradrenaline**—The main nerve chemical of the sympathetic nervous system and one of two major neurotransmitters in the brain that modulate the nerve activity of certain other cells; these in turn stimulate the behavioral (e.g., motivation) and physiological (e.g., heart rate, blood pressure, hormones) responses needed to cope with stress. Helps regulate sleep and responses to pain.

**obesity**—The condition of overfatness that increases the risk of morbidity and mortality (more than 25% body fat for men, more than 30% body fat for women).

**old**—Characterizing a person 65 to 84 years old.

**oncogenes**—Cancer-causing genes present in the body.

**one-repetition maximum (1-RM)**—The heaviest weight a person can successfully lift one time while maintaining proper form.

**osteoporosis**—An abnormal loss of bone mineral density—that is, beyond the normal loss that occurs with aging.

**overfat**—Referring to the accumulation of excess weight in the form of body fat. *Overweight* is typically a result of overfatness.

**overuse injury**—An injury that occurs as a result of excessive repetition of a movement or force.

**overweight**—The condition in which body weight exceeds (generally by 20%) an arbitrary figure according to height and frame size.

**periodization**—The planned progression of workouts over time. Each cycle emphasizes a different goal that contributes to the overall purpose of the training program.

**physical activity**—In simplest terms, moving about.

**plyometrics**—Exercises that involve rapid concentric muscle actions immediately after eccentric actions; they are designed to increase power.

**positive energy balance**—State in which more calories are consumed than are expended. A long-term positive energy balance leads to weight gain and obesity.

**power**—The amount of work performed in a given amount of time, often considered the product of strength and speed.

**proprioceptive neuromuscular facilitation**—A type of stretching that takes advantage of the body's reflex responses to enhance muscle relaxation and joint range of motion; it involves contracting the muscles around the joint to elicit reflex responses that contribute to enhanced range of motion.

**protein**—Consisting of carbon, oxygen, hydrogen, and nitrogen, proteins are a component of every living cell. Amino acids are the building blocks of proteins; the number and order of amino acids determines the type of protein.

**raphe nuclei**—Clusters of cells located along the midline of the brain stem in the region of the pons near the locus coeruleus. Neurons project from the raphe to the brain cortex, limbic system, cerebellum, and the brain stem where they help regulate sleep, appetite, pain, and cardiovascular and behavioral responses to stress.

**rating of perceived exertion (RPE)**—The rating of a person's perception of the sensations of effort during physical activity.

**recommended daily allowance (RDA)**—The recommended levels of intake for certain nutrients. The RDAs are set at levels high enough to take care of the nutrient needs of almost all healthy people.

**reinforcers**—Events added or removed in the environment that increase a behavior.

**reinforcement control**—A technique used in *behavior modification* to establish rewarding or punishing outcomes that are contingent on behavior change.

**relapse prevention**—A technique used in cognitive behavior modification to reduce the risk that a temporary slip during behavior change will lead to a complete failure or a return to old habits (i.e., a relapse).

**relaxin**—A hormone that softens ligaments, connective tissue, and the cervix of pregnant women to aid in the baby's delivery.

**repetition (rep)**—One complete movement of a weight-lifting exercise.

**resting metabolic rate (RMR)**—The metabolic rate (calories expended) during rest (plus the basal metabolic rate).

**risk factor**—A variable that is associated with an increased risk or probability that someone may develop morbidity (illness) or incur mortality (death) from a specific disease.

**saturated fat**—A type of fatty acid that is generally linked to an increased risk of elevated blood cholesterol; usually found in whole milk, cheese, meat, poultry, and other animal products, and in palm, palm kernel, and coconut oils.

**self-esteem**—The value people place on their conception or view of themselves.

**self-monitoring**—Keeping a record of your own behavior; a personal surveillance technique that is important for behavior change.

**self-motivation**—Similar to *willpower;* the ability to persist toward a goal without extrinsic reward.

**self-regulation**—Using behavioral skills such as self-monitoring, goal setting, cues, and rewards to prompt and sustain a personal behavior change.

**self-reinforcement**—The personal administration of rewards, contingent on a change in behavior.

**serotonin**—One of two major neurotransmitters in the brain that modulate the nerve activity of certain other cells; these in turn stimulate behavioral (e.g., motivation) and physiological (e.g., heart rate, blood pressure, hormones) responses needed to cope with stress. Also produced by blood platelets.

**set**—A series of repetitions of a weight-lifting exercise.

**simple carbohydrates**—The smallest form of carbohydrate, also referred to as sugars that occur naturally in milk, fruits, and other plant foods.

**skill-related fitness**—An aspect of fitness that refers to an ability to perform specific skills required to take part in various activities and sports.

**skinfold measurements**—Measures of subcutaneous fat at various sites on the body.

**social support**—Encouragement or other deeds that permit, facilitate, or reward someone's behavior.

**soft tissue injuries**—Musculoskeletal injuries that involve tissues such as ligaments, muscles, tendons, and bursa.

**soluble fiber**—A type of complex carbohydrate that binds with cholesterol in the intestines to keep it from being absorbed, thus reducing blood cholesterol.

**spot reduction**—The desire or attempt to eliminate body fat deposits in specific areas of the body, such as stomach, hips, and thighs.

**sprain**—An injury resulting from overstretching a ligament.

**state anxiety**—Feelings of anxiety that are temporary and fluctuate from moment to moment.

**static stretching**—Stretching either actively (i.e., with no assistance) or passively (i.e., with assistance) and holding the stretch at the end of the joint's range of motion for anywhere from 3 to 60 seconds.

**steady state**—The stage of aerobic exercise at which the heart rate and oxygen consumption remain stable (i.e., level) for a period of time.

**stimulus control**—A technique used in *behavior modification* to manipulate cues in the environment that prompt a behavior.

**strain**—An injury resulting from overstretching a muscle.

**strength**—The ability of a muscle to produce force, often represented by the 1-repetition maximum.

**stress fracture**—A type of fracture that comes from overtraining rather than acute trauma. Stress fractures occur from repetitive force on a bone.

**stroke**—A "brain attack" caused by a lack of blood flow to the brain.

**systolic blood pressure**—Blood pressure as measured when the heart is contracted.

**tendinitis**—Inflammation of a tendon.

**thermogenesis**—The caloric expenditure resulting from the body's attempt to digest food and maintain a constant body temperature.

**trait anxiety**—Condition in which feelings and symptoms of anxiety are constant and persistent.

**triglycerides**—A form of fat in the blood that is associated with an increased risk for coronary heart disease.

**tumor**—Mass of abnormal cells.

**type I diabetes**—A form of diabetes that requires daily injections of insulin. Also referred to as insulin-dependent diabetes mellitus or juvenile diabetes.

**type II diabetes**—The more common form of diabetes that can often be managed through diet, exercise, and weight control. Also referred to as noninsulin-dependent diabetes mellitus or adult onset diabetes.

**unsaturated fats**—There are two types of unsaturated fat: monounsaturated and polyunsaturated. Monounsaturated fats, found primarily in olive, canola, and peanut oils, have been shown to reduce "bad" (LDL-C) cholesterol levels while leaving "good" (HDL-C) cholesterol levels the same. Polyunsaturated fats, found primarily in corn, safflower, cottonseed, and fish oils, have been found to reduce both types of cholesterol.

**Valsalva maneuver**—Holding one's breath while performing a weight-lifting exercise; not recommended because it exaggerates the blood pressure response to exercise.

**values**—The valences or importance attached to a *belief.*

**very old**—Characterizing a person 85 years old or over.

**vitamins**—Food compounds that are needed in small amounts to regulate various metabolic reactions.

**waist circumference/hip circumference ratio**—The circumference of the waist divided by the circumference of the hips (used to detect android obesity).

**water-soluble vitamins**—Vitamins (B-complex and C) that dissolve easily in water and are absorbed directly from the intestines into the blood.

**willpower**—The strength of someone's ability to act on intentions.

# References

American Cancer Society. 1992. *How to do breast self-examination.* Austin, TX: American Cancer Society.

American Cancer Society. 1998. *Cancer facts and figures—1996.* New York: American Cancer Society.

American College of Obstetricians and Gynecologists. 1994. Exercise during pregnancy and the postpartum period. *ACOG Technical Bulletin* 189 (February): 1-5.

American College of Sports Medicine (ACSM). 1987. Position stand on the prevention of thermal injuries during distance running. *Medicine and Science in Sports and Exercise* 19: 529-533.

American College of Sports Medicine (ACSM). 1998. The recommended quantity and quality of exercise for developing and maintaining cardiorespiratory and muscular fitness, and flexibility in healthy adults. *Medicine and Science in Sports and Exercise* 30(6): 975-991.

American College of Sports Medicine (ACSM). 1998. ACSM position stand: Exercise and physical activity for older adults. *Medicine and Science in Sports and Exercise* 30 (6): 992-1008.

American Heart Association. 1993. Rationale of the Diet-Heart Statement of the American Heart Association. *Circulation* 88 (6): 3008-3029.

American Heart Association. 1994. *Heart and stroke facts.* Dallas: American Heart Association.

American Heart Association. 1996. *Heart and stroke facts.* Dallas: American Heart Association.

American Heart Association. 1998. *Heart and stroke statistical update.* Dallas: American Heart Association.

Andrew, G.M., B. Oldridge, J.O. Parker, D.A. Cunningham, et al. 1981. Reasons for dropout from exercise programs in post coronary patients. *Medicine & Science in Sports and Exercise* 13: 164-168.

Baechle, T.R., and B.R. Groves. 1998. *Weight training: Steps to success.* 2d ed. Champaign, IL: Human Kinetics.

Bassey, E.J., and S.J. Ramsdale. 1994. Increase in femoral bone density in young women following high-impact exercise. *Osteoporosis International* 4: 72-75.

Benson, H. 1975. *The relaxation response.* New York: Morrow.

Black, P.H. 1995. Psychoneuroimmunology: brain and immunity. *Scientific American: Science and Medicine* 2(6): 17.

Blair, S.N., H.W. Kohl III, R.S. Paffenbarger, D.G. Clark, K.H. Cooper, and L.W. Gibbons. 1989. Physical fitness and all-cause mortality: A prospective study of healthy men and women. *Journal of the American Medical Association* 262: 2395-2401.

Blair, S.N. 1993. C.H. McCloy Research Lecture: Physical activity, physical fitness, and health. *Research Quarterly for Exercise and Sport* 64: 365-376.

Blair, S.N., J.B. Kampert, H.W. Kohl III, C.E. Barlow, C.A. Macera, R.S. Paffenbarger, and L.W. Gibbons. 1996. Influences of cardiorespiratory fitness and other precursors on cardiovascular disease and all-cause mortality in men and women. *Journal of the American Medical Association* 276: 205-210.

Boissonnault, J., and M. Blaschak. 1988. Incidence of diastasis recti abdominis during the childbearing years. *Physical Therapy* 68: 1082.

Borg, G.A.V. 1998. *Borg's perceived exertion and pain scales.* Champaign, IL: Human Kinetics (47).

Bouchard, C., L. Perusse, C. Leblanc, A. Theriault, and G. Theriault. 1988. Inheritance of the amount and distribution of body fat. *International Journal of Obesity* 12: 205-215.

Breslow, L., and N. Breslow. 1993. Health practices and disability: Some evidence from Alameda County. *Preventive Medicine* 22 (1): 86-95.

Breus, M.J., and P.J. O'Connor. 1998. Exercise-induced anxiolysis: A test of the "time out" hypothesis in high anxious females. *Medicine and Science in Sports and Exercise* 30: 1107-1112.

Brody, D. 1993. Building bigger babies. *American Health,* November, 88.

Carlson, N.R. 1998. *Physiology of behavior,* 6ed. Needham Heights, MA: Allyn & Bacon.

Chu, D.A. 1998. *Jumping into plyometrics.* 2d ed. Champaign, IL: Human Kinetics.

Coggan, A.R., R.J. Spina, D.S. King, et al. 1992. Skeletal muscle adaptations to endurance training in 60- to 70-year old men and women. *Journal of Applied Physiology* 72 (5): 1780-1786.

Cohen, S., T. Kamarck, and R. Mermelstein. 1983. A global measure of perceived stress. *Journal of Health and Social Behavior* 24: 385-396.

Collings, C.A., L.B. Curet, and J.P. Mullin. 1983. Maternal and fetal responses to a maternal aerobic exercise program. *American Journal of Obstetrics and Gynecology* 145: 556-562.

Cooper Institute for Aerobics Research. 1992. The FITNESSGRAM. Dallas: Cooper Institute for Aerobics Research.

Desharnais, R., J. Jobin, C. Cote, et al. 1993. Aerobic exercise and the placebo effect: A controlled study. *Psychosomatic Medicine* 55: 149-154.

Dishman, R.K. 1988. *Exercise adherence: its impact on public health.* Champaign, IL: Human Kinetics.

Dishman, R.K. 1988. Supervised and free-living physical activity: No differences in former athletes and nonathletes. *American Journal of Preventive Medicine* 4: 153-160.

DuPont, R.L., D.P. Rice, L.S. Miller, S.S. Shiraki, C.R. Rowland, and H.J. Harwood. 1996. Economic costs of anxiety disorders. *Anxiety* 2 (4): 167-172.

Falls, H.B., A.M. Baylor, and R.K. Dishman. 1988. *Essentials of fitness.* Dubuque, IA: William C. Brown.

Farmer, M., B. Locke, E. Moscicki, A. Dannenberg, D. Larson, and L. Radloff. 1988. Physical activity and depressive symptoms: The NHANES I epidemiologic follow-up study. *American Journal of Epidemiology* 128 (6): 1340-1351.

Farrell, P.A., W.K. Gates, M.G. Maksud, and W.P. Morgan. 1982. Increases in plasma b-endorphin/b-lipoprotein immunoreactivity after treadmill running in humans. *Journal of Applied Physiology* 52: 1245-1249.

Fiatarone, M.A., E.F. O'Neill, N.D. Ryan, K.M. Clements, G.R. Solares, M.E. Nelson, S.B. Roberts, J.J. Kehayias, L.A. Lipsitz, and W.J. Evans. 1994. Exercise training and nutritional supplementation for physical frailty in very elderly people. *New England Journal of Medicine* 330: 1769-1775.

Fleck, S.J., and W.J. Kraemer. 1997. *Designing resistance training programs.* 2d ed. Champaign, IL: Human Kinetics.

Franklin, B.A., N.B. Oldridge, K.G. Stoedefalke, and W.F. Loechel. 1990. *On the ball.* Madison, WI: Brown & Benchmark.

Franks, B.D., and E.T. Howley. 1989. *Fitness facts.* Champaign, IL: Human Kinetics.

Frisch, R.E., G. Wyshak, N.L. Albright, T.E. Albright, L. Schiff, J. Witschi, and M. Marguglio. 1987. Lower lifetime occurrence of breast cancer and cancers of the reproductive system among former college athletes. *American Journal of Clinical Nutrition* 45: 328-335.

Gilliam, T.B., V.L. Katch, W. Thorland, and A.L. Weltman. 1977. Prevalence of cardiovascular disease risk factors in active children, 7 to 12 years of age. *Medicine and Science in Sports* 9: 21-25.

Goodman, C.C., and T.E. Snyder. 1995. *Differential diagnosis in physical therapy.* Philadelphia: Saunders.

Greenberg, P.E., L.E. Stiglin, S.N. Finkelstein, and E.R. Berndt. 1993. The economic burden of depression in 1990. *Journal of Clinical Psychiatry* 54: 405-418.

Hagberg, J.M., J.E. Graves, M. Limacher, D.R. Woods, S.H. Leggett, C. Cononie, J.J. Gruber, and M.L. Pollock. 1989. Cardiovascular responses of 70-79 year old men and women to exercise training. *Journal of Applied Physiology* 66: 2589-2594.

Hamermesh, D.S., and J.E. Biddle. 1994. Beauty and the labor market. *American Journal of Economics* 85 (March): 1174-1194.

Harvard Medical School. 1994. Losing weight: A new attitude emerges. *Harvard Health Letter* 4 (March): 1-6.

Haynes, S.G., S. Levine, N. Scotch, M. Feinleib, and W.B. Kannel. 1978. The relationship of psychosocial factors to coronary heart disease in the Framingham Study I: Methods and risk factors. *American Journal of Epidemiology* 107: 362-383.

*Healthy People 2000: National health promotion and disease prevention objectives.* 1990. Washington, DC: U.S. Department of Health and Human Services.

Heinzelmann, F., and R.W. Bagley. 1970. Response to physical activity programs and their effects on health behavior. *Public Health Reports* 86: 905-911.

Helmrich, S.P., D.R. Ragland, R.W. Leung, and R.S. Paffenbarger, Jr. 1991. Physical activity and reduced occurrence of non-insulin dependent diabetes mellitus. *New England Journal of Medicine* 325: 147-152.

Heyward, V. 1998. *Advanced exercise assessment and prescription.* 3d ed. Champaign, IL: Human Kinetics.

Howley, E.T., and B.D. Franks. 1992. *Health fitness instructor's handbook,* 2d ed. Champaign, IL: Human Kinetics.

Jackson, A.S., S.N. Blair, M.T. Mahar, L.T. Weir, R.M. Ross, and J.E. Stuteville. 1990. Prediction of functional aerobic capacity without exercise testing. *Medicine and Science in Sports and Exercise* 22: 863-870.

James, W.P. 1995. A public health approach to the problem of obesity. *International Journal of Obesity* 19: Supplement 3, S37-S45.

Katch, F.I., and W.D. McArdle. 1983. *Nutrition, weight control, and exercise.* Philadelphia: Lea & Febiger.

Kessler, R., K. McGonagle, S. Zhao, C. Nelson, M. Hughes, S. Eshleman, H. Wittchen, and K. Kendler. 1994. Lifetime and 12-month prevalence of DSM-III-R psychiatric disorders in the United States. *Archives of General Psychiatry* 51: 8-19.

Keyserling, W.M., G.D. Herrin, and D.B. Chaffin. 1980. Establishing an industrial strength testing program. *American Industrial Hygiene Association Journal* 41: 730-736.

King, A.C., W.L. Haskell, C.B. Taylor, H.C. Kraemer, and R.F. Debusk. 1991. Group- vs. home-based exercise training in healthy older men and women. *Journal of the American Medical Association* 266: 1535-1542.

King, A.C., R.F. Oman, G.S. Brassington, et al. 1997. Moderate-intensity exercise and self-rated quality of sleep in older adults: A randomized controlled trial. *Journal of the American Medical Association* 277 (1): 32-37.

Kline, G.M., J.P. Pocari, R. Hintermeister, P.S. Freedson, A. Ward, R.F. McCarron, J. Ross, and J.M. Rippe. 1987. Estimation of $\dot{V}O_2$max from a one-mile track walk, gender, age, and body weight. *Medicine and Science in Sports and Exercise* 19: 253-259.

Krall, E.A., and B. Dawson-Hughes. 1994. Walking is related to bone density and rates of bone loss. *American Journal of Medicine* 96: 20-26.

Manson, J.E., E.R. Rimm, M.J. Stampfer, G.A. Colditz, W.C. Willett, A.S. Krolewski, B. Rosner, C.H. Hennekens, and F.E. Spiezer. 1991. Physical activity and incidence of non-insulin dependent diabetes mellitus in women. *Lancet* 338: 774-778.

Morrow, J.R. Jr., A.W. Jackson, J.G. Disch, and D.P. Mood. 1995. *Measurement and evaluation in human performance.* Champaign, IL: Human Kinetics.

Nachemson, A., W.O. Spritzer, et al. 1987. Scientific approaches to the assessment and management of activity-related spinal disorders. A monograph for clinicians. Report of the Quebec Task Force on Spinal Disorders. *Spine* 12 (75, Suppl. 1): S1-559.

Nagle, F. and H. Montoye. 1981, *Exercise in health and disease*. Springfield, IL: Charles C. Thomas.

National Center for Health Statistics. 1996. *Health United States 1995*. Hyattsville, MD: Public Health Service.

National Research Council. 1989. *Recommended dietary allowances*. Washington, DC: National Academy Press.

National Strength and Conditioning Association. 1994. *Essentials of strength training and conditioning*, ed. T.R. Baechle. Champaign, IL: Human Kinetics.

Nieman, D.C. 1995. *Fitness and sports medicine: a health-related approach*. Mountain View, CA: Mayfield Publishing.

Nieman, D.C. 1998. *The exercise-health connection*. Champaign, IL: Human Kinetics.

NIH. 1984. *Optimal calcium intake*. NIH Consensus Statement. June 6-8; 12 (4): 1-31.

Noble, E. 1995. *Essential exercises for the childbearing year*. 4th ed. New Life Images.

Oldridge, N.B. 1979. Compliance of post-myocardial infarction patients to exercise programs. *Medicine and Science in Sports* 11: 373-375.

Paffenbarger, R.S., and E. Olsen. 1996. *LifeFit*. Champaign, IL: Human Kinetics.

Paffenbarger, R.S., Jr., I.M. Lee, and R. Leung. 1994. Physical activity and personal characteristics associated with depression and suicide in American College men. *Acta Psychiatrica Scandinavica* (Suppl. 377): 16-22.

Pate, R.R., and C.A. Macera. 1994. Risks of exercising: Musculoskeletal injuries. In *Physical activity, fitness, and health: International proceedings and consensus statement*, ed. C. Bouchard, R.J. Shepard, and T. Stephens. Champaign, IL: Human Kinetics.

Pate, R.R., M. Pratt, S.N. Blair, W.L. Haskell, C.A. Macera, C. Bouchard, D. Buchner, W. Ettinger, G.W. Heath, A.C. King, A. Kriska, A.S. Leon, B.H. Marcus, J. Morris, R.S. Paffenbarger, K. Patrick, M.L. Pollock, J.M. Rippe, J. Sallis, and J.H. Wilmore. 1995. Physical activity and the public health: A recommendation from the Centers for Disease Control and Prevention and the American College of Sports Medicine. *Journal of the American Medical Association* 273: 402-407.

Pivarnik, J.M. 1998. Potential effects of maternal physical activity on birth weight: brief review. *Medicine and Science in Sports and Exercise* 30 (3): 400-406.

Pollock, M.L., and J.H. Wilmore. 1990. *Exercise in health and disease: Evaluation and prescription for prevention and rehabilitation*. 2d ed. Philadelphia: Saunders.

President's Council on Physical Fitness and Sports. 1995. Osteoporosis and physical activity. *Physical Activity and Fitness Research Digest* 2(3): 1-8.

Prochaska, J.O., and B.H. Marcus. 1994. The transtheoretical model: Applications to exercise. In *Advances in exercise*

adherence, ed. R.K. Dishman, 161-180. Champaign, IL: Human Kinetics.

Radloff, L.S. 1977. The CES-D scale: A self-report depression scale for research in the general population. *Applied Psychological Measurement* 1: 385-401.

Sallis, J.F., W.L. Haskell, S.P. Fortmann, K.M. Vranizan, C.B. Taylor, and D.S. Solomon. 1986. Predictors of adoption and maintenance of physical activity in a community sample. *Preventive Medicine* 15: 331-346.

Sallis, J.F., M.F. Hovell, C.R. Hofstetter, J.P. Elder, M. Hackley, C.J. Caspersen, and K.E. Powell. 1990. Distance between homes and exercise facilities related to frequency of exercise among San Diego residents. *Public Health Reports* 105: 179-185.

San Diego State University Foundation. 1997. *What is your PACE score?* San Diego: San Diego State University Foundation.

Singh, N.A., K.M. Clements, and M.A. Fiatarone. 1997. A randomized controlled trial of the effect of exercise on sleep. *Sleep* 20 (2, February): 95-101.

Snook, S.H., R.A. Campanelli, and J.W. Hart. 1978. A study of three preventive approaches to low back injury. *Journal of Occupational Medicine* 20: 478-481.

Steinhardt, M., and R.K. Dishman. 1989. Reliability and validity of expected outcomes and barriers for habitual physical activity. *Journal of Occupational Medicine* 31: 536-546.

Stephens, T. 1988. Physical activity and mental health in the United States and Canada: Evidence from four population surveys. *Preventive Medicine* 17: 35-47.

Suzuki, N., and S. Endo. 1983. A quantitative study of trunk muscle strength and fatigability in the low-back-pain syndrome. *Spine* 8: 69-74.

U.S. Department of Health and Human Services. 1988. *The health consequences of smoking—nicotine addiction: A report of the Surgeon General*. Washington, DC: U.S. Department of Health and Human Services, Public Health Service, Centers for Disease Control, Center for Health Promotion and Education, Office on Smoking and Health.

U.S. Department of Health and Human Services. 1995. Nutrition and your health: Dietary guidelines for Americans, 4th ed. *Home Garden Bulletin No. 232*. Washington, D.C.: U.S. Department of Health and Human Services.

U.S. Department of Health and Human Services. 1996. *Physical activity and health: A report of the Surgeon General*. Atlanta, GA: U.S. Department of Health and Human Services, Centers for Disease Control and Prevention, National Center for Chronic Disease Prevention and Health Promotion.

Uusi-Rasi, K., C.-H. Nygard, P. Oja, M. Pasanen, H. Sievanen, and I. Vuori. 1994. Walking at work and bone mineral density of premenopausal women. *Osteoporosis International* 4: 336-340.

Varrassi, G., C. Bazzanno, and W. Edwards. 1989. Effects of physical activity on maternal plasma betaendorphin levels and perceptions of labor pain. *American Journal of Obstetrics and Gynecology* 160 (3): 707-712.

Wankel, L. 1984a. Decision-making approaches to increase exercise commitment. *Fitness Leader* 2 (10): 21.

Wankel, L. 1984b. Participant goals and leadership roles. *Fitness Leader* 2 (9): 17.

Webster, B.S., and S.H. Snook. 1994. The cost of 1989 worker's compensation low back pain claims. *Spine* 19: 1111-1116.

Weyerer, S. 1992. Physical inactivity and depression in the community: Evidence from the Upper Bavarian Field Study. *International Journal of Sports Medicine* 13: 492-496.

Wilmore, J.H., and D.L. Costill. 1999. *Physiology of sport and exercise.* 2d ed. Champaign, IL: Human Kinetics.

YMCA of the USA with Thomas Hanlon. 1995. *Fit for two: The official YMCA prenatal exercise guide.* Champaign, IL: Human Kinetics.

YMCA of the USA with Patricia Sammann. 1994. *YMCA healthy back book.* Champaign, IL: Human Kinetics.

## Internet Sources

Administration on Aging. 1998. Profile of older Americans 1997.
http://www.aoa.dhhs.gov/aoa/stats/profile

American Cancer Society
http://www.cancer.org

American College of Sports Medicine
http://www.acsm.org

American Diabetes Association
http://www.diabetes.org

American Heart Association
http://www.americanheart.org

Arby's
http://www.arby.com

Burger King
http://www.burgerking.com

Exercise, Fitness, and Sports Medicine
http://www.falk.med.pitt.edu/subjects/sportmed.html

Kentucky Fried Chicken food nutrient values [November 1998]
http://www.kfc.com/Townsquare/Cafe_Virtual_Tour/sanderscafe_nav.htm

Long John Silver's food nutrient values [November 1998]
http://www.longjohnsilvers.com/nutrit.htm

McDonald's food nutrient values [November 1998]
http://www.mcdonalds.com/food/nutrition/index.html

National Institute for Occupational Safety and Health. June 1997. Carpal Tunnel Syndrome factsheet. [November 1998]
http://www.cdc.gov/niosh/ctsfs.html

National Institute for Occupational Safety and Health. 1997. Work-related musculoskeletal disorders factsheet. [November 1998]
http://www.cdc.gov/niosh/muskdsfs.html

National Institute of Mental Health (NIMH)
http://www.nimh.org

Osteoporosis and Related Bone Diseases-National Resource Center. March 1998. [November 1998]
http://www.osteo.org/osteo.html

Osteoporosis NIH Consensus Development Conference Statement. 1998. [November 1998]
http://text.nlm.nih.gov/nih/cdc/www/43txt.html#Head6

Physical Activity [November 1998]
http://www.hkusa.com/infok/phylink.htm

Physical Activity and Health Network (PAHNet) [November 1998]
http://www1.pitt.edu/~pahnet/

Pizza Hut
http://www.pizzahut.com

Subway food nutrient values [November 1998]
http://www.subway.com/nguide

Taco Bell food nutrient values [November 1998]
http://www.tacobell.com/homepage/default1.asp

# Index

Note: Page numbers in bold type refer to tables, and page numbers in italics refer to figures.

# About the Authors

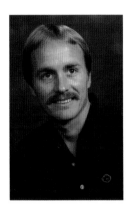

**Allen W. Jackson** is a professor of physical activity and health at the University of North Texas (UNT) in Denton. In more than nine years at the school, he has instructed over 10,000 students in a course entitled Health-Related Fitness. Jackson was also responsible for developing a website (http://courses.unt.edu/phed1000) and Internet instruction for the course. Selected as a Regents Professor at UNT, he is a Fellow of the American College of Sports Medicine (ACSM) and a member of the American Alliance for Health, Physical Education, Recreation and Dance (AAHPERD). Jackson received an EdD from the University of Houston in 1978. He has been an associate editor for *Medicine and Science in Sports*, section editor for the *Research Quarterly for Exercise and Sport*, and associate editor for the *National Strength and Conditioning Association Journal*. In his leisure time, Jackson enjoys exercising, surfing the Web, and hunting and fishing.

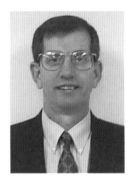

**James R. Morrow, Jr.** is a professor and chair of the Department of Kinesiology, Health Promotion, and Recreation at UNT. Dr. Morrow has authored more than 80 articles and chapters on exercise physiology, measurement, and computer use. He is coeditor of the Cooper Institute for Aerobics Research's *FITNESSGRAM Technical Reference Manual,* an innovative guide for using criterion reference standards in fitness tests. He also has produced four fitness-testing software packages, including the AAHPERD Health-Related Physical Fitness Test. In addition to teaching, Dr. Morrow was editor-in-chief of the *Research Quarterly for Exercise and Sport* from 1989 to 1993. He is an ACSM Fellow and an AAHPERD Research Fellow and has chaired the AAHPERD Measurement and Evaluation Council. He enjoys family activities and golf.

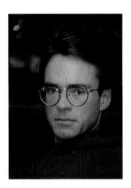

**David W. Hill** has taught exercise physiology for more than 10 years. He began at the University of North Carolina at Chapel Hill in 1987, and then in 1988 he moved to the University of North Texas, where he is currently an associate professor of exercise physiology and director of the exercise physiology lab. Prior to teaching, Hill spent nearly seven years working as a fitness program coordinator and as a researcher in adult fitness and cardiac rehabilitation. He received his PhD in physical education with an emphasis in exercise physiology from the University of Georgia in 1986. Hill is a Fellow of the ACSM and a member of the Canadian Society for Exercise Physiology. A former track and field athlete, Hill held the Canadian record in the mile from 1977 to 1994. Today he still enjoys running, as well as lifting weights, gardening, and traveling.

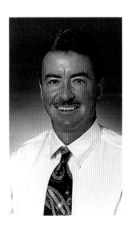

A professor of exercise science at the University of Georgia at Athens, **Rod K. Dishman** has served as a consultant on exercise adherence to numerous government agencies in the United States, Canada, and the United Kingdom, including the U.S. Department of Health and Human Services; the National Institute of Mental Health; the National Science Foundation; and the National Heart, Lung, and Blood Institute. Dr. Dishman has written two books on exercise adherence, and he coauthored the ACSM's position statement on *Achieving and Maintaining Physical Fitness in Healthy Adults.* He is also an editorial board member for ten exercise and health journals, including the ACSM's *Medicine & Science in Sports & Exercise* and *Exercise and Sport Sciences Reviews.* He's an ACSM Fellow and a member of the International Olympic Committee's Medical Commission Selection Committee, which awards the prestigious biannual Olympic prize for sport science. In his free time, Dr. Dishman enjoys running and boating.

# Related Resources from Human Kinetics

**Multimedia Workout**
Produced by Human Kinetics and Lifestyle Software
1996 • PC-Compatible CD-ROM
MLIF0241 • $39.95 ($59.95 Canadian)

Combining functional planning schedules and information databases with sound and live-action video, *Multimedia Workout* is a powerful tool for meeting your fitness goals.

**ACSM Fitness Book**
(Second Edition)
American College of Sports Medicine
Foreword by Steven N. Blair, PED, FACSM
1998 • Paper • 152 pp • Item PACS0783
ISBN 0-88011-783-4 • $13.95 ($19.95 Canadian)

A proven, step-by-step program from the leading experts in health and fitness.

**Nancy Clark's Sports Nutrition Guidebook**
(Second Edition)
Nancy Clark, MS, RD
1997 • Paper • 464 pp • Item PCLA0730
ISBN 0-87322-730-1 • $16.95 ($24.95 Canadian)

Includes 131 quick, delicious, and easy-to-prepare recipes to help you fuel an active lifestyle.

## Fitness Spectrum Series

Packed with workouts color-coded by level of difficulty, each of the following books features helpful information on selecting the proper equipment, using the right techniques, and performing effective warm-up and cool-down exercises. For information on other books in the series, call or visit our Web site.

**Fitness Swimming**
Emmett Hines
1999 • Paper • 192 pp • Item PHIN0656
ISBN 0-88011-656-0 • $17.95 ($26.95 Canadian)

**Fitness Cross-Country Skiing**
Steven E. Gaskill
1998 • Paper • 176 pp • Item PGAS0652
ISBN 0-88011-652-8 • $15.95 ($21.95 Canadian)

**Fitness In-Line Skating**
Susan Nottingham and Frank J. Fedel
1997 • Paper • 176 pp • Item PNOT0982
ISBN 0-87322-982-7 • $15.95 ($21.95 Canadian)

To request more information or to order, U.S. customers call 1-800-747-4457, e-mail us at *humank@hkusa.com*, or visit our Web site at *www.humankinetics.com*. Persons outside the U.S. can contact us via our Web site or use the appropriate telephone number, postal address, or e-mail address shown in the front of this book.

**HUMAN KINETICS**
*The Information Leader in Physical Activity*
2335